"With the compelling ascendance of psychotherapy integration into the mainstream of treatment approaches to psychological disorders, there is an ever-growing need to delineate, organize, compare, and contrast the array of specific integrative approaches that have been developed for different disorders. With striking comprehensiveness, Judy Koenigsberg has done precisely this in the realm of anxiety disorders—and thereby provided a precedent-setting contribution to the field. Reflecting state-of-the-art knowledge throughout, she lays the groundwork for this ambitious venture by articulating the meanings of different terms used under the rubric of 'psychotherapy integration' and, in my view, of particular importance, highlights key distinctions between integrated and the recently identified fifth pathway to integration—unified psychotherapies. Against this backdrop, in a separate chapter for each anxiety disorder, Koenigsberg synthesizes a multiplicity of vital information. Thus, she succinctly describes symptoms, diagnosis, prevalence, comorbidity, and heritability, followed by a theoretically and empirically based integrative account of the neurobiological, psychological, and social/interpersonal factors and processes involved in the etiological development and perpetuation of the specific anxiety disorder at hand. Crucially, the author then moves into the level of clinical application, concisely elucidating the specific integrated and unified treatment models that have been developed for that disorder, including a brief synopsis of each model's core conceptualization, primary intervention(s), and, when available, empirical evidence. Each chapter concludes with a brief case study demonstrating application of one specific integrated or unified approach to the anxiety disorder under discussion, valuably helping the reader to take the next step of implementing different models in their live clinical practice. Collectively, Koenigsberg's book is absolutely eye-opening in revealing the striking number and diversity of integrated and unified approaches that have been developed for treating the anxiety disorders; readers will come away with greater appreciation for and understanding of the truly complex multidimensionality of anxiety disorders as well as the strong likelihood of enhanced effectiveness in their clinical practice with this pervasive class of disorders by virtue of learning multiform ways of clinically thinking and working integratively. Fundamentally, this book is must reading for clinical practitioners and supervisors, researchers, and graduate students with a practical and/or academic interest in the anxiety disorders specifically—and indeed psychotherapy integration more generally."

Jack C. Anchin, Ph.D., Department of Counseling and Clinical Psychology, Medaille College Department of Psychology, University at Buffalo, SUNY

"Written for psychotherapists, researchers and students of mental health disciplines, this book, among other things, examines the critical relationship between the etiology of anxiety disorders and their treatment. In addition, Dr. Koenigsberg approaches this important task from integrative and unified therapy perspectives, both of which facilitate therapists' tailoring treatment to each individual. Conceptual, theoretical, and practical, *Anxiety Disorders: Integrated Psychotherapy Approaches* covers a great deal of important literature on anxiety disorders and integrative approaches, and thus is highly recommended."

Andre Marquis, Ph.D., University of Rochester, author of *Integral Psychotherapy: A Unifying Approach*

"In this exploration of integrated psychotherapy in the treatment of anxiety disorders Dr. Koenigsberg provides a comprehensive and scholarly review of these methods and their clinical relevance. Both beginning therapists and more experienced clinicians will find it a valuable reference. Humane in her approach to making formulations and prescribing treatments, Dr. Koenigsberg reminds us that effective psychotherapy begins and ends with the alliance and the flexibility needed to maintain it."

Judith Tanner, MD, clinical assistant professor of Psychiatry and Behavioral Sciences, Northwestern University

"Integrative approaches are surging, as are rates of anxiety disorders. This book offers an excellent review of the literature that exists at the intersection between these two domains. By helping to outline the literature, the domains of investigation, and the important references, it offers graduate students, practitioners, and scholars a valuable resource to survey the landscape of this complicated terrain and helps make sense of the pluralism."

Gregg Henriques, Ph.D., professor of Graduate Psychology, James Madison University and author of *A New Unified Theory of Psychology*

"Judy Koenigsberg has written a superbly referenced and scholarly book which nicely summarizes how different schools of psychologic treatment inform integrated psychotherapy. She makes a compelling case for why integrated psychotherapy is so helpful across the anxiety disorder spectrum. It is a great addition to the literature and is a must read for clinicians and academics alike."

Jack Dunietz, MD, clinical assistant professor of Psychiatry, Weill Cornell Medical School; assistant attending Psychiatrist, The New York Presbyterian Hospital

"Students, practitioners, and scholars alike struggle to develop an understanding of and a treatment model for the anxiety disorders. Developing a deep knowledge of the dynamic elements that undergird anxiety and an integrated or unified approach on which to base therapeutic interventions is central to this work. With an extensive and excellent review of the literature on the anxiety disorders and on integrating and unifying theoretical approaches, Dr. Koenigsberg provides an exceptional resource."

Marilyn Susman, Ph.D., professor emerita, Counseling Psychology Program, Loyola University Chicago; Senior Psychologist, The Evanston Psychological Group

"Dr. Judy Koenigsberg's text, *Anxiety Disorders: Integrated Psychotherapy Approaches*, is an innovative and comprehensive guide to the clinical application of integrated, integrative, and unified psychotherapy in the treatment of anxiety disorders. Dr. Koenigsberg's new work contributes to our understanding of integrative psychotherapy and the anxiety disorders through a scholarly elucidation of the complexities involved in the etiology and treatment of a common class of disorders, the anxiety disorders.

This book will serve as an invaluable resource across a variety of mental health practitioners. Experienced clinicians, behavioral researchers, academicians/theorists, seasoned supervisors, as well as graduate students in the social sciences will all no doubt refer time and again to *Anxiety Disorders: Integrated Psychotherapy Approaches* as it provides the kind of cohesive paradigm necessary to understand the interface between a common class of emotional disorders, the anxiety disorders, and integrated, integrative, integral, and unifying psychotherapy approaches. The book is essential for anyone who wishes to navigate the pluralism in the mental health profession and optimally apply evidence-based treatments to those struggling with anxiety."

Michelle Rodoletz, Ph.D., co-founder and director of HealthForumOnline.com; licensed clinical psychologist; assistant professor in the Department of Psychiatry at Philadelphia's Fox Chase Cancer Center (FCCC); adjunct faculty at the Temple University School of Medicine faculty; and former associate director of the Psychosocial and Behavioral Medicine Program at FCCC

Anxiety Disorders

This text provides integrated and unified treatment frameworks for anxiety disorders and examines how contemporary integrated psychotherapy treatment models from different therapeutic interventions can be used to help patients.

Dr. Koenigsberg provides a research-based overview of major themes that underlie these treatment models, then analyzes the symptoms and causes of specific anxiety disorders such as panic disorder, social anxiety disorder, and phobias, as well as obsessive-compulsive disorder, and posttraumatic stress disorder. Case studies of integrated or unified treatment approaches are provided for each disorder, along with the theoretical and technical factors that are involved in applying these approaches in clinical practice. Supplementary online materials include PowerPoint slides and test questions to help readers further expand their understanding of integrated and unified approaches for the anxiety disorders and assess their newfound knowledge.

Graduate and undergraduate students, novice and seasoned therapists, and researchers will learn the rationale for and the history of past and contemporary integrated and unified models of treatment to gain better insight into anxiety disorders.

Judy Z. Koenigsberg, Ph.D., is a clinical psychologist, licensed in Illinois, who has practiced integrated psychology for over 25 years. After earning her Ph.D. from Northwestern University in 1990, Dr. Koenigsberg was employed as a clinical psychologist at the University of Chicago. She has taught research design and methodology to graduate students in the social sciences at Loyola University. Dr. Koenigsberg's publications include articles in psychology and sociology which have been published in peer reviewed journals, chapters in an encyclopedia of mental disorders, a course in psycholinguistics designed for C.E. credit for mental health professionals, and a book. At present, she maintains an integrated psychology practice in Evanston, Illinois.

Anxiety Disorders

Integrated Psychotherapy Approaches

Judy Z. Koenigsberg

Routledge
Taylor & Francis Group
NEW YORK AND LONDON

First published 2021
by Routledge
52 Vanderbilt Avenue, New York, NY 10017

and by Routledge
2 Park Square, Milton Park, Abingdon, Oxon, OX14 4RN

Routledge is an imprint of the Taylor & Francis Group, an informa business

Library of Congress Cataloging-in-Publication Data
Names: Koenigsberg, Judy Z., author.
Title: Anxiety disorders: integrated psychotherapy approaches / Judy Z. Koenigsberg.
Description: New York, NY: Routledge, 2020. | Includes bibliographical references and index.
Identifiers: LCCN 2020009851 (print) | LCCN 2020009852 (ebook) | ISBN 9780367086633 (hbk) | ISBN 9780367086640 (pbk) | ISBN 9780429023637 (ebk)
Subjects: MESH: Anxiety Disorders–therapy | Psychotherapy
Classification: LCC RC531 (print) | LCC RC531 (ebook) | NLM WM 172 | DDC 616.85/22–dc23
LC record available at https://lccn.loc.gov/2020009851
LC ebook record available at https://lccn.loc.gov/2020009852

ISBN: 978-0-367-08663-3 (hbk)
ISBN: 978-0-367-08664-0 (pbk)
ISBN: 978-0-429-02363-7 (ebk)

Typeset in Bembo
by Deanta Global Publishing Services, Chennai, India

Visit the eResources: https://www.routledge.com/9780367086640

I dedicate the book, *Anxiety Disorders: Integrated Psychotherapy Approaches*, to David Koenigsberg, M.D.
I wish to express gratitude to my dear friend, Susan Solny, Design and Decorative Arts Historian, who has stood by me during periods of joy and grief. Thank you, Susan, my best friend, for your integrated wisdom, for your boundless intuition, and for your friendship.

Contents

Foreword

Anxiety is one of the most central concepts in psychotherapy. Many of the problems that bring individuals into the therapy room are maladaptive patterns of thinking, feeling, acting, and relating that have anxiety at their root. In particular, many individuals experience some threatening feeling and then have anxiety about those feelings and then move to avoid those feelings in a way that makes sense in the short term, but ultimately is maladaptive in the long term. Because of the central role anxiety plays in both the cause of psychopathology and the focus of psychotherapy, it has been a primary focus of the major approaches to intervention. Psychodynamic, cognitive-behavioral, existential humanistic, and systems theories and therapies have all devoted much effort to both understanding anxiety and developing adaptive strategies and ways of processing it. In addition, the anxiety disorders represent the largest cluster of diagnostic categories that are regularly addressed in psychotherapy. Moreover, rates of anxiety in children, adolescents, and young adults have been dramatically increasing in recent years and so the need to understand anxiety is more urgent than ever.

This is the context for Dr. Judy Koenigsberg's book, *Anxiety Disorders: Integrated Psychotherapy Approaches*. As students, practitioners, and scholars of psychotherapy know, the number of potentially viable perspectives in the field is enormous and it is often difficult to make sense out of the pluralism. Because the pluralism can be so great as to result in a disorienting maze of confusion, many practitioners and scholars have attempted to bring a more integrated lens to the field. Several psychological theorists have attempted to engage in a "deep dive" into the concepts and have generated metatheoretical perspectives that try to bring order. This has been my approach (see Henriques, 2011). Other more practitioner-oriented scholars have attempted to develop systematic integrative approaches to psychotherapy. These efforts have proliferated over the years and now the literature on eclectic approaches, psychotherapy integration, integrative psychotherapy, and even unified approach is growing and now represents an enormous body of work. Although there is some coherence among the various approaches, it nevertheless is the case that there is also now an increasing pluralism within the various approaches that are attempting to find some integrative or unified path.

Dr. Koenigsberg's *Anxiety Disorders: Integrated Psychotherapy Approaches* offers an excellent review of the literature that exists at the intersection between work in integrative psychotherapy and the anxiety disorders. In so doing, this work serves as a useful guide and shares with readers the complicated terrain and helps make sense of the pluralism. By helping to outline the literature, the domains of investigation, and the important references that are crucial to grasp in this important emerging domain of inquiry, this book offers graduate students, practitioners, and scholars a valuable resource to survey the landscape in this important area.

Gregg Henriques
Professor of Graduate Psychology
James Madison University

Preface

The book, *Anxiety Disorders: Integrated Psychotherapy Approaches,* elucidates the complexities involved in the etiology and treatment of a common class of disorders, the anxiety disorders. It shows the benefit of using integrated or unified treatments, rather than single-school interventions, to treat the anxiety disorders. It is a book that has spanned a dynamic career of 25 years of practice as a clinical psychologist.

Researchers have used different terms when referring to psychotherapy integration. Whether psychotherapy integration is called rapprochement, eclecticism, and/or assimilation, its goal is the same (Norcross, Goldfried, & Arigo, 2016). Although terms such as eclectic, integrated, and integrative have been used interchangeably, there are subtle distinctions among these terms. A defining goal of psychotherapy integration is its quest to expand on the benefits of therapy by addressing the particular needs of each client, and it encourages therapists to expand on single-school interventions in order for patients to learn from a variety of perspectives (Norcross et al., 2016). Psychotherapy integration, an ongoing process, calls for a therapist to have an extensive knowledge base and a variety of skills (Norcross & Halgin, 2005; Stricker, 1993). Integrationists focus on how pluralism can enhance the efficacy of psychotherapy, on the continuity of treatment, and on how varied treatments build upon and support each other (Comer, 2015; Norcross & Halgin, 2005; Scaturo, 1994).

Research verifies what practitioners have recognized for a long time, that is, that different kinds of patients call for different types of therapy (Norcross & Wampold, 2011). Are there many clinicians who have adopted psychotherapy integration? Recently, it was found that approximately 30% to 40% of therapists report that their approach is integrative (Norcross et al., 2016).

The book, *Anxiety Disorders: Integrated Psychotherapy Approaches,* is written for psychotherapists, researchers, and for undergraduate and graduate students in the mental health disciplines. Psychologists, psychiatrists, and social workers may use this book to learn about how to utilize eclectic, integrated, integrative, integral, and unified psychotherapy approaches in their practices. *Anxiety Disorders: Integrated Psychotherapy Approaches* seeks to provide psychotherapists with a broad range of conceptual, theoretical, and practical knowledge, gleaned from seemingly disparate sources, in order to assist them to more deeply recognize the presenting problems of their patients and to select an integrated psychotherapy approach tailored for each individual patient. Although several patients may be diagnosed with panic disorder, each requires an individualized treatment plan. A manualized step by step approach may work for one patient, but may not work for another individual because human beings are not machines. The book, *Anxiety Disorders: Integrated Psychotherapy Approaches*, seeks to describe the rationale and timing for the use of integrated psychotherapy models for the anxiety disorders. It shows how integrated and integral theory can be applied in a therapy practice that includes patients with anxiety disorders.

Different psychotherapeutic approaches may benefit different types of individuals (Leichsenring et al., 2018). A pain in the stomach can mean different things for different folks. The symptoms of patients with anxiety disorders may be the same, but the etiology and treatment of the disorder for each patient may be quite different. Thus, there is a need to devise an integrated approach that tailors interventions in a custom-made way, a perspective that depends upon the individuality of patients and their external contexts, e.g., culture, family. This book highlights the flexible way in which integrated therapy focuses on paying attention to the particular needs of each client. It explains how therapists can draw from a variety of therapy models to artfully devise a comprehensive treatment approach that goes beyond the limitations of a single intervention. The book, *Anxiety Disorders: Integrated Psychotherapy Approaches*, encourages therapists to select from a myriad of integrated psychotherapy models or to consider a unified framework, a metatheoretical or integral approach to psychotherapy (e.g., Marquis, 2018), as they plan interventions for their clients with anxiety disorders.

Rather than creating new psychotherapy models and setting one intervention orientation against another, *Anxiety Disorders: Integrated Psychotherapy Approaches* promotes efforts to bring clinicians and researchers of different perspectives together with a goal of enhancing psychotherapy approaches that are already in existence. Rather than focusing on the creation of new theoretical orientations, this book shows how integrated psychotherapy can progress in its own right by offering therapists an opportunity to develop their own flexible and ongoing integrations of already existing perspectives. The book, *Anxiety Disorders: Integrated Psychotherapy Approaches*, provides psychotherapists with an opportunity to delve into the way in which integrated psychotherapy treatments may be applied to specific types of anxiety disorders. It seeks to present course material and resources based on models of integrated treatment for graduate and undergraduate students, for novice and seasoned clinicians, and for psychologists as well for other mental health professionals.

Therapists have been distancing themselves from dualistic approaches of mind and brain and have been engaging a view of emotional disorders that considers an integration of both mental and biological processes (Busch, Oquendo, Sullivan, & Sandberg, 2010; Kendler, 2005). An integrated or a unified perspective that is applied to psychotherapy can help both novice and seasoned therapists to realize the advantages of considering the interaction among intrapsychic/biological, environmental, family, social, and cultural processes in the treatment of the anxiety disorders. Some mental health professionals are passionate about designing and using carefully selected integrated psychotherapy approaches that can facilitate the individual needs of clients; however, other psychiatrists, psychologists, and social workers find that integrated psychotherapy is confusing, ambiguous, and overly broad. Whereas some clinicians find that psychotherapy integration is quite natural, there are therapists who find integrated treatment to be both emotionally and cognitively problematic (Aafjes-van Doorn et al., 2018; Gold, 2005; Rihacek & Danelova, 2016). Integrated treatment approaches demand more from therapists and patients than do single-school models, and, indeed, both patients and therapists tend to be more active with integrated interventions (Stricker, 1993).

When do practitioners learn to integrate? The majority of therapists report that they learned to integrate only after they have attained licensure (Consoli & Jester, 2005). This book suggests to therapists in training that they need not wait until they become licensed to practice psychotherapy from an integrated or a unified vantage point. It is a call for psychotherapists to become aware, early on in their careers, that each theoretical approach has its advantages and disadvantages, and adherence to only one approach can limit their ability to bring about change. Therapists in training need to maintain an open and flexible perspective as the ability to integrate requires that a therapist maintain divergent points of view as well as a high level of ambiguity (Norcross, 1988). Therapists, at times, will experience failure as each perspective may hold weaknesses, and no one etiological approach or psychotherapy model may suffice (Norcross, 2005).

How do practitioners learn to integrate? Many training programs have incorporated an integrative framework (Castonguay, Eubanks, Goldfried, Muran, & Lutz, 2015; Norcross & Halgin, 2005). The key characteristics of an integrative supervisor, among others, include mental complexity and advanced theoretical knowledge along with an understanding that integrative work is not easy for novice therapists who may have difficulty approaching psychotherapy integration in a competent way (Norcross & Halgin, 2005). Supervisors who practice integrated psychotherapy need to custom-tailor the supervision experience to the needs of supervisees, to develop strategies that fit the unique characteristics of trainees, e.g., stage of development, cognitive style, and to model the goals of supervision by combining the techniques of a variety of theoretical orientations as they would in the practice of psychotherapy, e.g., directive, exploratory, so that a trainee feels understood and supported (Halgin, 1985–1986; Norcross & Halgin, 1997, 2005). Similar to integrative psychotherapy, which strives to develop a custom-tailored treatment for each patient, integrative supervision holds appeal in its aim to develop a unique plan of supervision for each supervisee while taking into consideration a supervisee's individual characteristics, e.g., developmental stage, style, sophistication, rather than coercing a trainee to accept a specific approach to psychotherapy, whether single-school or integrative (Norcross & Halgin, 2005). This book encourages psychologists, psychiatrists, social workers, counselors, and supervisors, over the course of their careers as their skills emerge and develop, to select their own clinical styles within the context of an individualized approach to psychotherapy.

What are the key characteristics of integrative therapy? Researchers suggest that rather than emphasizing an aggregate of symptoms, clinicians need to consider the patient's experience of distress as the focal point of therapy (Ingersoll & Marquis, 2014; Marquis, 2008). This book reminds therapists to maintain a humble approach as they explore themes and concepts that are meaningful for their patients with anxiety disorders. Therapists who adhere to only a single orientation without attending to the unique needs of their patients reinforce their own tunnel vision and are at risk for impeding their clients' progress. The integration model is a client-driven perspective that encourages therapists to develop humility in the face of human complexity as they become aware that it is the presenting problems of each individual that needs to suggest the orientation that therapists use to address their patients' suffering (Castonguay, 2005; Stricker & Gold, 1996; Trub & Levy, 2017).

To integrate is to be human. The book, *Anxiety Disorders: Integrated Psychotherapy Approaches*, emphasizes the need for therapists who treat anxiety disorders to familiarize themselves with different approaches, to savor different points of view in order to facilitate the best interest of their patients, and to access their potential to gracefully shift perspectives as they learn to use an integrated or a unified approach to psychotherapy for the anxiety disorders. For example, therapists need to recognize that treating only symptoms neglects the implicit nature of the source of the anxiety, that which triggers the anxiety (Alladin, 2014; Wolfe, 2003). At the same time, treating only the conflicts underlying the anxiety or recognizing only the meaning of a patient's anxiety may not alleviate the more explicit, immediate anxiety symptoms (Wolfe, 2003). Therapists who are integrated may need to shift methods after several sessions, when one approach may not be working, or within the same session; however, prior to each shift, a rationale or plan for such a shift in psychotherapeutic approach needs to carefully take into account the needs of a client (Halgin & McEntee, 1993). Psychotherapy integration requires that therapists expand their points of view (Fraser, 2018). A tribal mentality that negates the notion of integration can block therapists from focusing on more than one orientation in order to devise different ways to assist their clients (Lampropoulos & Dixon, 2007; Norcross & Goldfried, 2005).

The book, *Anxiety Disorders: Integrated Psychotherapy Approaches*, consists of three parts. The first part, "Integrated and Unified Psychotherapy," presents chapters that discuss integrated and unified psychotherapy treatments and the rationale for these treatments as well as a history of past and contemporary models of integrated and unified models of psychotherapy. The second part,

"Integrated and Unified Psychotherapy Approaches for the Anxiety Disorders," discusses the integrated and unified etiological and treatment models as they apply to specific anxiety disorders. The third part, "Integrated and Unified Psychotherapy Approaches for Obsessive-Compulsive Disorder (OCD) and Posttraumatic Stress Disorder (PTSD)," discusses the integrated and unified etiological and psychotherapy models as they apply to obsessive-compulsive disorder and posttraumatic stress disorder.

Part I, "Integrated and Unified Psychotherapy," opens with Chapter 1, "Integrated and Unified Psychotherapy Approaches." Chapter 1 defines and describes integrated and unified approaches to psychotherapy. Chapter 2, "The Need for Integrated and Unified Psychotherapy Approaches," explores the need and rationale for integrated and unified psychotherapy models. Chapter 3, "A Brief History of Integrated and Unified Psychotherapy Approaches," concludes with a history of past and contemporary models of integrated and unified approaches to psychotherapy.

Part II, "Integrated and Unified Psychotherapy Approaches for the Anxiety Disorders," begins with Chapter 4, "The Etiology of the Anxiety Disorders: Themes That Underlie Integrated Psychotherapy Models of the Anxiety Disorders." This chapter explores the etiology of the anxiety disorders, the concepts, themes, and thoughts that underlie integrated psychotherapy models for the anxiety disorders.

Chapter 5, "Generalized Anxiety Disorder (GAD)," focuses on the etiology and clinical practice applications of integrated and unified psychotherapy treatment models for generalized anxiety disorder (GAD). A case study is presented to demonstrate the implementation of a unified psychotherapy approach for generalized anxiety disorder (GAD). For this case study, the therapist treated a patient with generalized anxiety disorder by using Marquis' (2018) Integral, four quadrant psychotherapy approach (Upper Right, Upper Left, Lower Right, and Lower Left).

Chapter 6, "Panic Disorder (PD)," discusses the etiology and clinical practice applications of integrated and unified psychotherapy treatment models for panic disorder (PD). A case study is presented to demonstrate the implementation of an integrated psychotherapy treatment approach for panic disorder (PD). The case study shows how an integration of couples and individual as well as psychodynamic and cognitive-behavioral interventions is employed to enhance the therapy process. The case study relies, in part, on Busch, Oquendo, Sullivan, and Sandberg's (2010) psychoanalytic-neurobiological model and draws as well on Scaturo's (1994) integrative therapy work that integrates individual therapy with couples and family therapy.

Chapter 7, "Phobias: Social Anxiety Disorder (SAD) (Social Phobia) and Specific Phobia (SP)," presents the etiology and clinical practice applications of integrated and unified psychotherapy treatment models for social anxiety disorder (SAD) (social phobia) and specific phobia (SP). The first case study demonstrates the use of Magnavita and Anchin's (2014) unifying psychotherapy model for social anxiety, and the second case study employs an integrated psychotherapy approach that relies on Wolfe's (2006) integrative self-wound approach and incorporates Gold's (1993) model that derives from attachment theory (Bowlby, 1980; Guidano, 1987) for specific phobia.

Chapter 8, "Separation Anxiety Disorder (SAD) and Adult Separation Anxiety Disorder (ASAD)," explores the etiology and clinical practice applications of integrated and unified psychotherapy treatment models for separation anxiety disorder (SAD) and adult separation anxiety disorder (ASAD). A case study is presented to demonstrate how a therapist integrated attachment theory and individual cognitive-behavioral therapy (CBT) along with emotion-focused cognitive-behavioral group therapy in the treatment of a patient with separation anxiety disorder. The integrated treatment for the case study relies upon Weems and Carrion's (2003) framework, which incorporates attachment theory into a CBT model. The emotion-focused cognitive behavioral therapy (ECBT) component addresses the dysregulation of affect in youth with separation anxiety (Afshari et al., 2014; Suveg et al., 2006).

Part III, "Integrated and Unified Psychotherapy Approaches for Obsessive-Compulsive Disorder (OCD) and Posttraumatic Stress Disorder (PTSD)," begins with Chapter 9, "Obsessive-Compulsive Disorder (OCD)," and describes the etiology and clinical practice applications of integrated and unified psychotherapy treatment models for obsessive compulsive disorder (OCD). At the end of the chapter, a case study is presented to demonstrate the implementation of an integrated emotional schema therapy model along with cognitive therapy in the treatment of an adult with OCD. Basile, Luppino, Mancini, and Tenore (2018) proposed an integrated model which combines cognitive therapy (CT) and schema therapy (ST) for the treatment of OCD. The integrated psychotherapy treatment approach which relies on Basile et al.'s (2018) integrative framework of schema therapy can help patients to understand the emotional schemas comprising their OCD. The treatment for this case study relies as well on the integrative model of schema treatment of Sookman and Steketee (2007) which combines with exposure response prevention (ERP) to reinforce deeper learning.

Chapter 10, "Posttraumatic Stress Disorder (PTSD)," discusses the etiology and clinical practice applications of integrated and unified psychotherapy treatment models for posttraumatic stress disorder (PTSD). A case study is presented to demonstrate the implementation of an integrated psychotherapy approach for posttraumatic stress disorder (PTSD). The case study relies on Wolfe's (2005) integrative model of psychotherapy, and the psychotherapy integration includes self-psychology, cognitive-behavioral, and interpersonal themes along with hypnosis in the treatment of a young woman who returned from Vietnam and was diagnosed with PTSD. The final chapter, Chapter 11, provides a conclusion to the book, *Anxiety Disorders: Integrated Psychotherapy Approaches*. Supplementary materials can be found online including PowerPoint slides and test questions to help readers further expand their understanding of integrated and unified approaches for the anxiety disorders and assess their newfound knowledge.

References

Aafjes-van Doorn, K., Klinar Alfaro, D., Fialová, M., & Kamsteeg, C. (2018). Psychotherapy integration training around the globe: A personal and empirical perspective. *Journal of Psychotherapy Integration*. Advance online publication, *28*(4), 505–520. doi: 10.1037/int0000135

Afshari, A., Neshat-Doost, H. T., Maracy, M. R., Ahmady, M. K., & Amiri, S. (2014). The effective comparison between emotion-focused cognitive behavioral group therapy and cognitive behavioral group therapy in children with separation anxiety disorder. *Journal of Research in Medical Sciences*, *19*(3), 221–227.

Alladin, A. (2014). The wounded self: New approach to understanding and treating anxiety disorders. *American Journal of Clinical Hypnosis*, *56*(4), 368–388. doi: 10.1080/00029157.2014.880045

Basile, B., Luppino, O. I., Mancini, F., & Tenore, K. (2018). A theoretical integration of schema therapy and cognitive therapy in OCD treatment: Experiential techniques and cognitive-based interventions in action (Part III). *Psychology*, *9*(9), 2296–2311. doi: 10.4236/psych.2018.99131

Bowlby, J. (1980). *Attachment and loss, Vol. 3. Loss*. New York, NY: Basic Books.

Busch, F. N., Oquendo, M. A., Sullivan, G. M., & Sandberg, L. S. (2010). An integrated model of panic disorder. *Neuropsychoanalysis*, *12*(1), 67–79. doi: 10.1080/15294145.2010.10773631

Castonguay, L. G. (2005). Training issues in psychotherapy integration: A commentary. *Journal of Psychotherapy Integration*, *15*(4), 384–391. doi: 10.1037/1053-0479.15.4.384

Castonguay, L. G., Eubanks, C. F., Goldfried, M. R., Muran, J. C., & Lutz, W. (2015). Research on psychotherapy integration: Building on the past, looking to the future. *Psychotherapy Research*, *25*(3), 365–382. doi: 10.1080/10503307.2015.1014010

Comer, R. J. (2015). *Abnormal psychology*. New York, NY: Worth Publisher.

Consoli, S. J., & Jester, C. M. (2005). Training in psychotherapy integration II: Further efforts. *Journal of Psychotherapy Integration*, *15*(4), 355–357. doi: 10.1037/1053-0479.15.4.355

Fraser, J. (2018). *Unifying effective psychotherapies: Tracing the process of change*. Washington, DC: American Psychological Association.

Gold, J. (2005). Anxiety, conflict, and resistance in learning an integrative perspective on psychotherapy. *Journal of Psychotherapy Integration*, *15*, 374–383. doi: 10.1037/1053-0479.15.4.374

Gold, J. R. (1993). An integrated approach to the treatment of anxiety disorders and phobias. In G. Stricker & J. R. Gold (Eds.), *Comprehensive handbook of psychotherapy integration* (pp. 293–301). New York, NY: Plenum Press.

Guidano, V. (1987). *The development of the self*. New York, NY: Guilford.

Halgin, R. P. (1985–1986). Pragmatic blending of clinical models in the supervisory relationship. *The Clinical Supervisor*, *3*(4), 23–46. doi: 10.1300/J001v03n04_03

Halgin, R. P., & McEntee, D. J. (1993). Countertransference issues in integrative psychotherapy. In G. Stricker & J. R. Gold (Eds.), *Comprehensive handbook of psychotherapy integration* (pp. 513–522). New York, NY: Plenum Press.

Henriques, G. (2011). *A new unified theory of psychology*. New York: Springer Press.

Ingersoll, R. E., & Marquis, A. (2014). *Understanding psychopathology: An integral exploration*. Upper Saddle River, NJ: Pearson Education.

Kendler, K. S. (2005). Toward a philosophical structure for psychiatry. *American Journal of Psychiatry*, *162*(3), 433–440. doi: 10.1176/appi.ajp.162.3.433

Lampropoulos, G. K., & Dixon, D. N. (2007). Psychotherapy integration in internships and counseling psychology doctoral programs. *Journal of Psychotherapy Integration*, *17*(2), 185–208. doi: 10.1037/1053-0479.17.2.185

Leichsenring, F., Abbass, A., Hilsenroth, J., Luyten, P., Munder, T., Rabung, S., & Steinert, C. (2018). "Gold standards," plurality and monocultures: The need for diversity in psychotherapy. *Frontiers in Psychiatry, 9*, 159. doi: 10.3389/fpsyt.2018.00159

Magnavita, J. J., & Anchin, J. C. (2014). *Unifying psychotherapy: Principles, methods, and evidence from clinical science*. New York, NY: Springer.

Marquis, A. (2008). *The integral intake: A guide to comprehensive idiographic assessment in integral psychotherapy*. New York, NY: Routledge.

Marquis, A. (2018). *Integral psychotherapy: A unifying approach*. New York, NY: Routledge.

Norcross, J. C. (1988). Supervision of integrative psychotherapy. *Journal of Integrative and Eclectic Psychotherapy*, 7(2), 157–166.

Norcross, J. C. (2005). A primer on psychotherapy integration. In J. C. Norcross & M. R. Goldfried (Eds.), *Handbook of psychotherapy integration* (2nd ed., pp. 3–23). New York, NY: Oxford University Press.

Norcross, J. C., & Goldfried, M. R. (2005). The future of psychotherapy integration: A roundtable. *Journal of Psychotherapy Integration, 15*(4), 392–471. doi: 10.1037/1053-0479.15.4.392

Norcross, J. C., Goldfried, M. R., & Arigo, D. (2016). Integrative theories. In J. C. Norcorss, G. R. VandenBos & D. K. Freedheim (Eds.), *APA handbook of clinical psychology: Theory and research* (Vol. 2, pp. 303–332). Washington, DC: American Psychological Association. doi: 10.1037/14773-011

Norcross, J. C., & Halgin, R. P. (1997). Integrative approaches to psychotherapy supervision. In C. E. Watkins (Ed.), *Handbook of psychotherapy supervision* (pp. 203–222). New York, NY: Wiley.

Norcross, J. C., & Halgin, R. P. (2005). Training in psychotherapy integration. In J. C. Norcross & M. R. Goldfried (Eds.), *Handbook of psychotherapy integration* (2nd ed., pp. 439–458). New York, NY: Oxford University Press.

Norcross, J. C., & Wampold, B. E. (2011). What works for whom: Tailoring psychotherapy to the person. *Journal of Clinical Psychology, 67*(2), 127–132. doi: 10.1002/jclp.20764

Rihacek, T., & Danelova, E. (2016). The journey of an integrationist: A grounded theory analysis. *Psychotherapy: Theory, Research, and Practice, 53*(1), 78–89. doi: 10.1037/pst0000040

Scaturo, D. J. (1994). Integrative psychotherapy for panic disorder and agoraphobia in clinical practice. *Journal of Psychotherapy Integration, 4*(3), 253–266. doi: 10.1037/h0101261

Sookman, D., & Steketee, G. (2007). Directions in specialized cognitive behavior therapy for resistant obsessive-compulsive disorder: Theory and practice of two approaches. *Cognitive and Behavioral Practice, 14*(1), 1–17. doi: 10.1016/j.cbpra.2006.09.002

Stricker, G. (1993). The current status of psychotherapy integration. In G. Stricker & J. R. Gold (Eds.), *Comprehensive handbook of psychotherapy integration* (pp. 533–545). Boston, MA: Springer.

Stricker, G., & Gold, J. R. (1996). Psychotherapy integration: An assimilative, psychodynamic approach. *Clinical Psychology: Science and Practice, 3*(1), 47–58. doi: 10.1111/j.1468-2850.1996.tb00057.x

Suveg, C., Kendall, P. C., Comer, J. S., & Robin, J. (2006). *Contemporary Psychotherapy, 36*(2), 77–85. doi: 10.1007/s10879-006-9010-4

Trub, L., & Levy, D. (2017). Sowing the seeds for an assimilative integrationist stance toward psychotherapy. *Journal of Psychotherapy Integration, 27*(2), 172–185. doi: 10.1037/int0000056

Weems, C. F., & Carrion, V. G. (2003). The treatment of separation anxiety disorder employing attachment theory and cognitive behavior therapy techniques. *Clinical Case Studies, 2*(3), 188–198. doi: 10.1177/1534650103253818

Wolfe, B. E. (2003). Integrative psychotherapy of the anxiety disorders. In J. C. Norcross & M. R. Goldfried (Eds.), *Handbook of psychotherapy integration* (2nd ed., pp. 263–280). New York, NY: Oxford University Press.

Wolfe, B. E. (2005). *Understanding and treating anxiety disorders: An integrative approach to healing the wounded self.* Washington, DC: American Psychological Association.

Wolfe, B. E. (2006). An integrative perspective on the anxiety disorders. In G. Stricker & J. Gold (Eds.), *A casebook of psychotherapy integration* (pp. 65–77). Washington, DC: American Psychological Association.

Acknowledgments

I would like to thank Andre Marquis, Ph.D., for sharing his metatheoretical integral treatment approach, unified psychotherapy treatment. I am grateful to Marilyn Susman, Ph.D., for her integrated and flexible view of psychotherapy and for her genuine care for her students that inspired me to pursue a career in psychology many years ago. Thank you, Gregg Henriques, Ph.D., for writing the foreword.

Thank you, mentors, colleagues, and friends, Gloria Berkwits, M.D., John Crites, Ph.D. (deceased), and Michael Garet, Ph.D., for having taken an interest in me and my career. Thanks to my colleagues, Jo-Ann Hoeppner, Ph.D., Jack Dunietz, M.D., Judith Tanner, M.D., Rebecca Mermelstein, Ph.D., Barry Wolfe, Ph.D., Ali Mindel, Psy.D., Daniel Barnes, Ph.D., Michelle Rodoletz, Ph.D., and Bonnie Whyte, Ph.D., for their kindness. A special thank you to Nell Logan, Ph.D., and Thetis R. Cromie, Ph.D., for their deep insight and caring.

I am grateful to Nina Guttapalle, mental health editor at Routledge/Taylor & Francis, for recognizing the value of this project, for her sensible guidance, and for her gracious encouragement, support, and dedication throughout this project, to Daradi Patar, editorial assistant at Routledge/Taylor & Francis, to Grace McDonnell, editorial assistant at Routledge/Taylor & Francis, for her prompt support and for helping to make this book a reality, and to Stephen Riordan, project manager at Deanta Global Publishing Services, for assisting me with the copy editing process. Thank you to my clients who were served by a flexible approach to psychotherapy. Thank you, Mom (deceased) and Dad (deceased), for giving me the wherewithal and courage to pursue a path that women in my time and milieu were not encouraged to pursue.

Part I

Integrated and Unified Psychotherapy

Part I presents chapters that describe integrated and unified psychotherapy treatments, the rationale for integration, and offers a history of past and contemporary integrated and unified models of psychotherapy. The first chapter, "Integrated and Unified Psychotherapy Approaches," defines integrated psychotherapy and distinguishes between single-school, eclectic, integrated, integrative, and unified psychotherapy approaches. It aims to stimulate thoughts about how the reader may feel comfortable considering ways to integrate ideas and methods from various theoretical orientations. Chapter 2, "The Need for Integrated and Unified Psychotherapy Approaches," presents the rationale for integrated and unified frameworks and delineates various types of models of psychotherapy integration and unification. Part I, which ends with Chapter 3, "A Brief History of Integrated and Unified Psychotherapy Approaches," offers a brief history of integrated and unified psychotherapy perspectives.

1 Integrated and Unified Psychotherapy Approaches

Introduction

Chapter 1 describes the various types of psychotherapy models, e.g., single system or monotherapy, eclectic, integrated, integrative, and unified or integral. The chapter distinguishes one framework from another and offers examples of single-system, integrated, and unified psychotherapy models or frameworks.

Models of Psychotherapy and Supervision: Single-School, Eclectic, Integrated, Integrative, Integral, Unified

A goal of this chapter is to describe different types of therapy models and to explain how they influence the way in which practitioners practice and supervisors train. Models of psychotherapy include single-school or monotherapy, eclectic, integrated, integrative, and integral or unified. Although the chapter begins with single-school models, the primary focus is on psychotherapy integration and unified models of psychotherapy.

Single-School or Monotherapy Models of Psychotherapy

What is a single-school perspective? A single-system approach relies on one theoretical framework. Although there are several monotherapy perspectives, the following four are representative: Psychodynamic, existential/humanistic, cognitive-behavioral, and systemic (Fernández-Álvarez, 2001; Längle & Kriz, 2012; Wachtel, 2014). Whereas the aforementioned monotherapy orientations have contributed to psychotherapy integration, they, often, have been dismissive of each other (Fernández-Álvarez, Consoli, & Gómez, 2016; Wachtel, 2010). It is the integrated and unified perspectives that have contributed to the unity of psychotherapy while focusing on the particular needs of patients.

Distinctions Among Eclectic, Integrated, and Integrative Psychotherapy Models

What is the difference between eclectic psychotherapy, psychotherapy integration, and integrative psychotherapy? Terms such as eclectic, integrated, and integrative have been used interchangeably; however, there are differences among them. This section points out the distinctions among the aforementioned terms.

What is the difference between eclectic and integrated psychotherapy? The difference between the two involves the notion of theory. Eclectic psychotherapy draws ideas together without working to reconcile them, and appears to be a middle step towards integration (Forman, 2010). Whereas eclectic psychotherapy involves employing treatment techniques because of their effectiveness and without concern for a theoretical rationale, psychotherapy integration underscores the correlation between method and theory (Stricker, 1993). An eclectic psychotherapist applies divergent techniques; however, an integrated psychotherapist plans a synthesis of distinct theoretical orientations (Beitman, Goldfried, & Norcross, 1989). Both integrated therapy theories that are well-organized and systematic and eclectic psychotherapy perspectives that are less ordered aim towards a unified psychotherapy framework (Walder, 1993). According to Cutts (2011), although eclectic psychotherapy employs theoretical components, without referring to theory, the purpose of therapy integration is to achieve a unified approach. Macarthur (2013) argues that assimilative integration takes theory into account; however, its goal is not a unified model.

What is integrative psychotherapy, and how does it differ from psychotherapy integration? Integrative psychotherapy is represented as a bona fide treatment approach, as a psychotherapy school, rather than as a psychotherapy process that characterizes psychotherapy integration (Stricker, 1993). Stricker (1993) distinguishes between psychotherapy integration and integrative psychotherapy by describing psychotherapy integration as a process whose outcome is a myriad of integrations, both theoretical and technical, and defines integrative psychotherapy, on the other hand, as no more than an advanced single-school or monotherapy approach. Consistent with the aforementioned view, Wachtel (2010) distinguishes between psychotherapy integration and integrative psychotherapy by explaining that whereas therapy integration connotes an ongoing process, integrative therapy connotes a product or a method. The bottom line is that an integrative psychotherapy perspective challenges the idea that different treatment models cannot work together (Fernández-Álvarez et al., 2016).

Whereas an eclectic psychotherapist may employ a particular method, observe a positive change in a patient, and not analyze the reason that the positive change took place, an integrative psychotherapist would analyze the reason why, and the way in which, a patient changes (Jones-Smith, 2012). Therapists who adhere to an eclectic approach seem to not have much in common and do not adhere to a prior set of principles; however, therapists who opt for an integrated point of view consider both what works and the reason that something works (Jones-Smith, 2012).

The Meaning and Purpose of Psychotherapy Integration and Integrative Psychotherapy Models

Whereas the previous section explained the distinctions between eclecticism and integration, the next section discusses the meaning of integration. What does psychotherapy integration mean for patients and therapists? Psychotherapy integration refers to an investigation of the ways that different psychotherapy approaches can combine (Stricker & Gold, 2006). An integrated psychotherapy approach strives to improve psychotherapy by incorporating different perspectives and techniques (Castonguay & Goldfried, 1994). The essence of psychotherapy integration reflects alignment. Although the ideas and methods of models of psychotherapy vary, frequently, they are compatible (Comer, 2015). For example, it has been demonstrated that the positive effects for individuals who have engaged in psychodynamic treatments that are long-term are equal to the effects for interventions that are evidence-based, and clinicians who identify as other than psychodynamic tend to integrate psychodynamic concepts into their therapy sessions (Boulanger, 2011; Shedler, 2010).

Psychotherapy integration needs to include both an integration of a therapist's explicit theories or formal learning of orientations and implicit theories or conceptualizations about psychotherapy (Jones-Smith, 2012; Shoben, 1962). Whereas explicit theories involve the adoption of a formal orientation such as humanistic or cognitive, implicit theories involve notions on how to develop a therapeutic relationship with a client regardless of didactic or formal theoretical orientation (Jones-Smith, 2012).

Does psychotherapy integration occur within the treatment or within the therapist? Whereas some researchers propose that clinicians need to apply integration within the treatment in the way that a therapist employs several methods, others suggest that integration occurs within the therapist as each patient calls for a different perspective (Stricker, 1993). Psychotherapy integration is not a simple endeavor, and it seeks to recognize the complexity necessary to service a diversity of patient requirements (Fernández-Álvarez et al., 2016). For Stricker (2010), psychotherapy needs to include continuous integration.

How does integrated psychotherapy encompass a wider or broader view of human beings? How does integrated psychotherapy work to develop a complete view of a human being, a perspective that encompasses the physiological, psychological, and sociocultural elements of an individual's challenges? Biopsychosocial theories assert that deficits result from a broad range of communications among social, physiological, emotional, cognitive, developmental, genetic, cultural, and other domains (Calkins & Dollar, 2014; Comer, 2015; Pincus, 2012). Today, integration therapists blend treatment methods from distinct approaches, some of which are empirically supported (Comer, 2015; Norcross & Beutler, 2014). Prochaska and DiClemente's (2005) transtheoretical model is an example of a psychotherapy integration approach that has been empirically supported (Fernández-Álvarez et al., 2016).

What is the purpose of integrative psychotherapy? A goal of an integrative psychotherapy approach is to promote learning from a variety of standpoints in order to facilitate usefulness and productivity in a clinical context (Aafjes-van Doorn, Klinar Alfaro, Fialová, & Kamsteeg, 2018; Greben, 2004). A psychotherapist who is integrative is informed and flexible (Boulanger, 2011). For example, one type of integrative therapy involves pragmatic blending, which refers to the emergence of an emotional problem from a blend of learned, unconscious, and interpersonal sources that usually include interpersonal, Rogerian, psychodynamic, and behavioral intervention approaches (Halgin, 1985–1986; Halgin & McEntee, 1993). Integrative psychotherapists examine how patients benefit from treatments that are not restricted to one school of thought by drawing on methods across different orientations within an evidenced-based context (Norcross & Goldfried, 2005; Norcross & Popple, 2017).

Is there a connection between integrative psychotherapy and a common class of emotional disorders, the anxiety disorders? Evidence-based research has shown that integrative psychotherapy interventions (e.g., interpersonal, schema) can benefit patients with different anxiety disorders, e.g., generalized anxiety and social anxiety (Hamidpour, Dolatshai, Shahbaz, & Dadkhah, 2011; Stangier, Schramm, Heidenreich, Berger, & Clark, 2011; Zarbo, Tasca, Cattafi, & Compare, 2016).

What is the essence of patient integration? Critical to psychotherapy integration is the need for patients to have an opportunity to integrate. In his article, "Patient-Initiated Integration," Gold (2006) emphasized that shifting in an integrative way from one method or theoretical orientation to another may be initiated by the patient. He emphasized that it is important for a psychotherapist to try to match a patient's interest in a new approach with a method known by the therapist, that therapists who are secure will realize that integration that is initiated by a client may place greater demands upon them, and that this type of integration may induce anxiety in a therapist. It is suggested that therapists explore a patient's reasons for wanting to shift orientations and/or methods so as to facilitate the patient's confidence and a corrective affective experience (Alexander & French, 1946; Gold, 2006).

How does neuroscience advance the conceptualization of psychotherapy integration? In his "Pathways to Progress for Integrative Psychotherapy: Perspectives on Practice and Research," Wachtel (2017) suggests that neuroscience may facilitate further progress in integration. He recommends that integrated psychotherapists explore the connection between the body and the brain and the way in which trauma, which may not emerge verbally, can be stored in the body.

Wachtel (2017) suggests that integrated psychotherapists explore the theme of cognitive neuroscience that includes procedural memory and learning. For example, inherent knowing which is relational is a form of procedural knowledge which can be nonverbal (e.g., knowing how to use humor in social interactions) (Lyons-Ruth et al., 1998, Wachtel, 2017). The verbal part of therapy, at times, may impede procedural learning, and therapists need to learn how to be with human beings rather than what to speak about with them (Wachtel, 2017). Another theme that Wachtel (2017) suggests that integrated therapists explore with their clients includes the effect of economic, social, and cultural dimensions upon clients' lives. It is important for therapists to help clients understand how cultural underpinnings and values as well as their parents shape their lives (Wachtel, 2017).

Whereas many research studies examine integrative psychotherapy in terms of different models or investigate the process by which individuals become integrative psychotherapists, Finnerty and McLeod (2018) study how integrative psychotherapists understand their therapeutic work. Integrative clinicians in the aforementioned study conveyed that they tend to seek the totality of a patient's universe, are at ease with a synthesis during therapy sessions, and view integrative psychotherapy as a flexible, but complex, endeavor that blends different dimensions to fit the particular needs of patients while encouraging input from patients (Finnerty & McLeod, 2018). The integrative therapists promote a relational approach that highlights empathic attunement and active listening and seek to build an insightful, responsive, and ongoing working space for patients with multidimensional emotional issues (Finnerty & McLeod, 2018).

Integrated Models of Psychotherapy Supervision

More than three quarters of U.S. university directors of internships and supervision recognize that monotherapy models are not sufficient to treat the broad scope of issues brought by patients (Lampropoulos & Dixon, 2007). Although single-school psychotherapy approaches are practical, they are not sufficient to deal with the broad range of impairments that psychologists address on a daily basis (Magnavita, 2006). Indeed, it has been shown that therapists who have trained, at first, in a single-school perspective, generally shift towards integrative psychotherapy given the range of issues that they encounter in their clinical practices (Rønnestad & Skovholt, 2013).

Integration has informed psychotherapy supervision and training as well as psychotherapy itself. For example, in their model of integrative supervision, Lecomte, Castonguay, Cyr, and Sabourin, (1993) show how the theme of the "self" can be used to blend the concepts of Kohut (1971), Bandura (1986), and Rogers (1951). Whereas the concept of the "self" for Rogers (1951) refers to the self-concept and maladjustment can ensue unless there is congruence between the organism and the self, for Kohut (1971) and Kohut and Wolfe (1978) the concept of the "self" is deepened with the formulation of a self-object theory, and anxiety can ensue if the self becomes fragmented or regressed or if a patient's self-object experiences are not empathic (Lecomte et al., 1993). Bandura's (1986) social cognitive approach further extends on Rogers' (1951) and Kohut's (1971) approaches by viewing anxiety as an expectation that an individual may have difficulty self-regulating and may not possess the capacity to deal with a threat (Lecomte et al., 1993).

There has been controversy related to the use of psychotherapy integration during clinical training sessions with respect to the timing of how and when to teach an integrated approach (Aafjes-van Doorn et al., 2018; Trub & Levy, 2017). The type of integration, integration trend, or specific psychotherapy model (e.g., technical eclecticism, assimilative integration, discussed in Chapter 2) may suggest whether the timing of training takes place at the beginning or at a later stage of a supervisee's program (Aafjes-van Doorn et al., 2018; Lampropoulos, 2001).

The psychotherapy integration process can include several phases of a therapist's career beginning with a novice stage where a therapist adopts a single-school approach, the development of a middle phase where the therapist becomes dissatisfied because of limitations of the single-school perspective, and the emergence of a more advanced phase where integration takes place, making way for greater coherence (Fernández-Álvarez et al., 2016; Rihacek & Danelova, 2016). Training in psychotherapy integration needs to proceed slowly, with students acquiring mastery in the implementation of different approaches prior to training in actual integration (Castonguay, 2005; Stricker & Gold, 1996; Trub & Levy, 2017). Several researchers, on the other hand, are proponents of psychotherapy integration for novice therapists and assert that versatility allows clinicians to offer more extensive care than therapists who learn only one orientation at the outset (Schottenbauer et al., 2005).

How can integrated psychotherapy supervision be conceptualized throughout a therapist's lifespan? There is a need for integrated psychotherapy supervision that addresses therapists' needs throughout the life cycle. Jones-Smith (2012) explained that learning to be an integrative therapist is a process that continues throughout one's lifespan, and she suggests using the integrative psychotherapy helping skills model of Hill (2004) to train students. Hill (2004) described the stages of the helping skills model – exploration, insight, and action – and their accompanying theoretical orientations. Whereas the exploration stage is based on the theory of Rogers (1951), insight is based on psychoanalytic theory, and the action stage on cognitive-behavioral theory (Hill, 2004; Jones-Smith, 2012).

Unified Psychotherapy Models

The current or fifth wave of psychotherapy integration has, at its core, the notion of unification. What characterizes a unified approach? Unified approaches strive to offer maps that can help psychologists conceptualize clearly (Henriques, 2013). For example, character adaptation systems theory (CAST) (Henriques, 2017), based on the unified approach of Henriques (2011), offers the discipline of psychology a bridge between contemporary integrative perspectives of personality and therapy. A later section of this chapter discusses justification, the fifth system of Henriques (2017), and shows how it relates to the concept of minute-to-minute states described by Marquis (2018), who developed his own integral or unified psychotherapy approach.

What is a unified psychotherapy approach, and is there a difference between integration and unification? There is a distinction between "psychotherapy integration" and "unified psychotherapy" (Knoblauch, 2008; Magnavita, 2008). Whereas psychotherapy integration merges single-school therapies without the loss of meaning for any one school, "unified psychotherapy" dissolves the parts into a new entity and highlights the core meaning that is universal to human functioning (Knoblauch, 2008; Magnavita, 2008; Marquis, 2018). Examples of unified models include Barlow et al.'s (2011, 2018) unified framework for the treatment of the psychiatric disorders, the unification approach of Henriques (2011), and Magnavita's (2012) system framework for broadening family treatment with psychotherapy that is unified. Clinical science and psychotherapy that are unified need to rely on a broad range of perspectives that are evidence-based (Magnavita, 2012).

What is unique about unified models of psychotherapy? According to Allen (2007), models of unified metatheories of psychology (e.g., Magnavita, 2005; Mahoney, 2003; Scaturo, 2005) include the following three elements that are common to metatheories: (1) Interrelated levels, (2) a notion of agency, and (3) a friction between consistency versus change and between bonding versus individuation. For example, with respect to the first element – level– an integral component of unified metatheories of psychology is the notion of an interactive, complex level system (Allen, 2007). The biopsychosocial model of Engel (1980) is a metatheoretical paradigm that includes the interactions of levels, e.g., gene, organ, and therapists can use many treatments on several levels simultaneously (Allen, 2007; Magnavita, 2005). Generally, psychotherapy treatment from the different single-school or unitary approaches targets change at only one or two levels (Allen, 2007). For example, although most psychoanalysts would agree that relationships are important, the focus seems, for the most part, to be at the level of intrapsychic dynamics, and, similarly, interpersonal therapists seem to focus on the level of relationships between two individuals rather than on other levels, e.g. families (Allen, 2007). It is a unified metatheory of psychology that suggests a variety of interventions that can influence many different levels, e.g., individual, family, culture, and others (Allen, 2007).

Building blocks of unified psychotherapy include treatment modalities, e.g., individual, group, settings, treatment lengths, principles, and a strong therapeutic alliance that enhances treatment (Castonguay & Beutler, 2006; Magnavita & Anchin, 2014). How does attachment theory and the therapeutic alliance relate to a unified psychotherapy framework? Attachment theory, a developmental and an emotional regulation theory, is at the core of a unified psychotherapy approach (Johnson, 2019; Magnavita & Anchin, 2014). A critical building block of unified psychotherapy includes relational factors that focus on the curative aspect of the working alliance or patient–therapist match (Magnavita & Anchin, 2014). Attachment theory, an integrative force, can offer a cohesive framework that targets both the reduction of symptoms and character growth within an interpersonal context (Johnson, 2019; Magnavita & Anchin, 2014). The combination of an attachment approach, with emotion as an outgrowth, and an experiential perspective can offer a psychotherapeutic intervention that includes both the intrapsychic and interpersonal (Johnson, 2019). A shift towards the meaning of a psychotherapist's relational presence requires a deeper attunement with patients in order to recognize the importance of patients' needs as human beings, and this process relies on more than mechanistic interventions, symptom management, and coping methods, interventions that have been considered the gold standard for treatment, but have been challenged (Johnson, 2019; Leichsenring & Steinert, 2018).

Integral Psychotherapy Models

What is an integral framework, and what is its goal? Integral theory is a metatheoretical or comprehensive unification of various fields of study which can be used in different contexts given its comprehensive and cohesive character (Esbjörn-Hargens, 2009; Marquis & Elliot, 2015; Wilber, 2003). The unified framework of integral theory considers psychological complexity, is aware of therapists' stages of training, and is a unified model that facilitates the use of a broad scope of theories and orientations (Forman, 2010; Marquis & Elliot, 2015). A goal of integral theory is to recognize that different sides of human structures such as physiological makeup, cultural perspective, intrapsychic dynamics, and social systems contribute equally (Marquis & Elliot, 2015). Unlike single school or unitary theories or models (e.g., psychodynamic, cognitive-behavioral) that compete with each other, integral psychotherapy relies on integral theory to integrate various subsystems (Marquis, 2018; Wilber, 1999, 2000). Marquis' (2018) unifying psychotherapy approach, which derives from Wilber's integral theory (Marquis & Wilber, 2008; Wilber, 1999, 2000), draws on several domains, e.g., existential-humanistic, neuroscientific, developmental, that are in conflict with each other.

Proponents of integral psychotherapy assert that it is possible for therapists to view the life of a patient from the following four sides: Individual-objective, individual-subjective, collective-objective, and collective-subjective (Forman, 2010; Marquis, 2018). Marquis (2018) developed a parsimonious unifying model of psychotherapy, a metatheoretical perspective, based on an integral framework of four quadrants, e.g., interior–exterior, individual–system. For example, according to the metatheoretical perspective of Marquis (2018), a therapist who views the patient from the interior makes use of an existential lens, and a therapist who views the patient from the exterior uses a behavioral lens. The quadrants or reality dimensions convey that phenomena can be understood from an inside and exterior view and from an individual and plural view (Esbjörn-Hargens, 2009; Marquis, 2018). Esbjörn-Hargens (2009) offers the following example: If one wishes to increase productivity at a work meeting, one examines psychological insights and cultural opinions (the interior of individuals and systems) as well as behavioral observations and organizational subtleties (the exterior of individuals and systems).

The integral model of psychotherapy, based on integral theory embraces a quadratic perspective (Ingersoll & Marquis, 2014; Wilber, 2000). The four quadrant framework of Marquis (2018) includes an integration of psychological, behavioral–physiological, cultural, and social perspectives in therapy. The Upper Left quadrant (subjective-individual) includes, among other perspectives, the cognitive, existential, and psychodynamic; the Upper Right quadrant (objective-individual) contains, among others perspectives, the physiological, behavioral, and genetic; the Lower Left (subjective-collective) consists of, among other perspectives, the culture; and the Lower Right (objective-collective) includes, among other perspectives, the family and other social systems (Forman, 2010; Marquis, 2018). The integral model can reveal the complexity of a patient's realms or dimensions of reality in that it preserves the conceptualizations of the quadrants rather than reduces, as many frameworks do, each quadrant into another quadrant (Esbjörn-Hargens, 2009). Integral therapists recognize that the quadrants facilitate an initial assessment of a client's issue along with an attempt to present an issue from multiple views, and if one of the quadrants is removed, a perspective of the integral is lost from understanding (Esbjörn-Hargens, 2009).

Vignette That Applies to the Integral Quadrant Model of Marquis (2018)

The following vignette contains an example of a therapist who uses the four quadrants of Marquis (2018) to begin to elicit the whole or the integral portion of a 33-year-old female patient's issue:

Patient: [Somewhat anxious and angry.] This afternoon, I will need to get over to the university hospital and teach the residents.

Therapist: How do you feel about getting to the hospital to teach the residents this afternoon?

(Therapist in the Upper Left [UL] quadrant: Does the patient cognitively think about the time needed to get to the hospital, about the time it takes to teach the residents? How does the patient feel about teaching the residents? Is there anxiety about whether the patient can impart her skills?)

The therapist's question, related to the Upper Left (UL) quadrant, attempts to elicit the patient's cognitive, experiential, and/or psychodynamic feelings.

Patient: I'm somewhat anxious and angry. [Silence]

Therapist: Can you tell me more?

(Therapist in the Upper Right [UR] quadrant: Does the patient take a bus or drive to go to the hospital?)

The therapist's second question reflects her broad recognition that the anxiety might be related to the Upper Right quadrant and attempts to elicit material from the physiological, behavioral, and/or genetic dimensions (e.g., behaviors that are related to the patient's getting to the hospital, such as getting on a train or bus).

Patient: [Patient is angry and close to tears.] My husband says that I need to take the bus because he needs to take our children in the car this afternoon to shop. He often says that he needs the car when he knows that Tuesday afternoon is my turn to use the car so that I can get to the hospital and share carpool grant and research discussions with colleagues from the hospital!

Therapist: So you are feeling bad because you and your husband disagree about transportation, and your colleagues are depending upon you. Are there other areas of disagreement with your husband that you find difficult and/or that impede the work ethos culture with your colleagues?

(Therapist in the Lower Right [LR] and Lower Left [LL] quadrants: Is the patient's relationship with her husband causing her concern? Are there other family issues that need attention? What is the work ethos culture expressed by the patient?)

The therapist's questions, related to the Lower Right (LR) and Lower Left (LL) quadrants, attempt to elicit information about the patient's family, other social systems, and the patient's culture at the university hospital.

Patient: The other physicians carpool to work and then drive to a café for about an hour to discuss grants and other projects after rotations at the hospital. When I have nothing to offer my colleagues in terms of shared discussions on the way to and from work, I am anxious that it will be difficult for me to make the connections that I need in the hospital.

Therapist: It is the culture of the physicians to share their work projects while at the hospital as well as to extend outside the boundaries of the hospital.

Patient: Exactly.

Had the therapist speaking to the patient in this vignette lapsed into an empirically supported treatment plan such as cognitive-behavioral therapy rather than embraced the material related to the four quadrants, she may have missed the nuances of what the patient was trying to convey in her minute-to-minute states.

In addition to the four quadrants – the experiential, behavioral, cultural, and social – the unified approach of Marquis (2018) includes clients' minute-to-minute states of consciousness, which he considers to be more clinically important than clients' developmental stages. For example, it is important for therapists to assess their patients' minute-to-minute anxiety levels so that they understand whether to present challenges to a patient's defenses or to help a patient regulate the anxiety so that the anxiety does not surpass the ability to manage the anxiety (Fredrickson, 2013; Marquis, 2018). Although the integral model of Marquis (2018) includes patients' developmental levels of ego development (conveyed by the model's levels and lines) (Loevinger, 1976), he points out that it is more important for therapists to offer treatments that correspond to patients' states than to patients' levels of ego development. In the aforementioned vignette, the therapist responded to the patient's minute-to-minute states and learned the source of her concerns.

How important are the fluid states? With respect to states, Bassett-Short and Hammel (2008) explain that, often, therapists in training lose sight of the individuality of the client when they don't pay attention to the immediacy of an individual's experiences. For example, subtle changes in a client's verbal and nonverbal expressions, e.g., intensity, facial shifts, gestures, quality of utterances, can represent core client disclosures (Bassett-Short & Hammel, 2008). The unified approach of Henriques (2011, 2013) suggests that whereas some animals have the ability to generate nonverbal symbols, only human beings have the ability to produce language replete with syntactic elements, meaning, and reason-giving. It is the fifth system of character adaptation, the linguistic justification system of Henriques (2017), that describes the synthesis of human language, awareness of self, the ability to reason, and culture. In "Listening to the Language of Your Patients: Integrating Psycholinguistic Concepts Into Clinical Practice," Koenigsberg (2017) discusses how the study of psycholinguistics can facilitate the diagnosis of anxiety disorders and enhance psychotherapy treatment. An existential or humanistic perspective can help student clinicians to stay attuned to fluid states, thereby getting to know the client and deepening the therapeutic alliance (Bassett-Short & Hammel, 2008; May, 1958).

Integral psychotherapy seeks to integrate several orientations, e.g., psychodynamic, pharmacological, behavioral (Forman, 2010). How are therapy approaches represented within the quadrants? Whereas the biological/pharmacological and behavioral approaches are upper-right perspectives of psychotherapy, the cognitive, humanistic, existential, and transpersonal approaches represent upper-left perspectives of psychotherapy, the multicultural approach represents a lower-left perspective of psychotherapy, the psychodynamic approach represents upper-left and lower-left perspectives of psychotherapy, the feminist approach represents lower-left and lower-right perspectives of psychotherapy, and the somatic approach represents upper-left and upper-right perspectives of psychotherapy (Forman, 2010). It has been demonstrated that patients' states (e.g., affective, cognitive) affect therapists' selection of interventions more than do other integral concepts, e.g., quadrants (Marquis & Elliot, 2015).

A guiding principal of unified psychotherapy is that assessment needs to occur across four levels (intrapsychic, dyadic, triadic, and sociocultural) of the biopsychosocial system (Magnavita & Anchin, 2014). Magnavita and Anchin (2014) propose that unified psychotherapy treatment includes several building blocks, with the first block being treatment approaches. They explain that the advantages of a formalized intervention or an evidence-based treatment (EBT; Chambless, 1996) are that it has undergone empirical investigation and is a critical tool for skill training; however, the disadvantages are that an evidence-based intervention that is a manualized intervention usually targets only one domain level, e.g., intrapsychic, and may not be sufficiently flexible to address multifaceted systems, e.g., dyadic and so on. Unified psychotherapy calls for therapists to familiarize themselves with several treatment approaches so they can effect a shift to another level when an approach that targets one domain is not attaining beneficial results for a patient (Magnavita & Anchin, 2014). Chapters 5 through 10 on the anxiety disorders demonstrate clinical illustrations of therapists' implementations of these shifts.

Another block or component that comprises unified psychotherapy consists of treatment methods that include techniques such as cognitive, affective, and defensive restructuring (Magnavita & Anchin, 2014). For example, techniques can include heightening anxiety or distress, e.g., confrontation, questions, or lowering arousal or anxiety, e.g., reassurance, relaxation (Beutler & Clarkin, 1990; Magnavita & Anchin, 2014).

Integrated and unifying psychotherapy models are here to stay (Norcross & Beutler, 2019). They are the fifth trend or the wave of the future (Henriques, 2011; Jones-Smith, 2012; Marquis, 2018). Given the multidimensional nature of human beings (e.g., individuals' distress can be traced to different sources), it is necessary for therapists to devise interventions that are integrated so that the specific needs of each individual are addressed (Marquis, 2018). For example, the combination of different approaches can improve treatment if a therapist who is using one intervention to help regulate a client's emotion then begins to use a different treatment approach that focuses on trauma (Magnavita & Anchin, 2014).

Summary

Contemporary psychotherapy calls for approaches beyond the confines of single-school perspectives, and highlights the clinician's treatment of a variety of patients, each of whom seek relief in a different context, while underscoring the need for criteria such as efficacy and application (Norcross & Beutler, 2019). The chapter, "Integrated and Unified Psychotherapy Approaches," provided an overview of single-system, eclectic, integrated, integrative, integral, and unified approaches to psychotherapy, pointed out differences among the perspectives, and offered examples of single-system, integrated, and unified psychotherapy models or frameworks (see Table 1.1).

Table 1.1 Models of Psychotherapy

Single-School	*Eclectic*	*Integrated*	*Integrative*	*Integral or Unified*
Relies on one theoretical framework	Employs treatment techniques without concern for a theoretical rationale[a]	Refers to how different psychotherapy frameworks combine,[b] and underscores the correlation between method and theory[a]	Refers to a bona fide treatment framework or a school of psychotherapy[a]	Offers maps in order to conceptualize[c]

[a]Stricker (1993). [b]Stricker & Gold (2006). [c]Henriques (2013).

The psychotherapy approaches discussed in the chapter convey the need for clinicians to keep an open mind as different issues call for answers that suit individual patients. Practitioners need to take care to avoid being blind to alternative treatments, and theorists, therapists, and researchers are encouraged to welcome the unification of divergent points of view.

References

Aafjes-van Doorn, K., Klinar Alfaro, D., Fialová, M., & Kamsteeg, C. (2018). Psychotherapy integration training around the globe: A personal and empirical perspective. *Journal of Psychotherapy Integration, 28*(4), 505–520. doi: 10.1037/int0000135

Alexander, F., & French, T. (1946). *Psychoanalytic therapy*. New York, NY: Ronald Press.

Allen, D. M. (2007). The search for a unified metatheory of personality, psychopathology, and psychotherapy: Grand or grand illusion? A book review essay. *Journal of Psychotherapy Integration, 17*(3), 274–286. doi: 10.1037/1053-0479.17.3.274

Bandura, A. (1986). *Social foundations of thought and action: A social cognitive theory*. Englewood Cliffs, NJ: Prentice-Hall.

Barlow, D. H., Farchione, T. J., Fairholme, C. P., Ellard, K. K., Boisseau, C. L., Allen, L. B., & Ehrenreich-May, J. (2011). *Unified protocol for transdiagnositic treatment of emotional disorders*. New York, NY: Oxford Press.

Barlow, D. H., Farchione, T. J., Sauer-Zavala, S., Murray-Latin, H., Ellard, K. K., Bullis, J. R., ... Cassiello-Robbins, C. (2018). *Unified protocol for transdiagnostic treatment of emotional disorders: Therapist guide* (2nd ed.). New York, NY: Oxford University Press.

Bassett-Short, A., & Hammel, G. A. (2008). A student point of view: Existential psychotherapy from within the training process. In K. I. Schneider (Ed.), *Existential-integrative psychotherapy* (pp. 23–29). New York, NY: Routledge.

Beitman, B. D., Goldfried, M. R., & Norcross, J. C. (1989). The movement toward integrating the psychotherapies: An overview. *American Journal of Psychiatry, 146*(2), 138–147. doi: 10.1176/ajp.146.2.138

Beutler, L. E., & Clarkin, J. (1990). *Systematic treatment selection: Toward targeted therapeutic interventions*. New York, NY: Brunner/Mazel.

Boulanger, G. (2011). Arguing with myself: Thoughts on taking an integrative approach. *Clinical Social Work Journal, 39*(2), 201–203. doi: 10.1007/s10615-010-0277-2

Calkins, S. D., & Dollar, J. M. (2014). Emotion: Commentary: A biopsychosocial perspective on maternal psychopathology and the development of child emotion regulation. *Journal of Personality Disorders, 28*(1), 70–77. doi: 10.1017/S0954579413000680

Castonguay, L. G. (2005). Training issues in psychotherapy integration: A commentary. *Journal of Psychotherapy Integration, 15*(4), 384–391. doi: 10.1037/1053-0479.15.4.384

Castonguay, L. G., & Beutler, L. E. (Eds.). (2006). *Principles of therapeutic change that work: Integrating relationship, treatment, client, and therapist factors*. New York, NY: Oxford University Press.

Castonguay, L. G., & Goldfried, M. R. (1994). Psychotherapy integration: An idea whose time has come. *Applied and Preventative Psychology, 3*(3), 159–172. doi: 10.1016/S0962-1849(05)80068-X

Chambless, D. L. (1996). In defense of dissemination of empirically supported psychological interventions. *Clinical Psychology: Science and Practice, 3*(3), 230–235. doi: 10.1111/j.1468-2850.1996.tb00074.x

Comer, R. J. (2015). *Abnormal psychology*. New York, NY: Worth Publisher.

Cutts, L. (2011). Integration in counselling psychology: To what purpose? *Counselling Psychology Review, 26*(2), 38–48.

Engel, G. L. (1980). The clinical application of the biopsychosocial model. *American Journal of Psychiatry, 137*(5), 535–544. doi: 10.1176/ajp.137.5.535

Esbjörn-Hargens, S. (2009). An overview of integral theory: An all-inclusive framework for the 21st century. *Integral Institute, Resource Paper, 1*(1), 1–24.

Fernández-Álvarez, H. (2001). *Fundamentals of an integrated model of psychotherapy* (A. L. Labruzza, Trans.). New York, NY: Jason Aronson.

Fernández-Álvarez, H., Consoli, A. J., & Gómez, B. (2016). Integration in psychotherapy: Reasons and challenges. *American Psychologist, 71*(8), 820–830. doi: 10.1037/amp0000100

Finnerty, M., & McLeod, J. (2019). A qualitative study of the principles that self-defined integrative therapists in Ireland perceive as underpinning their practice. *Journal of Psychotherapy Integration, 29*(4), 345–358. doi: 10.1037/int0000128

Forman, M. D. (2010). *A guide to integral psychotherapy: Complexity, integration, and spirituality in practice*. Albany, NY: SUNY Press.

Fredrickson, J. (2013). *Co-creating change. Effective dynamic therapy techniques*. Kansas City, MO: Seven Leaves Press.

Gold, J. (2006). Patient-initiated integration. In G. Stricker & J. Gold (Eds.), *A casebook of psychotherapy integration* (pp. 253–260). Washington, DC: American Psychological Association.

Greben, D. H. (2004). Integrative dimensions of psychotherapy training. *The Canadian Journal of Psychiatry, 49*(4), 238–248. doi: 10.1177/070674370404900404

Halgin, R. P. (1985–1986). Pragmatic blending of clinical models in the supervisory relationship. *The Clinical Supervisor, 3*(4), 23–46. doi: 10.1300/J001v03n04_03

Halgin, R. P., & McEntee, D. J. (1993). Countertransference issues in integrative psychotherapy. In G. Stricker & J. R. Gold (Eds.), *Comprehensive handbook of psychotherapy integration* (pp. 513–522). New York, NY: Plenum Press.

Hamidpour, H., Dolatshai, B., Shahbaz, A. P., & Dadkhah, A. (2011). The efficacy of schema therapy in treating women's generalized anxiety disorder. *Iranian Journal of Psychiatry and Clinical Psychology, 16*, 420–431.

Henriques, G. (2011). *A new theory of psychology*. New York, NY: Springer Press. doi: 10.1007/978-1-4614-0058-5

Henriques, G. (2013). Evolving from methodological to conceptual unification. *Review of General Psychology, 17*(2), 168–173. doi: 10.1037/a0032929

Henriques, G. (2017). Character adaptation systems theory: A new big five for personality and psychotherapy, *21*(1), 9–22. doi: 10.1037/gpr0000097

Hill, C. (2004). *Helping skills: Facilitating exploration, insight, and action* (2nd ed.). Washington, DC: American Psychological Association.

Ingersoll, R. E., & Marquis, A. (2014). *Understanding psychopathology: An integral exploration*. Upper Saddle River, NJ: Pearson Education.

Johnson, S. M. (2019). *Attachment theory in practice: Emotionally focused therapy (EFT) with individuals, couples, and families*. New York, NY: Guilford.

Jones-Smith, E. (2012). *Theories of counseling and psychotherapy: An integrative approach*. Thousand Oaks, CA: Sage.

Knoblauch, F. W. (2008). Some disparate thoughts on the idea of a unified psychotherapy. *Journal of Psychotherapy Integration, 18*(3), 301–309. doi: 10.1037/a0013558

Koenigsberg, J. (2017). Listening to the language of your patients: Integrating psycholinguistic concepts into clinical practice. *Health Forum Online (HFO, a nationally-approved APA provider of continuing education (CE) for psychologists)*. Retrieved from https://www.healthforumonline.com/ce-course-detail/course--12033/ April 2, 2020.

Kohut, H. (1971). *The analysis of the self.* New York, NY: International Universities Press.

Kohut, H., & Wolf, E. S. (1978). The disorders of the self and their treatment: An outline. *International Journal of Psycho-Analysis, 59*, 413–425.

Lampropoulos, G. K. (2001). Bridging technical eclecticism and theoretical integration: Assimilative integration. *Journal of Psychotherapy Integration, 11*(1), 5–19. doi: 10.1023/A:1026672807119

Lampropoulos, G. K., & Dixon, D. N. (2007). Psychotherapy integration in internships and counselling psychology doctoral programs. *Journal of Psychotherapy Integration, 17*(2), 185–208. doi: 10.1037/1053-0479.17.2.185

Längle, A. A., & Kriz, J. (2012). The renewal of humanism in European psychotherapy: Developments and applications. *Psychotherapy: Theory, Research, and Practice, 49*(4), 430–436. doi: 10.1037/a0027397

Lecomte, C., Castonguay, L. G., Cyr, M., & Sabourin, S. (1993). Supervision and instruction in doctoral psychotherapy integration. In G. Stricker & J. R. Gold (Eds.), *Comprehensive handbook of psychotherapy integration* (pp. 483–498). New York, NY: Plenum Press.

Leichsenring, F., & Steinert, C. (2018). Towards an evidence-based unified psychodynamic protocol for emotional disorders. *Journal of Affective Disorders, 232*, 400–416. doi: 10.1016/j.jad.2017.11.036

Loevinger, J. (1976). *Ego development.* San Francisco, CA: Jossey-Bass Publishers.

Lyons-Ruth, K., Bruschweiler-Stern, N., Harrison, A. M., Morgan, A. C., Nahum, J. P., Sander, L., … Tronick, E. Z. (1998). Implicit relational knowing: Its role in development and psychoanalytic treatment. *Infant Mental Health Journal: Official Publication of The World Association for Infant Mental Health, 19*(3), 282–289. doi: 10.1002/(SICI)1097-0355(199823)19:3<282::AID-IMHJ3>3.0.CO;2-O

Macarthur, J. (2013). An integrative approach to addressing core beliefs in social anxiety. *Journal of Psychotherapy Integration, 23*(4), 386–396. doi: 10.1037/a0035043

Magnavita, J. J. (2005). *Personality-guided relational psychotherapy: A unified approach.* Washington, DC: American Psychological Association.

Magnavita, J. J. (2006). In search of the unifying principles of psychotherapy: Conceptual, empirical, and clinical convergence. *American Psychologist, 61*(8), 882. doi: 10.1037/0003-066X.61.8.882

Magnavita, J. J. (2008). Toward unification of clinical science: The next wave in the evolution of psychotherapy? *Journal of Psychotherapy Integration, 18*(3), 264–291. doi: 10.1037/a0013490

Magnavita, J. J. (2012). Advancing clinical science using system theory as the framework for expanding family psychology with unified psychotherapy. *Couple and Family Psychology: Research and Practice, 1*(1), 3–13. doi: 10.1037/a0027492

Magnavita, J. J., & Anchin, J. C. (2014). *Unifying psychotherapy: Principles, methods, and evidence from clinical science.* New York, NY: Springer.

Mahoney, M. J. (2003). *Constructive psychotherapy: A practical guide.* New York, NY: Guilford Press.

Marquis, A. (2018). *Integral psychotherapy: A unifying approach.* New York, NY: Routledge.

Marquis, A., & Elliot, A. (2015). Integral psychotherapy in practice, Part 2: Revisions to the metatheory of Integral Psychotherapy based on therapeutic practice. *Journal of Unified Psychotherapy and Clinical Science, 3*(1), 1–40.

Marquis, A., & Wilber, K. (2008). Unification beyond eclecticism and integration: Integral psychotherapy. *Journal of Psychotherapy Integration, 18*(3), 350–358.

May, R. (1958). Contributions of existential psychotherapy. In R. May, E. Angel & H. F. Ellenberger (Eds.), *Existence: A new dimension in psychiatry and psychology* (pp. 37–91). New York, NY: Basic Books.
Norcross, J. C., & Beutler, L. E. (2014). Integrative psychotherapies. In D. Wedding & R. J. Corsini (Eds.), *Current psychotherapies* (10th ed., pp. 499–532). Belmont, CA: Brooks/Cole, Cengage.
Norcross, J. C., & Beutler, L. E. (2019). Integrative psychotherapies. In D. Wedding & R. J. Corsini (Eds.), *Current psychotherapies* (11th ed., pp. 527–560). Boston, MA: Cengage.
Norcross, J. C., & Goldfried, M. R. (2005). The future of psychotherapy integration: A roundtable. *Journal of Psychotherapy Integration, 15*(4), 392–471. doi: 10.1037/1053-0479.15.4.392
Norcross, J. C., & Popple, L. M. (2017). *Supervision essentials for integrative psychotherapy.* Washington, DC: American Psychological Association.
Pincus, D. (2012). Self-organizing biopsychosocial dynamics and the patient-healer relationship. *Research in Complementary Medicine, 19*(1) Suppl. 1, 22–29. doi: 10.1159/000335186
Prochaska, J. O., & DiClemente, C. C. (2005). The transtheoretical approach. In J. C. Norcross & M. R. Goldfried (Eds.), *Handbook of psychotherapy integration* (2nd ed., pp. 147–171). New York, NY: Oxford University Press.
Rihacek, T., & Danelova, E. (2016). The journey of an integrationist: A grounded theory analysis. *Psychotherapy: Theory, Research, and Practice, 53*(1), 78–89. doi: 10.1037/pst0000040
Rogers, C. R. (1951). *Client-centered therapy*. Boston, MA: Houghton Mifflin.
Rønnestad, M. H., & Skovholt, T. (2013). *The developing practitioner: Growth and stagnation of therapists and counselors*. London, UK: Routledge.
Scaturo, D. J. (2005). *Clinical dilemmas in psychotherapy: A transtheoretical approach to psychotherapy integration*. Washington, DC: American Psychological Association.
Schottenbauer, M. A., Glass, C. R., & Arnkoff, D. B. (2005). Eclectic psychotherapy: A common factors approach. In J. C. Norcross & M. R. Goldfried (Eds.), *Handbook of psychotherapy integration* (2nd ed., pp. 459–493). New York, NY: Oxford University Press.
Shedler, J. (2010). The efficacy of psychodynamic psychotherapy. *American Psychologist, 65*(2), 98–109. doi: 10.1037/a0018378
Shoben, E. J., Jr. (1962). The counselor's theory as personal trait. *Personnel and Guidance Journal, 40*(7), 617–621. doi: 10.1002/j.2164-4918.1962.tb02171.x
Stangier, U., Schramm, E., Heidenreich, T., Berger, M., & Clark, D. M. (2011). Cognitive therapy vs interpersonal psychotherapy in social anxiety disorder: A randomized controlled trial. *Archives of General Psychiatry, 68*(7), 692–700. doi: 10.1001/archgenpsychiatry.2011.67
Stricker, G. (1993). The current status of psychotherapy integration. In G. Stricker & J. R. Gold (Eds.), *Comprehensive handbook of psychotherapy integration* (pp. 533–545). Boston, MA: Springer.
Stricker, G. (2010). A second look at psychotherapy integration. *Journal of Psychotherapy Integration, 20*(4), 397–405. doi: 10.1037/a0022037
Stricker, G., & Gold, J. R. (1996). Psychotherapy integration: An assimilative, psychodynamic approach. *Clinical Psychology: Science and Practice, 3*(1), 47–58. doi: 10.1111/j.1468-2850.1996.tb00057.x
Stricker, G., & Gold, J. (2006). Introduction: An overview of psychotherapy integration. In G. Stricker & J. Gold (Eds.), *A casebook of psychotherapy integration* (pp. 3–16). Washington, DC: American Psychological Association.

Trub, L., & Levy, D. (2017). Sowing the seeds for an assimilative integrationist stance toward psychotherapy. *Journal of Psychotherapy Integration, 27*(2), 172–185. doi: 10.1037/int0000056

Wachtel, P. L. (2010). Psychotherapy integration and integrative psychotherapy: Process or product? *Journal of Psychotherapy Integration, 20*(4), 406–416. doi: 10.1037/a0022032

Wachtel, P. L. (2014). On the limits of theoretical fundamentalism. *Journal of Psychotherapy Integration, 24*(2), 95–98. doi: 10.1037/a0036973

Wachtel, P. L. (2017, May 8). Pathways to progress for integrative psychotherapy: Perspectives on practice and research. *Journal of Psychotherapy Integration.* Advance online publication. doi: 10.1037/int0000089

Walder, E. H. (1993). Supervision and instruction in postgraduate psychotherapy integration. In G. Stricker & J. R. Gold (Eds.), *Comprehensive handbook of psychotherapy integration* (pp. 499–512). New York, NY: Plenum Press.

Wilber, K. (1999–2000). *The collected works of Ken Wilber.* Boston, MA: Shambhala.

Wilber, K. (2000). *Integral psychology: Consciousness, spirit, psychology, therapy.* Boston, MA: Shambala.

Wilber, K. (2003). Foreword. In F. Visser (Ed.), *Ken Wilber: Thought as passion* (pp. xii–xiii). Albany, NY: SUNY Press.

Zarbo, C., Tasca, G. A., Cattafi, F., & Compare, A. (2016). Integrative psychotherapy works. *Frontiers in Psychology, 6*, 2021. doi: 10.3389/fpsyg.2015.02021

2 The Need for Integrated and Unified Psychotherapy Approaches

Introduction

Do therapists identify as proponents of single-school or monotherapy or as integrated? An investigation of the theoretical orientation used by more than 1000 psychotherapists in their practice indicated that 15% of therapists employed only one theoretical approach, and that the median number of theoretical approaches used was four (Tasca et al., 2015; Zarbo, Tasca, Cattafi, & Compare, 2016). The aforementioned finding that therapists identify as integrated lends support to the fact that psychotherapy integration has emerged as a prominent movement for clinicians. Although psychotherapy integration exerts an important effect on clinical practice, it has not had as influential an effect on psychotherapy research (Castonguay, Eubanks, Goldfried, Muran, & Lutz, 2015).

Chapter 2 discusses the need for an integrated or unified approach to psychotherapy and supervision within the context of five waves or trends (see Figure 2.1). Practitioners use integrated psychotherapy approaches because they recognize that some patients are hard to treat and may not respond to single-school interventions, and they concur with the need to offer empirically supported perspectives for patients with complex problems (Fernández-Álvarez, Consoli, & Gómez, 2016; Norcross, 2005; Schottenbauer, Glass, & Arnkoff, 2005). The chapter presents the rationale for integrated and unified frameworks, delineates various types of models of psychotherapy integration and unification, and suggests that clinicians design and/or adapt unified frameworks, which can help them to organize information from different sources. Vignettes are provided to demonstrate the application of integrated psychotherapy models.

The Need for Integrated Psychotherapy

Is there a need for integrated theory and therapy? According to Feixas and Botella (2004), the purpose of an integrative psychotherapy model is to formulate a context for dialogue among a variety of psychotherapy approaches. An integrated psychotherapy approach can be custom tailored to suit different

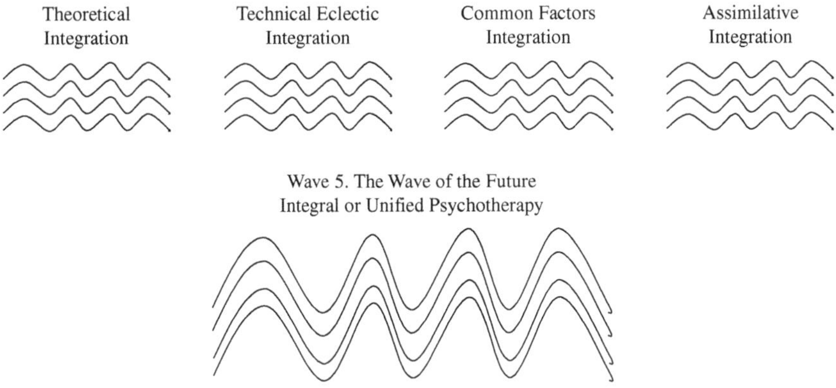

Figure 2.1 Integrated and unified psychotherapy. This figure illustrates five waves or trends of integrated or unified psychotherapy.

patients with a myriad of problems. Therapists who employ an integrative psychotherapy approach need to learn to adjust their treatment based on the individualized makeup of a particular client.

Although many clinicians in the United States describe themselves as employing an eclectic or integrative approach to psychotherapy (Norcross, 2005), only within the last few decades has integration emerged as a distinct field of interest (Glock, Hilsenroth, & Curtis, 2018). Whereas different types of single-school psychotherapy treatments have been shown to be equally effective, integrated psychotherapy approaches have been used as alternatives to single-school treatments, and the exploration of these integrated models of psychotherapy have been found to benefit outcome (Cutts, 2011). There is a paucity of research that shows the superiority of one single-school treatment over another for most disorders (Marquis, 2018). An exception to the aforementioned is the case of specific phobias (SP) where exposure models of psychotherapy have been found to be superior to other treatments (Marquis, 2018). At the same time, exposure rarely heals the phobias (Wolfe, 2005).

Single-school psychotherapy approaches such as cognitive behavioral therapy, e.g., the meta-analytic studies on anxiety of Stewart & Chambless (2009), the research on obsessive-compulsive disorder of Olatunji, Davis, Powers, and Smits (2013) and of Eddy, Dutra, Bradley, & Westen (2004), have been found to be effective in treating emotional disorders (Haverkampf, 2017). Similarly, psychodynamic therapy has been shown to be effective in treating social anxiety (Leichsenring et al., 2013). At the same time, there is no one psychotherapy treatment that has been found to be the gold standard for the emotional disorders, and cognitive-behavioral therapy, given rates of response that are approximately 50% and rates of remission that are less than 50%, is not the only cure (Fisher, & Wells, 2005; Leichsenring et al., 2018; Loerinc et al., 2015). Other psychotherapy treatments do not fare better (Cuijpers et al., 2014; Leichsenring et al., 2018).

Is there a need for more than one perspective? There is a need for plurality or an integrated psychotherapy perspective, particularly for patients who do not respond to one therapy approach (Leichsenring et al., 2018). Several researchers have integrated a cognitive-behavioral approach with psychodynamic therapy in the treatment of anxiety and obsessive-compulsive disorder (Bram & Björgvinsson, 2004; McFall & Wollersheim, 1979), and Haverkampf (2017) suggests that cognitive-behavioral therapy and psychodynamic interventions need to be considered complementary. In fact, it has been shown that the greater the utilization of a combination of psychodynamic-interpersonal and cognitive-behavioral psychotherapy, the greater the changes in patients' views of the working alliance (Owen, Hilsenroth, & Rodolfa, 2013).

Much has been said about the effect of the therapeutic alliance upon therapy outcome. The literature has shown that the relational component is a unifying tenet of psychotherapy, which affects an individual's function and maladaptive behaviors (Magnavita, 2006). Psychotherapy employs a relational component to facilitate therapeutic progress, and it is the working alliance that is critical to a therapeutic result (Magnavita, 2006; Norcross, 2002). Consistent with the conceptualization of integrated psychotherapy is Moursund and Erskine's (2004) approach, which is focused on the relationship, with a recognition that a wide range of human activity is involved including emotion, behavior, along with bodily and thought processes. More recently, Erskine (2013) proposed philosophical principles of a relational integrative therapy, a non-pathological approach to behavior, that underscores the therapeutic alliance as primary to a patient's growth. He considers the alliance within the context of a relational integrative therapy where a therapist promotes concepts such as authenticity, communication that individuals share, and vulnerability.

Researchers and clinicians have resorted to integrated psychotherapy approaches in an attempt to offer interventions that are empirically supported to patients who are complex, and/or who are hard to treat, and/or who do not respond to unitary interventions (Fernández-Álvarez et al., 2016; Norcross, 2005; Schottenbauer et al., 2005). In fact, there are endorsements for an integrative psychotherapy approach both in the U.S. and abroad (Liu et al., 2013; Norcross, Karpiak, & Santoro, 2005).

According to the APA Presidential Task Force on Evidence-Based Practice (2006), therapists who offer evidence-based practice need to integrate the best research and clinical findings depending on their clients' characteristics and needs (Fernández-Álvarez et al., 2016). The principles recommended by the APA Presidential Task Force on Evidence-Based Practice (2006) are not connected to a single-school orientation, can be common across a variety of emotional disorders, and lend themselves towards psychotherapy integration (Fernández-Álvarez et al., 2016).

The purpose of an integrated psychotherapy approach is to include different manners of psychotherapy practice rather than to promote uniformity where one clinician becomes identical to another (Schottenbauer et al., 2005; Zarbo, Tasca, Cattafi, & Compare, 2016). Whereas therapists are encouraged to develop an individual style and maintain a specific approach, awareness of the limitations of that approach as they interact with clinicians with other points of view will facilitate their recognition of when a patient is a good match for another therapist but a poor match for their own orientation (Schottenbauer et al., 2005).

Integrated Psychotherapy Models

How have integrated theories and therapy models evolved, why are they needed, and are they empirically supported? Researchers have delineated four types of integration or four integration trends (Castonguay et al., 2015; Norcross, 2005). The various types of integration – theoretical, technical eclectic, common factors, and assimilative – expand on the single-school approaches and rely on different means to enhance the effectiveness of psychotherapy (Norcross, Goldfried, & Arigo, 2016). Common factors integration has received the most empirical backing (Castonguay et al., 2015).

Theoretical Integration

What is theoretical integration, why is it needed, how did it evolve, how does it differ from assimilative integration, and which theorists provide examples of theoretical integration? The first type of integration, theoretical integration, is a sophisticated framework that refers to the integration of two or more therapy methods and theories into a new therapeutic model (Castonguay et al., 2015; Norcross, 2005; Marquis, 2018). The goal of theoretical integration is a theoretical formulation and the creation of a unified approach rather than a technical merging of methods (Cutts, 2011; Norcross, 2005). Theoretical integration is an advanced and complex type of integration as it aims to draw different theoretical ideas from contrasting perspectives (Jones-Smith, 2012; Stricker & Gold, 2006). The cyclical psychodynamic theory along with its integrative psychotherapy of Wachtel (1977) can be considered the first mature type of theoretical integration (Stricker & Gold, 2006).

How is theoretical integration different from other integration trends? Theoretical integration differs from assimilative integration in that it may develop from a combination of several theories rather than originate from one kind of typical psychotherapy approach (Schottenbauer et al., 2005). What is the goal of theoretical integration? The purpose of the aforementioned pure type of integration, theoretical integration, is to develop a richer and broader perspective that promotes the nuances of different theories (Norcross & Goldfried, 2005; Safran & Messer, 1997; Trub & Levy, 2017). Although there is a myriad of perspectives, a theoretical integration approach, generally, integrates only a few of the orientations (Marquis, 2018). Examples of a theoretical integration perspective are the works of Wachtel (1977, 1997,

2014), Ryle's (1990) Cognitive Analytic Therapy (CAT), Wachtel, Kruk, and McKinney's (2005) cyclical psychodynamics and integrative relational psychotherapy, Prochaska and DiClemente's (2005) transtheoretical model (TTM), and Constantino and Westra's (2012) expectancy-based model, which integrates psychodynamic theory, cognitive therapy, and social psychology.

How do integrated theorists and therapists approach theoretical integration? In its reliance on cyclical psychodynamics, for example, integrative relational therapy aims to integrate family-systems, psychodynamic, and behavioral orientations (Wachtel et al., 2005). Wachtel and colleagues (2005) contrast the systematic perspective of cyclical psychodynamics, which aims to design a comprehensive theoretical framework to guide a therapist's clinical decisions, with a technical eclectic approach that helps therapists select methods that work for clients with similar features. Cyclical psychodynamics can be viewed as both theoretical and assimilative integration (Wachtel et al., 2005). Wachtel and colleagues (2005) explain that although the core of cyclical psychodynamics derives from classical psychoanalytic concepts, it incorporates interpersonal notions (e.g., Sullivan, 1953), sociocultural ideas (e.g., Fromm, 1949), and relational conceptualizations (e.g., Mitchell, 1988) in its focus on the way in which past circumstances and relationships contribute to vicious circles that are projected into the present (e.g., Wachtel, 1982). Cyclical psychodynamic theory, which derives from an interpersonal psychodynamic orientation and method as well as an integration of cognitive-behavioral and systems perspectives, and integrative relational therapy have frequently been used as treatments for anxiety and interpersonal problems (Gold & Wachtel, 1993; Wachtel et al., 2005).

How do multi-theoretical models integrate? Prochaska and DiClemente (2005) approach theoretical integration by proposing a multi-theoretical framework, a transtheoretical model (TTM), which appeals to therapists who promote a broader approach. TTM emphasizes the examination of behavior change including the change process, the stages, the advantages and disadvantages, and levels of change, and the integration of processes, levels, and stages (Prochaska & DiClemente, 2005). It has been found that a patient's stage prior to treatment can predict the outcome of treatment (Norcross, Krebs, & Prochaska, 2011).

Another multi-theoretical framework includes the approach of Brooks-Harris (2008). This model integrates experiential, biopsychosocial, psychodynamic, systemic, multicultural, cognitive, and behavioral theoretical orientations and describes the way in which various therapy systems, e.g., actions, feelings, thoughts, interact (Brooks-Harris, 2008; Jones-Smith, 2012).

Vignette

The following is an example that uses a vignette to illustrate a multidimensional survey within the context of the multi-theoretical psychotherapy model of Brooks-Harris (2008):

Rebecca is a female, age 92, in good physical health, who has lost most of her support system. She has one son who lives out of the U.S. who calls her twice a week. Most of her friends have died, and there is a neighbor who looks in on her every so often. When Rebecca was 5, she saw an SS officer shoot her father in the head in Dachau. Recently she has been feeling more anxious and has trouble calming herself down. She is the oldest of three children, her husband died about 20 years ago, and she lives alone.

Thoughts: I am having problems relaxing, and I feel somewhat traumatized.
Social: Rebecca's friends have died. She remembers a good relationship with her father. After the war, her mother was too depressed to engage her.
Actions: Avoidance of crowds, family, and social events.
Cultural: In her culture, children respect their parents. They listen, but do not speak.
Feelings: Anxiety, worry, nervousness.
Biology: Aches and pains.
Interpersonal: Not wishing to talk to people.

A psychotherapist may select a theoretical orientation for each of the aforementioned dimensions (e.g., thought, social); however, it is suggested that initially the psychotherapist focus on two or three dimensions (Brooks-Harris, 2008; Jones-Smith, 2012).

Technical Eclectic Integration

What is the focus of technical eclectic integration, why is it needed, and how does it differ from theoretical integration? Technical eclectic integration involves the use of methods from different psychotherapy perspectives without the need to reconcile theoretical differences and without integrating them into a new psychotherapeutic model (Castonguay et al., 2015; Lazarus, 2005; Norcross, 2005). The focus of technical eclectic integration (related to eclectic therapy) is on techniques rather than on a rapprochement of theory (Norcross, 2005; Stricker & Gold, 2006). At the same time, technical eclectic integration employs a systematic approach in its selection of treatment techniques (Castonguay, Reid, Halperin, & Goldfried, 2003).

Technical eclectic integration underscores empirically supported techniques that facilitate patient change rather than theories (Lampropoulos, 2001; Lazarus & Beutler, 1993; Trub & Levy, 2017). Unlike the goal of theoretical integration, which has the formulation of a unified theory as an end goal, the purpose of technical eclecticism in therapy is the use of tested methods rather than the advancement of a unified theory, and therapists who are technical eclectics do not adhere to the theories from which the methods originate (Cutts, 2011; Lazarus, 1989, 2005). For example, the multimodal therapy (MMT) of Lazarus (2005) and Beutler's systematic treatment selection (STS)

(Beutler, Consoli, & Lane, 2005) focus on a patient's problems or characteristics and the choice of a particular relevant therapeutic method (Ziv-Beiman & Shahar, 2015).

Unlike Rogerian therapy which is unimodal and viewed by Lazarus as the antithesis of multimodal therapy, MMT selects techniques from a variety of disciplines, does not include or merge theories, and relies on a social-cognitive learning orientation (Lazarus, 2005). Experiential and cognitive techniques, as well as methods based on imagery are added to behavioral treatment (Lazarus, 2005; Stricker & Gold, 2006). Lazarus (2005) advocates the use of a myriad of selected technical eclectic methods that have an empirical basis, and he applies these techniques to provide a broad and flexible psychotherapy approach for each individual patient. The emphasis of technical eclectic integration is on the choice of the best type of intervention for a patient's issues or on methods that are selected because they are the best match for the needs of a particular client (Stricker & Gold, 2006; Ziv-Beiman & Shahar, 2015).

In their article, "Systematic Treatment Selection and Prescriptive Psychotherapy: An Integrative Eclectic Approach," Beutler, Consoli, and Lane (2005) describe a model of intervention, Systematic Treatment Selection (STS) (Beutler, Clarkin, & Bongar, 2000), that includes intervention planning and the matching of clients to specific interventions. The use of STS facilitates an interaction among client, therapist, working alliance, intervention, and the fit of a particular treatment (Beutler, Consoli, & Lane, 2005). The emphasis is on techniques or procedures that best fit the client rather than on the theories that are connected to those methods, and the focus is on expanding the therapists' clinical decision formulations rather than on etiology (Beutler, Consoli, & Lane, 2005).

Beutler et al. (2005) identify the following client dimensions and intervention qualities that influence prognosis: The complexity and chronicity of the patient's issues, the level of the patient's impairment, distress, reactance or resistance to the control of others, and the patient's coping style (e.g., internalizing or externalizing). For example, although a high level of patient impairment is associated with a better response to interpersonal psychotherapy and medication, a low level of patient impairment suggests that medication is not necessary (Elkin et al., 1989).

Beutler's (1979) research targets the matching of treatment to the individual patient, and the Systematic Treatment Selection (STS) approach (Beutler, Clarkin, & Bongar, 2000) posits tenets such as patient features, e.g., the patient's reactance and style of coping (Beutler, Harwood, Michelson, Song, & Holman, 2011; Castonguay et al., 2015). Whereas patients with a high degree of reactance to the control of others will improve more with therapists who have low levels of directiveness, patients with a low degree of reactance will do better with treatments where therapists are more directive (Beutler, Harwood, Michelson, Song, & Holman, 2011; Castonguay et al., 2015).

Vignette

Based on the match between reactance and directive treatment (Beutler et al., 2011; Castonguay et al., 2015), the following vignette conveys the therapist's work with a patient with social anxiety disorder who has a low level of reactance to the control of others:

Margaret: I need to play the cello at the school orchestra this week. I am really anxious about my position in the school orchestra. We need to play for each other together this week. I don't know whether I will be able to get up in front of the others and play my part.
Therapist: Divide the music that you will be playing for the members of the orchestra into small parts. Practice a small part of the music at a time in front of a close friend. Stand in front of the mirror, imagine the whole orchestra is there, and play a small part of the music. Before you play for the members of the band, think of your most relaxing place (sitting with the books in the stacks of a library).
Margaret: Sounds relaxing.
Therapist: So when can you start?
Margaret: Today, I can start with my friend, Mia. I'll play a short piece of the music for her.
Therapist: Let me know how you felt during the practice session with Mia.

The following week, Margaret let the therapist know that it went well with Mia. Margaret seemed open to the therapist's offering brief homework exercises each week. The therapist proceeded to ask her what she thought and how she felt during each therapy session and to adjust the homework exercises based on Margaret's feedback. Margaret seemed to maintain a low level of resistance, and, at the end of a few cello practice sessions with Mia and in front of the mirror along with imagining that she was in the library looking through the book stacks, she was able to play her cello part in front of the members of the orchestra.

Whereas patients with an externalizing coping style, patients with a tendency to blame others, are a better match for treatments that target the decrease of symptoms (e.g., cognitive-behavioral therapy), patients with an internalizing style, patients with obsessive-compulsive behaviors who tend to ruminate and blame themselves, are a better match for interventions that focus on the exploration of the self (e.g., psychodynamic or interpersonal therapy) (Castonguay & Beutler, 2006; Castonguay et al., 2015; Fernández-Álvarez et al., 2016).

Do cognitive therapists need to abandon their ways of practice when treating different types of patients? It is not necessary for cognitive clinicians to discontinue their use of their favored manner of practice when they treat patients with an internalizing coping style or a high level of resistance; however, it is suggested that cognitive therapists modify their use of their cognitive-behavioral treatments to fit or match their patients' specific style (Castonguay, 2000; Castonguay et al., 2015; Goldfried & Castonguay, 1992).

The takeaway from the section on technical eclectic therapy principles is that it is possible to use methods from different psychotherapy orientations and that treatment needs to be matched to the individual patient (Beutler, 1983; Schottenbauer et al., 2005). The emphasis of technical eclectic integration is on methods rather than on theories (Cutts, 2011; Lazarus, 1989; 2005).

Common Factors Integration

What is the origin of the common factors integration perspective? The founder of the common factors perspective is Rosenzweig whose 1936 article, "Some Implicit Common Factors in Diverse Methods of Psychotherapy," was the first integrative one to be published (Duncan, 2002; Stricker & Gold, 2006). Rogers's (1951) core conditions to facilitate change influenced the common factors approach (Jones-Smith, 2012).

Why is the common factors integration approach needed, and what is its purpose? Common factors integration aims at discerning the key components that various treatments share with the goal of developing more effective interventions based on the shared components (Norcross, 2005). The aforementioned perspective relies on the idea that common elements, rather than differentiating factors, contribute to effectiveness in therapy (Norcross, 2005). Proponents of common factors promote the idea that rather than focusing on a single school's correct theory or technique, therapists need to assess their patients' perceptions of the working alliance and treatment progress to direct the therapeutic endeavor (Norcross, Goldfried, & Arigo, 2016). They explain that the therapeutic alliance, a committed patient, and a therapist who is empathic are more important for treatment outcome than the specific treatment technique employed. Although researchers have proposed that it is possible to classify the common factors according to patients' characteristics, e.g., working alliance, qualities of the psychotherapist (Bickman, 2005), there has not been agreement on the specific delineations of the common factors (Cutts, 2011; Lampropoulos, 2000).

What is the focus of common factors integration? Common factors integration emphasizes the shared factors (relational or non-relational) contributing to change across different psychotherapy perspectives and the influence of these shared principles over distinctive treatment dimensions (Castonguay et al., 2015; Fernández-Álvarez et al., 2016; Norcross, 2005). Proponents of common factors assert that these shared factors contribute a greater amount to psychotherapy than do factors that distinguish among therapeutic approaches (Norcross et al., 2016). Consistent with the aforementioned research, psychotherapists who follow a common factors approach inquire about the specific common factors that are critical for developing interventions for each specific patient (Stricker & Gold, 2006). The therapeutic approaches of Frank (1973) and Garfield (1992) are examples of the common factors perspective.

An innovative example of the common factors approach is the psychotherapy model of Beitman, Soth, and Bumby (2005), a framework with an orientation towards the future. They rely on a common integrative concept of a future-focused psychotherapy reflected across different psychotherapy approaches. For example, with respect to the interpersonal psychotherapy approach, maladaptive interpersonal schemas may lead patients to hold unrealistic expectations of their future functioning, e.g., that if, in the future, they go to a meeting, nobody will want to talk to them, that if, in the future, they communicate in the wrong way their significant other will break off the relationship (Beitman et al., 2005). From a psychodynamic perspective, for example, patients' motives are viewed as future projections, e.g., wishes, psychodynamic principles such as unconscious conflicts that incorporate a notion of the future, a patient's unconscious conflicts being met with interpretations to negotiate between two futures (Beitman et al., 2005). In their model, Beitman et al. (2005) describe psychotherapy techniques of change with a future perspective. One can conceive of this approach as both etiological and teleological as it connects etiology or cause to a teleological direction, future or destiny.

How does common factors integration compare to other integration approaches? Common factors approaches predict that models are more similar than dissimilar (D'Aniello, 2015). Similar to eclectic perspectives, common factors approaches are missing an underlying logical core for offering different psychotherapeutic interventions to different patients, and these common factors approaches do not strive to create a unified theory (Cutts, 2011; Marquis, 2018). There are researchers who have suggested that common factors be integrated into training in marriage and family therapy (D'Aniello, 2015; Weeks & Chad, 2004).

Assimilative Integration

What is the origin of the fourth type of integration, assimilative integration, and how does it differ from other forms of integration? The fourth type of integration, assimilative integration, differs from the aforementioned three types in that it anchors itself to a single psychotherapy approach while incorporating methods and tenets from other psychotherapy frameworks (Castonguay et al., 2015; Norcross, 2005). For technical eclectic integration and assimilative integration, the integration occurs at the point of practice rather than theory, and both types of integration incorporate therapeutic methods from a variety of approaches (Norcross, 2005).

Who is the founder of assimilative integration? It was Messer (1992) who first addressed the notion of assimilation as related to therapy integration (Stricker & Gold, 2006). Theoretical integration and technical eclecticism have influenced assimilative integration (Messer, 1992; Stricker & Gold, 2002). Assimilative integration offers psychotherapists the opportunity to integrate methods from other therapy schools into their own model, thus allowing them to keep their preferred approach to psychotherapy (Wolfe, 2008). The majority of integrative psychotherapy models may be classified as assimilative integration frameworks (Wolfe, 2008).

What are examples of assimilative integration, and how does it work in practice? Examples of assimilative integration include Stricker and Gold's (2005) assimilative psychodynamic therapy and Castonguay, Newman, Borkovec, Holtforth, and Maramba's (2005) cognitive-behavioral assimilative psychotherapy. Stricker and Gold (2005), in their use of assimilative psychodynamic therapy, identify several clinical situations, e.g., a patient's severe anxiety, where it can be beneficial for a psychodynamically oriented therapist to be flexible, to make an assimilative shift, and to incorporate more active approaches to treatment (cognitive-behavioral, experiential, family-systems). They point out that in these situations, it is the therapist's commitment to be more active, rather than to interpret, that can serve as a deeper curative emotional experience for the patient. They found that patients whose order of treatment is psychodynamic-behavioral benefited more than patients who received a behavioral intervention prior to psychodynamic psychotherapy.

Whereas Stricker and Gold (2005) suggested that a psychodynamically oriented therapist make an assimilative shift and incorporate more active approaches to treatment, Castonguay et al. (2005) developed a treatment approach for generalized anxiety disorder, a cognitive-behavioral assimilative integration, that attempts to enhance cognitive-behavioral therapy, by incorporating or assimilating methods, e.g., emotionally focused and interpersonal strategies, from other perspectives (interpersonal, humanistic, psychodynamic). Castonguay and colleagues (2005) realize that standard cognitive-behavioral therapy (CBT) methods do not sufficiently consider the nuances of their patients' lives, and their goal was to improve on CBT by employing a cohesive assimilation of interventions from other theoretical approaches in order to address the distress of their patients, enhance their patients' interpersonal skills, and deepen their patients' emotions. For example, the way in which obstacles have been addressed in the therapeutic alliance during CBT have been found to decrease the effectiveness of CBT interventions (Castonguay et al., 2005). Castonguay, Goldfried, Wiser, Raue, and Hayes (1996) showed that cognitive therapists tend to increase their use of techniques when problems related to the working relationship emerge, and this treatment strategy tends to increase the rupture in the therapeutic alliance. Rather, what may be needed is a willingness on the part of therapists to shift to a new strategy, a more comprehensive assimilation of treatments from other theoretical orientations, in an effort to address difficulties in the client–therapist relationship (Castonguay et al., 2005). The aforementioned work of Castonguay et al. (2005) is consistent with the assimilative integration work of Safran (1990), Safran and Segal (1990), and Young, Klosko, and Weishaar (2003) who show how the cognitive notion of schema can be broadened by introducing concepts from gestalt, developmental, and interpersonal therapy, e.g., ruptures in the therapeutic relationship (Castonguay et al., 2015).

Whereas earlier examples of assimilative integration include Safran and Segal's (1990, 1996) interpersonal and cognitive assimilative therapy, West's (2000) humanistic approach, and O'Leary and Barry's (2006) gestalt reminiscence therapy, more recent examples of assimilative integration include Alladin's (2012) assimilative model of integrated psychotherapy, cognitive hypnotherapy (CH) or cognitive-behavioral hypnotherapy (CBH), and Trub and Levy's (2017) example of a practicum. Alladin's (2012) cognitive hypnotherapy (CH) or cognitive-behavioral hypnotherapy (CBH) is an example of an integrated model that combines hypnotherapy with cognitive behavioral therapy (CBT). In practice, Alladin (2014) combines cognitive hypnotherapy (CH) with Wolfe's (2005, 2006) integrated model of therapy for the anxiety disorders. Alladin (2012) shows how cognitive hypnotherapy can help patients trace their self-wounds to their origin and provides a framework for patients to heal their self-wounds or past emotional damage to the self that has not been resolved. Trub and Levy's (2017) perspective is a more recent example of an approach towards a practicum that facilitates an orientation towards assimilative integration.

Wolfe (2001) explains that integrationists who are assimilative need to incorporate an accommodative approach by adjusting their anchor theory when they employ treatment methods from another perspective. The accommodation will then contribute towards greater internal consistency of the new theory (Wolfe, 2008). For example, researchers such as Safran and Segal (1996) modified their initial anchor theory, their cognitive perspective, to accommodate the results from process research as they expanded CBT to encompass the interpersonal interactions between client and psychotherapist, integrated interpretive methods of a psychodynamic approach based on the interpersonal, and incorporated emotion-focused methods of the humanistic orientation (Wolfe, 2008).

Whereas some researchers assert that assimilative integration paves the way for the fifth wave or trend, unified psychotherapy, others view assimilative integration as preferable to a unified approach because of its inherent heuristic worth for theory building and clinical application (Fisch, 2001; Wolfe, 2008). Although Magnavita's (2008) integrative or unified approach is comprehensive, it does not include a humanistic perspective (Wolfe, 2008). When assimilative integrationists consider the construction of a unified psychotherapy theory, they need to include the primary therapy approaches along with an experiential perspective given that processes based on meaning and emotion are critical in the understanding of emotional disorders such as anxiety (Wolfe, 2008).

How do researchers and clinicians who rely on the five waves or trends seek to build integrative psychotherapy frameworks? When one sets out to design a new integrative psychotherapy model, one needs to know the reason and how to select the correct strategy for doing so (Krupnik, 2018). Krupnick suggests an approach to integration, nested hierarchy (NH), that connects the interventions in a hierarchical nest, a strategy where the interventions are directed by theories that buttress the interventions. According to her organizational strategy, theories that are general reside at the top, and subsidiary theories that are specific can be found on the lower steps of the hierarchy. According to Krupnik (2018), therapy integration routes, themselves, e.g., technical eclecticism, common factors, and so on, have been organized in a hierarchical arrangement, with theoretical integration on the top rung, assimilative integration on the second rung down, common factors on the next to lowest, and eclecticism on the lowest step. NH can be conceptualized as a framework that can be used to build integrated psychotherapy treatments (Krupnik, 2018).

This section discussed the need for four types of integration or four integration trends or waves – theoretical, technical eclectic, common factors, and assimilative. Whereas the end goal of technical eclectic and common factors is not the formation of a unified model, theoretical integration and assimilative integration aim towards the development of a unified theory (Cutts, 2011).

A Unified Psychotherapy Approach: The Fifth Wave

What is unified psychotherapy, and why is it needed? The fifth wave or trend, unified or integral therapy or integration that is metatheoretical, derives from the prior four waves of therapy integration, e.g., theoretical, technical eclectic, common factors, and assimilative integration (Anchin & Magnavita, 2008; Critchfield, Mackaronis, & Benjamin, 2017; Magnavita & Anchin, 2014). To help mental health professionals who are overloaded with information from extensive sources, Magnavita (2006) called for a unified framework that organizes the material as it applies to psychotherapy with individuals, families, and systems with multiple impairments. According to Magnavita (2006), a psychotherapist who uses a unified approach needs to integrate several levels of deep knowledge while cultivating a recognition of complex domains. He recommended a model or framework of unified treatment that facilitates domains of the biopsychosocial universe to be expanded by the use of neuroscience, statistics of a nonlinear nature, and technology. Therapeutic efficacy is further enhanced by pulling together seemingly disparate perspectives of psychotherapy (Magnavita, 2008). The Integral Intake (Marquis, 2008) and Integral Taxonomy of Therapeutic Interventions (Marquis, 2009) can assist therapists to sort out how to conceptualize their cases and to decide on the selection of interventions that are suited to their patients' states.

Wolfe (2008) recognized that the development of a unified theory would be the next wave of the psychotherapy integration movement, and he viewed Magnavita's (2008) unified psychotherapy approach along with its integration of family systems and the interpersonal as a step towards unification. He predicted that the vacillation between assimilated integration and accommodative integration would inspire the emergence of the next wave of psychotherapy integration.

How can the fifth trend be characterized? The fifth wave of psychotherapy integration consists of a metatheoretical integration or a unified integral model or framework (Marquis, 2018). The integral model of psychotherapy, based on integral theory (Wilber, 2000), emphasizes the need for understanding a human being from different points of view, e.g., biological cultural, rather than adhering to one theoretical approach (Ingersoll & Marquis, 2014; Marquis & Elliot, 2015). The model includes a quadratic perspective with lines and levels of development, states of consciousness, and psychological types or styles (Wilber, 2000; Ingersoll & Marquis, 2014). The four quadrants constitute the basic elements (interiors, exteriors, individuals, and groups) of human experience (Ingersoll, 2007). Whereas the Upper Left quadrant (UL) consists of the psychological or the interior of an individual and the Upper Right quadrant (UR) consists of the medical or the exterior of an individual, the Lower Left (LL) consists of the culture or the intersubjective component of a group and the Lower Right (LR) consists of the social or the exterior of a group (Ingersoll & Marquis, 2014; Marquis & Elliot, 2015). For example, the lines of development that include various aspects, e.g., cognitive, moral, develop at different rates within each individual, and the levels or stages of development make up the developmental dynamics, e.g., patient's level of cognition signifying what the patient can recognize (Ingersoll & Marquis, 2014). Another line of development is comprised of ego development (Ingersoll, 2007). The integral approach includes states of consciousness, e.g., a depressed state, and states are not permanent (Ingersoll & Marquis, 2014). Finally, the integral model includes types or styles which represent the client's personality (Ingersoll & Marquis, 2014). For example, types refer to how humans filter their experiences (Ingersoll, 2007).

When utilizing a unified psychotherapy approach that is holistic or broader than existing theoretical approaches, therapists can employ particular methods from any perspective so that the treatment engages principles or change mechanisms that are related to theory (Critchfield et al., 2017). A recent unified model was developed by Henriques, Kleinman, and Asselin (2014) who described a Nested Model (NM) of well-being, based on a unified metatheoretical orientation of psychology (Henriques, 2011) with subjective, biological-psychological, social context, and values elements, four domains, which interact to establish a holistic notion of well-being. An individual enjoys authentic well-being when the aforementioned domains align (Henriques et al., 2014). The well-being of individuals is elevated when they are pleased with their lives, when they function effectively in the biological and psychological domain, when they maintain sufficient social relationships, and have a life filled with meaning and purpose (Henriques et al., 2014).

Recently, Henriques (2017) extended the aforementioned work by developing a systems theory (Henriques, 2016) that connects integrative conceptualizations of personality theory and unified approaches to psychotherapy. According to Henriques (2017), CAST, or character adaptation systems theory (described in Chapter 1), extends from Henriques' (2011) unified perspective of psychology, and includes five character adaptation systems, i.e., habit, experiential, relational, defensive, justification, that correspond to physiological, developmental, and sociocultural contexts. CAST facilitates a holistic view of a human being, can help clinicians to develop interventions, and promotes a unified approach (Henriques, 2017). For example, whereas a psychodynamic approach may correspond to the relational system, a cognitive perspective may be in line with the justification system (Henriques, 2017). Chapter 1 described the linguistic justification system that delineates the integration of language, self-awareness, reasoning capacity, meaning, and culture, and suggests that therapists pay attention to the immediacy of a patient's states or experiences (Bassett-Short & Hammel, 2008; Henriques, 2017; Marquis, 2018).

Are there other unified approaches that share similar characteristics to the holism of Henriques et al. (2014)? Similar to Henriques et al.'s (2014) notion of holism, Magnavita and Anchin's (2014) unifying perspective for psychotherapy relies on a holistic paradigm. According to Magnavita and Anchin (2014), it is difficult to aim towards a unified approach towards psychotherapy without a metatheory. The metatheory of the biopsychosocial system can unify as it relies on a holistic framework where inherent notions of analysis and synthesis interact (Engel, 1977; Magnavita & Anchin, 2014). Magnavita and Anchin (2014) advocated the use of a holistic approach and suggested a biopsychosocial perspective of human development that can facilitate psychotherapy unification. They proposed the following four categories of human development: (1) Intrapsychic-biological, (2) interpersonal-dyadic, (3) relational-triadic, and (4) sociocultural-familial, and they demonstrated that it is possible for clinicians who are flexible to recognize the interrelationships among the four levels of the unified model in their use of the unified framework to navigate levels of an ecological system that complement each other. Magnavita and Anchin (2014) offer the following example: Suppose a therapist is working with a patient on Level 1, intrapsychic defenses, at the same time as the therapist is working at Level 2, the interpersonal-dyadic, or the therapeutic alliance; and while the therapist is targeting a patient's defenses (Level 1), there are communications that ensue between the therapist and patient that affect the working alliance (Level 2). It is a unified clinician who can effect a smooth and flexible shift in perspective so that different angles are elicited (Magnavita & Anchin, 2014).

How do other researchers approach unification? According to Tryon (2014), theoretical unification constitutes an agreement among psychologists to work together in sharing a common vocabulary and key concepts. He suggested that with greater theoretical unification, the competitive hostility that characterizes many settings in the field of psychology will dissolve. In his text, *Cognitive Neuroscience and Psychotherapy*, Tryon (2014) used a Bio Psychology Network framework to show how neuroscience can explain the way in which emotion and cognition influence behavior, and he demonstrated the notion of emergence, e.g., the emergence of psychology from biology. He explained that the concept of emergence includes transcendence, and he offers the following example of the properties of water: Although water emerges from the combination of oxygen and hydrogen, water is different from these two gases, or a new reality occurs with the emergence of water which is different from the parts, oxygen and hydrogen. In a similar vein, one can think of human science as an investigation of the properties of individuals who transcend or emerge from their own biology (Tryon, 2014). Tryon (2014) illustrated how his unified theory along with its network principles integrates different clinical orientations, e.g., psychodynamic, cognitive. The major contribution of his book is the elucidation of how the core network principle, transformation, explains the way in which mind derives from brain.

In a study that investigated how integral psychotherapists used a unified approach to psychotherapy (integral metatheory), Marquis, Short, Lewis, and Hubbard (2015) found that a multi-quadrant system that includes interpersonal, neurobiological, and phenomenological concepts assisted therapists to facilitate experiential awareness, a key issue that promotes change for patients in therapy. Whereas Wilber (2000) emphasized cognitive awareness, therapists in Marquis et al.'s (2015) study highlighted experiential change, the notion of being in tune with the physical body and its accompanying emotions. According to Marquis and colleagues (2015), an approach to integral psychotherapy guided by principles has been shown to facilitate custom tailored clinical practice for each patient. Novice therapists may find it difficult to practice integral psychotherapy (Ingersoll & Zeitler, 2010; Marquis & Wilber, 2008) because it offers a conceptual framework that is more abstract than monotherapy orientations or integrative therapeutic perspectives and does not offer novice therapists concrete rules as to what to do during therapy sessions (Marquis et al., 2015).

Recently, Marquis (2018) developed a cohesive model, an organizing framework, that underscores the need for a unified approach to psychotherapy. Chapters 1 and 3 describe his metatheoretical integral or unifying model in detail.

Summary

This chapter discussed the need for psychotherapy integration or unification, presented five waves or trends of integrated and unified psychotherapy, and provided examples of integrated and unified psychotherapy models that are representative of the different trends (see Table 2.1). It is suggested that

Table 2.1 The Need for Integrated or Unified Psychotherapy: Five Waves or Trends

Theoretical Integration	*Technical Eclectic*	*Common Factors*	*Assimilative*	*Integral or Unified*
A theoretical formulation and the creation of a unified approach rather than a technical merging of methods[a,b]	Techniques rather than a rapprochement of theory[b,c]	Key components that various treatments share with the goal of developing effective interventions based on the shared components[b]	Anchors itself to a single approach while incorporating methods from other frameworks[d,b]	A holistic framework that suggests a biopsychosocial perspective of human development and encourages psychotherapy unification[e]

[a]Cutts (2011). [b]Norcross (2005). [c]Stricker and Gold (2006). Castonguay, Eubanks, Goldfried, Muran, and Lutz, 2015. [e]Magnavita and Anchin (2014).

integrative therapists consider the entirety of the domains of their patients' reality and that they value knowledge attained from a reflection on life events as much as recognized courses of research study (Finnerty & McLeod, 2018).

References

Alladin, A. (2012). Cognitive hypnotherapy: A new vision and strategy for research and practice. *American Journal of Clinical Hypnosis, 54*(4), 249–262. doi: 10.1080/00029157.2012.654528

Alladin, A. (2014). The wounded self: New approach to understanding and treating anxiety disorders. *American Journal of Clinical Hypnosis, 56*(4), 368–388. doi: 10.1080/00029157.2014.880045

Anchin, J. C., & Magnavita, J. J. (2008). Toward the unification of psychotherapy: An introduction to the journal symposium. *Journal of Psychotherapy Integration, 18*(3), 259–263. doi: 10.1037/a0013556

APA Presidential Task Force on Evidence-Based Practice. (2006). Evidence-based practice in psychology. *American Psychologist, 61*(4), 271–285. doi: 10.1037/0003-066X.61.4.271

Bassett-Short, A., & Hammel, G. A. (2008). A student point of view: Existential psychotherapy from within the training process. In K. I. Schneider (Ed.), *Existential-integrative psychotherapy* (pp. 23–29). New York, NY: Routledge.

Beitman, B. D., Soth, A. M., & Bumby, N. A. (2005). The future as an integrating force through the schools of psychotherapy. In J. C. Norcross & M. R. Goldfried (Eds.), *Handbook of psychotherapy integration* (2nd ed., pp. 65–83). New York, NY: Oxford University Press.

Beutler, L. E. (1979). Toward specific psychological therapies for specific conditions. *Journal of Consulting and Clinical Psychology, 47*(5), 882–897. doi: 10.1037/0022-006X.47.5.882

Beutler, L. E. (1983). *Eclectic psychotherapy: A systematic approach*. Elmsford, NY: Pergamon Press.

Beutler, L. E., Clarkin, J., & Bongar, B. (2000). *Guidelines for the systematic treatment of the depressed patient*. New York, NY: Oxford University Press.

Beutler, L. E., Consoli, A. J., & Lane, G. (2005). Systematic treatment selection and prescriptive psychotherapy. In J. C. Norcross & M. R. Goldfried (Eds.), *Handbook of psychotherapy integration* (2nd ed., pp. 121–144). New York, NY: Oxford University Press.

Beutler, L. E., Harwood, T. M., Michelson, A., Song, X., & Holman, J. (2011). Reactance/resistance level. In J. C. Norcross (Ed.), *Psychotherapy relationships that work: Evidence-based responsiveness* (pp. 261–278). New York, NY: Oxford University Press. doi: 10.1093/acprof:oso/9780199737208.003.0013

Bickman, L. (2005). A common factors approach to improving mental health services. *Mental Health Services Research*, 7(1), 1–4. doi: 10.1007/s11020-005-1961-7

Bram, A., & Björgvinsson, T. (2004). A psychodynamic clinician's foray into cognitive-behavioral therapy utilizing exposure-response prevention for obsessive-compulsive disorder. *American Journal of Psychotherapy, 58*(3), 304–320. doi: 10.1176/appi.psychotherapy.2004.58.3.304

Brooks-Harris, J. E. (2008). *Integrative multitheoretical psychotherapy*. Boston, MA: Houghton Mifflin.

Castonguay, L. G. (2000). A common factors approach to psychotherapy training. *Journal of Psychotherapy Integration, 10*(3), 263–282. doi: 10.1023/A.1009496929012

Castonguay, L. G., & Beutler, L. E. (Eds.). (2006). Common and unique principles of therapeutic change: What do we know and what do we need to know? In L. G. Castonguay & L. E. Beutler (Eds.), *Principles of therapeutic change that work* (pp. 353–369). New York, NY: Oxford University Press.

Castonguay, L. G., Eubanks, C. F., Goldfried, M. R., Muran, J. C., & Lutz, W. (2015). Research on psychotherapy integration: Building on the past, looking to the future. *Psychotherapy Research*, *25*(3), 365–382. doi: 10.1080/10503307.2015.1014010

Castonguay, L. G., Goldfried, M. R., Wiser, S., Raue, P. J., & Hayes, A. H. (1996). Predicting outcome in cognitive therapy for depression: A comparison of unique and common factors. *Journal of Consulting and Clinical Psychology*, *64*(3), 497–504. doi: 10.1037/0022-006X.64.3.497

Castonguay, L. G., Newman, M. G., Borkovec, T. D., Holtforth, M. G., & Maramba, G. G. (2005). Cognitive–behavioral assimilative integration. In J. C. Norcross & M. R. Goldfried (Eds.), *Handbook of psychotherapy integration* (pp. 241–260). New York, NY: Oxford University Press. doi: 10.1093/med:psych/9780195165791.003.0011

Castonguay, L. G., Reid, J. J., Jr., Halperin, G. S., & Goldfried, M. R. (2003). Psychotherapy integration. In G. Stricker & T. A. Widiger (Eds.), *Handbook of psychology: Clinical psychology*, (Vol. 8, pp. 327–366). New York, NY: Wiley.

Constantino, M. J., & Westra, H. A. (2012). An expectancy-based approach to facilitating corrective experiences in psychotherapy. In L. G. Castonguay & C. E. Hill (Eds.), *Transformation in psychotherapy: Corrective experiences across cognitive behavioral, humanistic, and psychodynamic approaches* (pp. 121–139). Washington, DC: American Psychological Association.

Critchfield, K. L., Mackaronis, J. E., & Benjamin, L. S. (2017). Characterizing the integration of CBT and psychodynamic techniques in interpersonal reconstructive therapy for patients with severe and comorbid personality pathology. *Journal of Psychotherapy Integration*, *27*(4), 460–475. doi: 10.1037/int0000092

Cuijpers, P., Karyotaki, E., Weitz, E., Andersson, G., Hollon, S. D., & van Straten, A. (2014). The effects of psychotherapies for major depression in adults on remission, recovery and improvement: A meta-analysis. *Journal of Affective Disorders*, *159*, 118–126. doi: 10.1016/j.jad.2014.02.026

Cutts, L. (2011). Integration in counselling psychology: To what purpose? *Counselling Psychology Review*, *26*, 38–48.

D'Aniello, C. (2015). Common factors as a road map to MFT model integration: Implications for training therapists. *Contemporary Family Therapy*, *37*(2), 176–182. doi: 10.1007/s10591-015-9338-6

Duncan, B. L. (2002). The legacy of Saul Rosenzweig: The profundity of the dodo bird. *Journal of Psychotherapy Integration*, *12*(1), 32–57. doi: 10.1037/1053-0479.12.1.32

Eddy, K. T., Dutra, L., Bradley, R., & Westen, D. (2004). A multidimensional meta-analysis of psychotherapy and pharmacotherapy for obsessive-compulsive disorder. *Clinical Psychology Review*, *24*(8), 1011–1030. doi: 10.1016/j.cpr.2004.08.004

Elkin, I., Shea, M. T., Watkins, J. T., Imber, S. D., Sotsky, S. M., Collins, J. F., … Parloff, M. B. (1989). National Institute of Mental Health Treatment of Depression Collaborative Research Program: General effectiveness of treatments. *Archives of General Psychiatry*, *46*(11), 971–982. doi: 10.1001/archpsyc.1989.01810110013002

Engel, G. (1977). The need for a new medical model: A challenge for biomedicine. *Science*, *196*(4286), 129–136. doi: 10.1126/science.847460

Erskine, R. G. (2013). Vulnerability, authenticity, and inter-subjective contact: Philosophical principles of integrative psychotherapy. *International Journal of Integrative Psychotherapy*, *4*(2), 1–9.

Feixas, G., & Botella, L. (2004). Psychotherapy integration: Reflections and contributions from a constructivist epistemology. *Journal of Psychotherapy Integration, 14*(2), 192–222. doi: 10.1037/1053-0479.14.2.192

Fernández-Álvarez, H., Consoli, A. J., & Gómez, B. (2016). Integration in psychotherapy: Reasons and challenges. *American Psychologist, 71*(8), 820–830.

Finnerty, M., & McLeod, J. (2018). A qualitative study of the principles that self-defined integrative therapists in Ireland perceive as underpinning their practice. *Journal of Psychotherapy Integration, 29*(4), 345–358. doi: 10.1037/int0000128

Fisch, E. S. (2001). What is the end point of psychotherapy integration: A commentary. *Journal of Psychotherapy Integration, 11*(1), 117–122. doi: 10.1023/A:1026685109845

Fisher, P. L., & Wells, A. (2005). How effective are cognitive and behavioral treatments for obsessive-compulsive disorder? A clinical significance analysis. *Behaviour Research and Therapy, 43*(12), 1543–1558. doi: 10.1016/j.brat.2004.11.007

Frank, J. D. (1973). *Persuasion and healing: A comparative study of psychotherapy* (2nd ed.). Baltimore: Johns Hopkins University Press.

Fromm, E. (1949). Psychoanalytic characterology and its application to the understanding of culture. In S. S. Sargent & M. W. Smith (Eds.), *Culture and personality* (pp. 1–12). New York, NY: Viking Fund. doi: 10.1037/11254-001

Garfield, S. L. (1992). Eclectic psychotherapy: A common factors approach. In J. C. Norcross & M. R. Goldfried (Eds.), *Handbook of psychotherapy integration* (pp. 169–201). New York, NY: Basic Books.

Glock, G., Hilsenroth, M., & Curtis, R. (2018). Therapeutic interventions patients with anxiety problems find most helpful: A case for integration? *Journal of Psychotherapy Integration, 28*(2), 233–241. doi: 10.1037/int0000075

Gold, J. R., & Wachtel, P. L. (1993). Cyclical psychodynamics. In G. Stricker & J. R. Gold (Eds.), *Comprehensive handbook of psychotherapy integration* (pp. 59–72). New York, NY: Plenum Press.

Goldfried, M. R., & Castonguay, L. G. (1992). The future of psychotherapy integration. *Psychotherapy, 29*(1), 4–10. doi: 10.1037/0033-3204.29.1.4

Haverkampf, C. J. (2017). CBT and psychodynamic psychotherapy - A comparison. *Journal of Psychiatry Psychotherapy Communication, 6*(4), 61–67.

Henriques, G. (2011). *A new unifying theory of psychology*. New York, NY: Springer.

Henriques, G. (2016). Teaching clinical decision-making. In J. Magnavita (Ed.), *Clinical decision-making in behavioral and mental health practice* (pp. 273–307). Washington, DC: American Psychological Association. doi: 10.1037/14711-011

Henriques, G. (2017). Character adaptation systems theory: A new big five for personality and psychotherapy. *Review of General Psychology, 21*(1), 9–22. doi: 10.1037/gpr0000097

Henriques, G., Kleinman, K., & Asselin, C. (2014). The nested model of well-being: A unified approach. *Review of General Psychology, 18*(1), 7–18. doi: 10.1037/a0036288

Ingersoll, R. E. (2007). Perspective and psychotherapy: Applying integral theory to psychotherapy practice. *The Journal of Transpersonal Psychology, 39*(2), 175–198.

Ingersoll, R. E., & Marquis, A. (2014). *Understanding psychopathology: An integral exploration*. Upper Saddle River, NJ: Pearson Education.

Ingersoll, R. E., & Zeitler, D. M. (2010). *Integral psychotherapy: Inside out/outside in*. Albany, NY: State University of New York Press.

Jones-Smith, E. (2012). *Theories of counseling and psychotherapy: An integrative approach*. Thousand Oaks, CA: Sage.

Krupnik, V. (2018). Nested hierarchy for therapy integration: Integrating the integrative. *International Journal of Integrative Psychotherapy, 8*, 40–78.

Lampropoulos, G. K. (2000). Definitional and research issues in the common factors approach to psychotherapy integration: Misconceptions, clarifications, and proposals. *Journal of Psychotherapy Integration, 10*(4), 415–438. doi: 10.1023/A:1009483201213
Lampropoulos, G. K. (2001). Bridging technical eclecticism and theoretical integration: Assimilative integration. *Journal of Psychotherapy Integration, 11*(1), 5–19. doi: 10.1023/A:1026672807119
Lazarus, A. A. (1989). Why I am an eclectic (not an integrationist). *British Journal of Guidance and Counselling, 17*(3), 248–258. doi: 10.1080/03069888900760241
Lazarus, A. A. (2005). Multimodal therapy. In J. C. Norcross & M. R. Goldfried (Eds.), *Handbook of psychotherapy integration* (2nd ed., pp. 105–120). New York, NY: Oxford University Press.
Lazarus, A. A., & Beutler, L. E. (1993). On technical eclecticism. *Journal of Counseling and Development, 71*(4), 381–385. doi: 10.1002/j.1556-6676.1993.tb02652.x
Leichsenring, F., Abbass, A., Hilsenroth, M. J., Luyten, P., Munder, T., Rabung, S., & Steinert, C. (2018). "Gold standards," plurality and monocultures: The need for diversity in psychotherapy. *Frontiers in Psychiatry, 9*, 159. doi: 10.3389/fpsyt.2018.00159
Leichsenring, F., Salzer, S., Beutel, M. E., Herpertz, S., Hiller, W., Hoyer, J., ... Leibing, E. (2013). Psychodynamic therapy and cognitive-behavioral therapy in social anxiety disorder: A multicenter randomized controlled trial. *American Journal of Psychiatry, 170*(7), 759–767. doi: 10.1176/appi.ajp.2013.12081125
Liu, X., Cao, Y., Shi, Q., Jiang, C., Liu, J., Wei, H., ... Zhang, Y. (2013). National survey of therapeutic orientation and associated factors of counselors and psychotherapists in China. *Experimental and Therapeutic Medicine, 5*(4), 1075–1082. doi: 10.3892/etm.2013.929
Loerinc, A. G., Meuret, A. E., Twohig, M. P., Rosenfield, D., Bluett, E. J., & Craske, M. G. (2015). Response rates for CBT for anxiety disorders: Need for standardized criteria. *Clinical Psychology Review, 42*, 72–82. doi: 10.1016/j.cpr.2015.08.004
Magnavita, J. J. (2006). In search of the unifying principles of psychotherapy: Conceptual, empirical, and clinical convergence. *American Psychologist, 61*(8), 882. doi: 10.1037/0003-066X.61.8.882
Magnavita, J. J. (2008). Psychoanalytic psychotherapy. In J. L. Lebow (Ed.), *Twenty-first century psychotherapies: Contemporary approaches to theory and practice* (pp. 206–236). Hoboken, NJ: John Wiley & Sons.
Magnavita, J. J., & Anchin, J. C. (2014). *Unifying psychotherapy: Principles, methods, and evidence from clinical science*. New York, NY: Springer.
Marquis, A. (2008). *The integral intake: A guide to comprehensive idiographic assessment in integral psychotherapy*. New York: Routledge.
Marquis, A. (2009). An integral taxonomy of therapeutic interventions. *Journal of Integral Theory and Practice, 4*(2), 13–42.
Marquis, A. (2018). *Integral psychotherapy: A unifying approach*. New York, NY: Routledge.
Marquis, A., & Elliot, A. J. (2015). Integral psychotherapy in practice, Part 2: Revisions to the metatheory of integral psychotherapy based on therapeutic practice. *Journal of Unified Psychotherapy and Clinical Science, 3*(1), 1–40.
Marquis, A., Short, E. B., Lewis, J. L., & Hubbard, S. T. (2015). Integral psychotherapy in practice, Part 3: Three case studies illustrating the differential use of integral metatheory in informing unified treatment. *Journal of Unified Psychotherapy and Clinical Science, 3*(1), 41–79.
Marquis, A., & Wilber, K. (2008). Unification beyond eclecticism and integration: Integral psychotherapy. *Journal of Psychotherapy Integration, 18*(3), 350–358.

McFall, M. E., & Wollersheim, J. P. (1979). Obsessive-compulsive neurosis: A cognitive-behavioral formulation and approach to treatment. *Cognitive Therapy and Research, 3*(4), 333–348. doi: 10.1007/BF01184447
Messer, S. (1992). A critical examination of belief structures in integrative and eclectic psychotherapy. In J. C. Norcross & M. R. Goldfried (Eds.), *Handbook of psychotherapy integration* (2nd ed., pp. 130–168). New York, NY: Basic Books.
Mitchell, S. A. (1988). *Relational concepts in psychoanalysis.* Cambridge, MA: Harvard University Press.
Moursund, P. J., & Erskine, R. G. (2004). *Integrative psychotherapy: The art and science of relationship.* San Francisco, CA: Brooks/Cole.
Norcross, J. C. (2002). Empirically supported therapy relationships. In J. C. Norcross (Ed.), *Psychotherapy relationships that work: Therapist contributions and responsiveness to patients* (pp. 3–16). New York, NY: Oxford University Press.
Norcross, J. C. (2005). A primer on psychotherapy integration. In J. C. Norcross & M. R. Goldfried (Eds.), *Handbook of psychotherapy integration* (2nd ed., pp. 3–23). New York, NY: Oxford University Press.
Norcross, J. C., & Goldfried, M. R. (2005). The future of psychotherapy integration: A roundtable. *Journal of Psychotherapy Integration, 15*(4), 392–471. doi: 10.1037/1053-0479.15.4.392
Norcross, J. C., Goldfried, M. R., & Arigo, D. (2016). Integrative theories. In J. C. Norcross, G. R. VandenBos & D. K. Freedheim (Eds.), *APA handbook of clinical psychology: Theory and research*, (Vol. 2, pp. 303–332). Washington, DC: American Psychological Association. doi: 10.1037/14773-011
Norcross, J. C., Karpiak, C. P., & Santoro, S. O. (2005). Clinical psychologists across the years: The division of clinical psychology from 1960 to 2003. *Journal of Clinical Psychology, 61*(12), 1467–1483. doi: 10.1002/jclp.20135
Norcross, J. C., Krebs, P. M., & Prochaska, J. O. (2011). Stages of change. *Journal of Clinical Psychology, 67*(2), 143–154. doi: 10.1002/jclp.20758
O'Leary, E., & Barry, N. (2006). Gestalt reminiscence therapy. In E. O'Leary & M. Murphy (Eds.), *New approaches to integration in psychotherapy* (pp. 50–60). New York, NY: Routledge.
Olatunji, B. O., Davis, M. L., Powers, M. B., & Smits, J. A. (2013). Cognitive-behavioral therapy for obsessive-compulsive disorder: A meta-analysis of treatment outcome and moderators. *Journal of Psychiatric Research, 47*(1), 33–41. doi: 10.1016/j.jpsychires.2012.08.020
Owen, J., Hilsenroth, M. J., & Rodolfa, E. (2013). Interaction among alliance, psychodynamic- interpersonal and cognitive-behavioural techniques in the prediction of post-session change. *Clinical Psychology and Psychotherapy, 20*(6), 513–522. doi: 10.1002/cpp.1792
Prochaska, J. O., & DiClemente, C. C. (2005). The transtheoretical approach. In J. C. Norcross & M. R. Goldfried (Eds.), *Handbook of psychotherapy integration* (2nd ed., pp. 147–171). New York, NY: Oxford University Press.
Rogers, C. R. (1951). *Client-centered therapy.* Boston, MA: Houghton-Mifflin.
Rosenzweig, S. (1936). Some implicit common factors in diverse methods of psychotherapy. *American Journal of Orthopsychiatry, 6*(3), 412–415. doi: 10.1111/j.1939-0025.1936.tb05248.x
Ryle, A. (1990). *Cognitive analytic therapy: Active participation in change.* Chichester, UK: Wiley.
Safran, J. D. (1990). Towards a refinement of cognitive therapy in light of interpersonal theory: II. Practice. *Clinical Psychology Review, 10*(1), 107–121. doi: 10.1016/0272-7358(90)90109-N

Safran, J. D., & Messer, S. B. (1997). Psychotherapy integration: A postmodern critique. *Clinical Psychology: Science and Practice, 4*(2), 140–152. doi: 10.1111/j.1468-2850.1997.tb00106.x

Safran, J. D., & Segal, Z. V. (1990). *Interpersonal process in cognitive therapy*. Lanham, MD: Jason Aronson.

Safran, J. D., & Segal, Z. V. (1996). *Interpersonal process in cognitive therapy*. Lanham, MD: Jason Aronson.

Schottenbauer, M. A., Glass, C. R., & Arnkoff, D. B. (2005). Eclectic psychotherapy: A common factors approach. In J. C. Norcross & M. R. Goldfried (Eds.), *Handbook of psychotherapy integration* (2nd ed., pp. 459–493). New York, NY: Oxford University Press.

Stewart, R. E., & Chambless, D. L. (2009). Cognitive–behavioral therapy for adult anxiety disorders in clinical practice: A meta-analysis of effectiveness studies. *Journal of Consulting and Clinical Psychology*, 77(4), 595–606. doi: 10.1037/a0016032

Stricker, G., & Gold, J. (2002). An assimilative approach to integrative psychodynamic psycho-therapy. In J. Lebow (Ed.), *Comprehensive handbook of psychotherapy, Vol. 4: Integrative/eclectic* (pp. 295–316). New York, NY: Wiley.

Stricker, G., & Gold, J. (2005). Assimilative psychodynamic psychotherapy. In J. C. Norcross & M. R. Goldfried (Eds.), *Handbook of psychotherapy integration* (pp. 221–240). New York, NY: Oxford University Press. doi: 10.1093/med:psych/9780195165791.003.0010

Stricker, G., & Gold, J. (2006). *Introduction: An overview of psychotherapy integration*. In G. Stricker & J. Gold (Eds.). *A casebook of psychotherapy integration* (pp. 3–16). Washington, DC: American Psychological Association.

Sullivan, H. S. (1953). *The interpersonal theory of psychiatry*. New York, NY: Norton.

Tasca, G. A., Sylvestre, J., Balfour, L., Chyurlia, L., Evans, J., Fortin-Langelier, B., ... Wilson, B. (2015). What clinicians want: Findings from a psychotherapy practice research network survey. *Psychotherapy, 52*(1), 1–11. doi: 10.1037/a0038252

Trub, L., & Levy, D. (2017). Sowing the seeds for an assimilative integrationist stance toward psychotherapy. *Journal of Psychotherapy Integration, 27*(2), 172–185. doi: 10.1037/int0000056

Tryon, W. W. (2014). *Cognitive neuroscience and psychotherapy: Network principles for a unified theory*. New York: Academic Press.

Wachtel, P. L. (1977). *Psychoanalysis and behaviorism: Toward an integration*. New York, NY: Basic Books.

Wachtel, P. L. (1982). Vicious circles: The self and the rhetoric of emerging and unfolding. *Contemporary Psychoanalysis, 18*(2), 259–273. doi: 10.1080/00107530.1982.10746582

Wachtel, P. L. (1997). *Psychoanalysis, behavior therapy, and the relational world*. Washington, DC: American Psychological Association. doi:10.1037/10383-000

Wachtel, P. L. (2014). On the limits of theoretical fundamentalism. *Journal of Psychotherapy Integration, 24*(2), 95–98. doi: 10.1037/ a0036973

Wachtel, P. L., Kruk, J. C., & McKinney, M. K. (2005). Cyclical psychodynamics and integrative relational psychotherapy. In J. C. Norcross & M. R. Goldfried (Eds.), *Handbook of psychotherapy integration* (2nd ed., pp. 172–195). New York, NY: Oxford University Press.

Weeks, G. R., & Chad, C. L. (2004). The intersystem model of psychotherapy: An integrated systems treatment approach. *Guidance and Counseling, 19*, 57–64. doi: 10.1177/ 1066480708323205.

West, W. (2000). Eclecticism and integration in humanistic therapy. In S. Palmer & R. Wolfe (Eds.), *Integrative and eclectic counselling and psychotherapy* (pp. 218–232). London, England: Sage. doi: 10.4135/9781446280409.n12

Wilber, K. (2000). *Integral psychology: Consciousness, spirit, psychology, therapy*. Boston, MA: Shambala.

Wolfe, B. E. (2001). A message to assimilative integrationists: It's time to become accommodative integrationists: A commentary. *Journal of Psychotherapy Integration, 11*(1), 123–131.

Wolfe, B. E. (2005). *Understanding and treating anxiety disorders: An integrative approach to healing the wounded self*. Washington, DC: American Psychological Association.

Wolfe, B. E. (2006). An integrative perspective on the anxiety disorders. In G. Stricker & J. Gold (Eds.). *A casebook of psychotherapy integration* (pp. 65–77). Washington, DC: American Psychological Association.

Wolfe, B. E. (2008). Toward a unified conceptual framework of psychotherapy. *Journal of Psychotherapy Integration, 18*(3), 292–300. doi: 10.1037/1053-0479.18.3.292

Young, J. E., Klosko, J. S., & Weishaar, M. E. (2003). *Schema therapy: A practitioner's guide*. New York, NY: Guilford Press.

Zarbo, C., Tasca, G. A., Cattafi, F., & Compare, A. (2016). Integrative psychotherapy works. *Frontiers in Psychology, 6*, 2021. doi: 10.3389/fpsyg.2015.02021

Ziv-Beiman, S., & Shahar, G. (2015). Psychotherapy integration. In R. L. Cautin & S. O. Lilienfeld (Eds.), *The encyclopedia of clinical psychology* (pp. 1–6). New York, NY: Wiley. Advanced online publication. doi: 10.1002/9781118625392.wbecp189

3 A Brief History of Integrated and Unified Psychotherapy Approaches

Introduction

What was it like to learn psychotherapy at the beginning of the 1900s? In the first half of the twentieth century, mental health professionals drew rigid boundaries around the different theoretical orientations and single school tribes, e.g., cognitive, psychodynamic, and viewed their specific orientation as the truth while competing vigorously with each other (Norcross, 2005; Zarbo, Tasca, Cattafi, & Compare, 2016). The psychotherapists of today who promote integration and unification point out that therapists of previous generations displayed intolerance towards the treatment approaches of others (Marquis, 2018). Recently, many training programs have incorporated an integrative framework (Castonguay, Eubanks, Goldfried, Muran, & Lutz 2015; Norcross & Halgin, 2005).

This chapter offers a brief history of integrated and unified psychotherapy approaches. Examples of past and contemporary models of psychotherapy integration are provided. Rather than offering a comprehensive treatment of the vast range of extant integrated and unified therapy models, this chapter offers a sampling by the decade (see Figure 3.1.) Furthermore, although some integrated and unified models may not be mentioned or may be included only briefly in this chapter, they may be noted or more fully discussed in earlier or later chapters of this book. For example, although emotion-focused therapy is mentioned only briefly in this chapter, the section in Chapter 5, "Emotion-Focused Therapy (EFT): An Integrated Treatment for Generalized Anxiety Disorder (GAD)," shows in detail how this integrated psychotherapy model relates specifically to the anxiety disorders. Case studies of integrated and unified treatment are offered in Chapters 5 through 10 when there is specific application to the anxiety disorders.

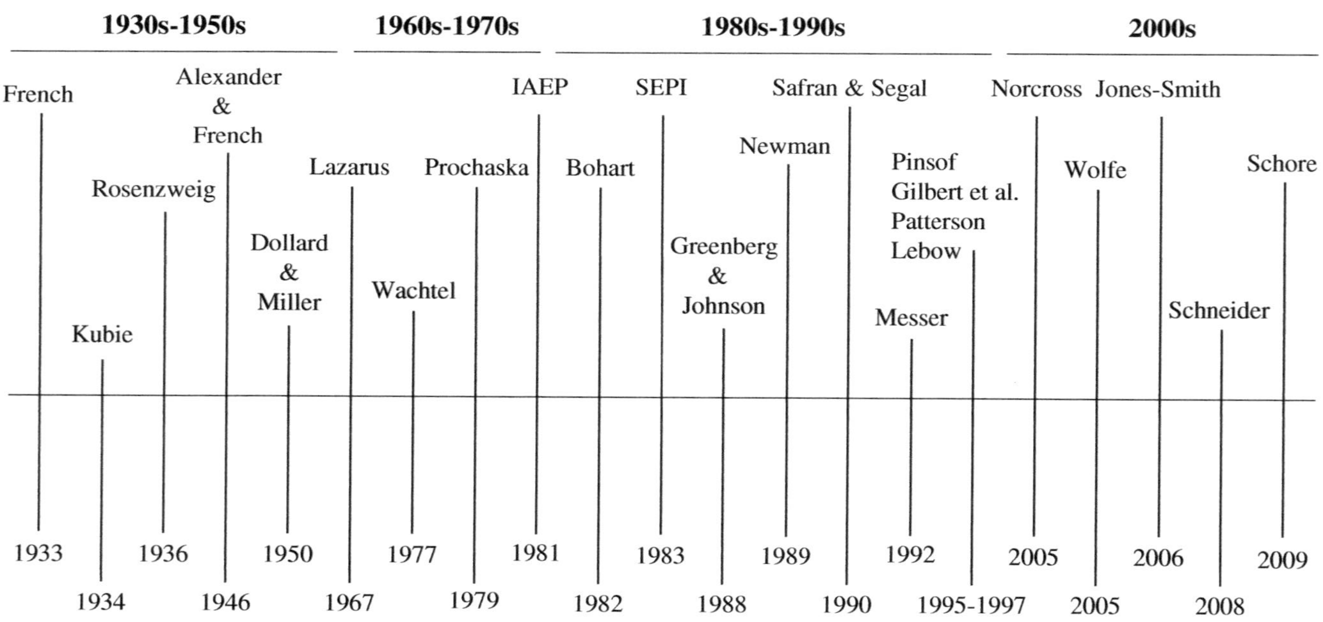

Figure 3.1 Integrated psychotherapy. This figure illustrates a timeline that represents a brief history of integrated psychotherapy from the 1930s until 2013.

Integrated and Unified Treatment Models from the 1930s to 2013

Integrated Psychotherapy Perspectives

1930s–1950s

When did attempts to integrate begin? Integration in the 1930s through the 1950s was characterized by beginning attempts to combine psychoanalytic and cognitive frameworks and to recognize common themes in the different approaches. These early attempts served as important contributions in the field of integration. For example, the beginning efforts to integrate psychotherapy began to emerge early in the work of French (1933) who suggested the integration of conditioning and the free association of psychoanalysis (Fernández-Álvarez, Consoli, & Gómez, 2016; Goldfried, Pachankis, & Bell, 2005; Tryon, 2014). Kubie's (1934) work extends the aforementioned integration in that it describes the association between psychoanalysis and conditioning for the purpose of demonstrating that psychoanalysis is based in principles of physiology. In 1936, Rosenzweig's research on common factors contributed to the psychotherapy integration movement by proposing that psychotherapy interventions are similar in the processes that result in change, but can be distinguished by the different names for the processes (Fernández-Álvarez et al., 2016; Stricker & Gold, 2006). The work of Alexander and French (1946) extends integration in its depiction of the experience of emotion as a common factor present in all therapies (Tryon, 2014). Researchers such as Dollard and Miller (1950) whose work integrated psychoanalytic theories and learning concepts and Wachtel (1977, 1997) who extended the influence of integration by formulating a model of psychotherapy that combined psychodynamic, behavioral, and systems orientations made important contributions in psychotherapy integration (Fernández-Álvarez et al., 2016; Magnavita, 2008).

1960s–1970s

The 1960s and the 1970s were characterized by the emergence of approaches that underscored the importance of different types of integration, e.g., technical eclecticism (Lazarus, 1967), theoretical integration (Wachtel, 1977), and a transtheoretical framework (Prochaska, 1979). (Chapter 2 distinguishes between the aforementioned types of integration.) In the 1960s and 1970s, researchers highlighted aspects of therapeutic change such as learning, cognition changes, and the working alliance, and they underscored the need to reduce discouragement across different therapies (Frank, 1961; Ziv-Beiman & Shahar, 2015). Researchers such as Lazarus (1967), Wachtel (1977), and Prochaska (1979) contributed towards the integration movement in different ways. For example, whereas Lazarus (1967, 2005), with his presentation of a broad or multimodal approach, considered theoretical integration to be a failed attempt to blend concepts that do not fit together, and, instead, recommended the use of technical eclecticism, Wachtel's (1977) work, "Psychoanalysis and Behavior Therapy: Toward an Integration," promoted theoretical integration (Stricker & Gold, 2006). It was Prochaska (1979) who was the first to try to develop a broad or transtheoretical psychotherapy model (Jones-Smith, 2012).

1980s–1990s

Psychotherapy integration was a hidden theme that only began to emerge into a specific focal point of interest starting in the 1980s (Goldfried, Pachankis, & Bell, 2005). Commencing as eclectic (Norcross, 1986, 1987), psychotherapy integration began to refresh itself in the 1980s (Fernández-Álvarez et al., 2016). In 1981, the International Academy of Eclectic Psychotherapists (IAEP) was founded; in 1983, the Society for the Exploration of Psychotherapy Integration (SEPI; www.sepiweb.org), an international society, was founded; and in 1985, the first conference of SEPI took place (Muse, Moore, & Stahl, 2013; Stricker, 2010). The *International Journal of Eclectic Psychotherapy*, later named the *Journal of Integrative and Eclectic Psychotherapy*, was published in 1982 (Jones-Smith, 2012).

Psychotherapy integration in the 1980s included the following four key roads: A technical eclectic approach, a common factors orientation, theoretical integration, and assimilative integration, which influenced treatment for over three decades (Magnavita & Anchin, 2014). Chapter 2 described the aforementioned four trends or waves. Psychotherapy integration decreased dogma, promoted the diversification of ideas, and encouraged flexibility in therapists (Magnavita & Anchin, 2014). In 1982, Bohart showed how an integrated perspective can be applied to client-centered therapy by outlining a common factors approach. In 1988, Greenberg and Johnson developed Emotion-Focused Therapy (EFT) for couples. EFT integrates the humanistic approach of Rogers (1951), systemic perspectives of Minuchin and Fishman (1981), and Bowlby's (1973, 1977, 1988) notion of attachment, and focuses on the way in which emotions that are expressed result in communication patterns that repeat themselves (Greenberg & Johnson, 1988; Ventura & Stavrianopoulos, 2014). What type of model is EFT? This empirically supported model is an assimilative integration psychotherapy framework because its source is experiential, and the features of family therapy have been modified extensively (Greenberg & Johnson, 1988; Simon, 2004). In the latter part of the 1980s, psychodynamic and cognitive-behavioral perspectives on the therapeutic alliance began to merge (Goldfried et al., 2005). An example of the aforementioned integration is Newman's (1989) exploration of the countertransference reflected from the vantage point of a cognitive-behavioral approach.

Psychotherapy integration began to pick up new momentum as the 1990s approached. Whereas during the 1980s, integration first became a formal movement, in the 1990s, the concepts of the integration movement were, in actuality, adopted by researchers and therapists (Goldfried et al., 2005). For example, researchers showed how cognitive therapy could be improved by integrating methods related to interpersonal principles (Safran & Segal, 1990).

In 1990, researchers found that most therapists endorsed eclectic and/or integrative types of therapy (Goldfried et al., 2005; Jensen, Bergin, & Greaves, 1990). In 1991, the *Journal of Psychotherapy Integration* was published by the Society for the Exploration of Psychotherapy Integration (SEPI) (Goldfried et al., 2005). In 1992, Messer further contributed to the psychotherapy integration movement with his work on assimilated integration. Chapter 2 discussed several assimilated integration approaches.

In the mid and latter part of the 1990s, researchers showed how different theoretical approaches could be applied to therapeutic treatment beyond individual interventions. Goldfried et al. (2005) consider the following to be examples of integration beyond individual treatments: (1) Pinsof's (1995) text, *Integrative Problem-Centered Therapy*, which includes a perspective that integrated a variety of theoretical approaches that are related to individual, family, and biological treatments, (2) Gilbert and Shmukler's (1996) description of an integrative approach that showed how humanistic, psychodynamic, and behavioral orientations could be applied to couples intervention, and (3) Patterson's (1997) inclusion of an integrative approach for family therapy. Lebow's (1987, 1997) integrative therapy focuses on the couple as well, has a basis in a generic, biopsychosocial perspective that employs interventions from psychodynamic, systemic, cognitive, and behavioral sources, and aims to assist patients to achieve their goals.

2000s

During the past few decades, integrated treatment has emerged into a defined area of study (Norcross, 2005). The concept of rapprochement has emerged since the 1990s, and psychotherapists were encouraged to assimilate clinical designs that were, at one time, considered irregular (Norcross, 2005). In 2005, Wolfe developed a model aimed at offering an integrative view of the nature, formulation, and continuance of the anxiety disorders, and worked with both common and distinct characteristics of cognitive-behavioral, existential-humanistic, biomedical, and psychodynamic concepts. In 2006, Jones-Smith developed a strength-based psychotherapy model that integrates positive psychology and resilience theory and focuses on patients' strengths within a multicultural context.

Progress towards integration continued in the twenty-first century. Schneider (2008) asserted that although, for decades, there had existed a large divide between the behavioral and humanistic perspectives, researchers suggested integration. Since the 1990s, an integrative approach to psychotherapy, a more inclusive perspective towards the various theoretical models, has been increasingly favored among mental health professionals (Greben, 2004; Norcross, 2005; Zarbo et al., 2015). For example, Schneider (2008) proposed his existential-integrative psychology, an artistic, visionary statement that employs a phenomenological technique for approaching a recognition of human existence with an emphasis on the internally felt rather than the external experience. Existential-integrative psychology blends a standard existential perspective with existential psychodynamic and humanistic existential approaches (Schneider, 2008). In his book, *Existential-Integrative Psychotherapy,* Schneider (2008) distinguished between existential psychoanalysis, which highlights the unconscious and change that is somewhat gradual, and a humanistic existential approach, which emphasizes optimism and change that is somewhat more rapid. Existential-integrative psychotherapy utilizes elements from a combination of the aforementioned perspectives (Schneider, 2008).

Consistent with the integration between the neurobiological and the psychological is Schore's (2009) synthesis of neuroscience and self-psychology related to the effects of neuropsychoanalytic ideas on the self's interpersonal neurobiological foundations. Schore (2009) suggested that a rapprochement between neuroscience and psychoanalysis can benefit psychotherapy treatment models, and he developed a model of relational trauma where there is an integration between neurobiology and self psychology. He explained that parents who traumatize have an effect on the relational security of their child along with the child's development of the right brain and the mature emergence of self. The common element shared by neuroscience and psychoanalytic self psychology is the notion that mistreatment at an early age is related to negative effects on a child's mind, brain, and body, and will change the pathway of the self in the future (Schore, 2009). The integration of self psychology with biology can help to explain how early childhood trauma mediates the transmission of impairments in emotional regulation that occur when the self begins to experience an emotional disorder (Schore, 2009).

Unified or Integral Psychotherapy Approaches

How did unification begin? (see Figure 3.2.) Whereas Angyal (1941, 1982), who was advanced for his time, promoted holism, the language of Staats (1983) was one of unification (Magnavita, 2008, 2012). It was Angyal (1941) who laid the groundwork for a unified, holistic, metatheoretical framework of personality that continues today (Magnavita & Anchin, 2014). When there is a lack of unity or an excess of specialization, the universe of knowledge can become fragmented, and connections and interrelatedness are frequently lost (Magnavita, 2006; Staats, 1983).

In 2000, Wilber's text, *Integral Psychology*, described a unified framework, and in 2001, Sternberg and Grigorenko continued the call for unification (Magnavita, 2008). Magnavita (2008) promoted the idea that neuroscience needs to be a guiding force for unified psychotherapy, which seeks to understand the brain–behavior relationships that emerge in a psychotherapy practice. In fact, neuroscientific studies have begun to verify notable views of psychotherapy, e.g., the character of the unconscious (Hassin, Uleman, & Bargh, 2005; Magnavita, 2006).

Unified approaches tend to include complex systems that mirror the intricate nature of human beings. For example, Magnavita's (2008) is a unified

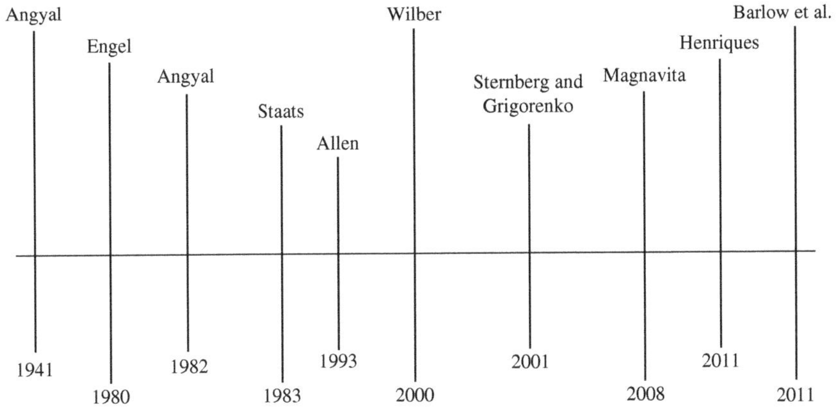

Figure 3.2 Unified or integral psychotherapy. This figure illustrates a timeline that represents a brief history of unified or integral psychotherapy from the 1940s until 2013.

psychotherapy approach that includes four subsystems of restructuring. Magnavita's (2008) subsystems include the following: (1) The intrapsychic-biological with a focus on the hereditary, the neurobiological, and the internal relational and cognitive systems, (2) the interpersonal-dyadic with its focus on the relationship, which includes verbal and nonverbal linguistic cues and the notion of attachment, (3) the relational-triadic with its focus on the relational structure of two or more and the notion of triangulation (Bowen, 1976), and (4) the sociocultural-familial or the mesosystem, which includes the interrelationship among the sociopolitical, the family, and the individual.

How do the subsystems of a unified framework work? The first domain of restructuring, the intrapsychic-biological, is concerned with the inner level of health needed to adapt to the external environment and with the coping defenses needed to regulate affect (Magnavita, 2008). Magnavita's (2008) first subsystem, which includes patients' hereditary tendencies, considers the following: How cohesive (or fragmented) is the self? At what point does an individual develop symptoms? For example, can an individual with an anxiety disorder complete a specific task that involves others without developing symptoms?

The second, the interpersonal-dyadic, is concerned with the ability of an individual to develop relationships (Magnavita, 2008). Here, the focus is on a system that involves two individuals in a relationship (Magnavita & Anchin, 2014). In short, Magnavita's (2008) second subsystem considers the following: What is an individual's capacity to attach to others? To what extent can an individual understand derivative communication?

Magnavita's (2008) third domain, the relational triadic, focuses on relationships that consist of more than two, is concerned with the level of triangulation in the context of a dyad, and considers the following: What is the frequency of the emergence of these triadic relationships over time? Magnavita's (2008) fourth domain, the mesosystem, concerns itself with how the family transmits memes (Dawkins, 1982) or cultural rather than genetic codes, and concerns itself with the following: How do parents and grandparents transmit the sociocultural context to the next generation?

According to Magnavita (2012), the personality is a system that is comprised of elements of the four subsystems such as individual, interpersonal, and family processes, genetic aspects, and sociocultural effects. The four domains are equal, one category is not more important than another, and each of the categories interact with each other (Magnavita, 2008; Quinn, 2003; Wilber, 2000). Magnavita (2008) suggests that, in their therapeutic work, mental health professionals incorporate a unified, holistic psychotherapy approach rather than focus on only one of the categories, e.g., intrapsychic-biological. Magnavita (2012) views his system model as one of several models that represents the unified clinical science and therapy approach. He recognizes that there are other models that include unified psychotherapy approaches, e.g.. Engel's (1980) biopsychosocial model, Allen's (1993) unified psychotherapy, Barlow, Ellard et al.'s (2011) unified protocol, and Henrique's unifying framework (2011).

Contemporary Integrated and Unified Treatment Models (2013 to Present)

How have integrated and unified models developed more recently, from the time of the publication of the DSM-5 (American Psychiatric Association, 2013) until the present? (see Figure 3.3.) Psychotherapy integration can expand the horizon of therapists who seek modes of practice beyond the use of one theoretical model (McWilliams, 2017). Within an evidence-based context, integrative psychotherapists have continued to investigate the advantages of interventions that are not limited to monotherapies by considering methods across various perspectives (Norcross & Goldfried, 2005; Norcross & Popple, 2017). Since the emergence of the DSM-5 (APA, 2013), new integrated and unified models of psychotherapy have been developed. Unified therapy treatments that are transdiagnostic and that emphasize the similarities among disorders have been developed both for psychodynamic therapy and for cognitive-behavioral therapy (Leichsenring & Steinert, 2018). Chapter 5 describes how Barlow, Farchione, Fairholme et al.'s cognitive-behavioral unified protocol (UP) (2004, 2011, 2017, 2018) and the unified psychodynamic psychotherapy (UPP-ANXIETY) model of Leichsenring and Salzer (2014) relate to the anxiety disorders. Since the emergence of DSM-5 (APA, 2013), researchers have continued to develop integrated and unified models of psychotherapy such as Magnavita and Anchin's (2014) unified psychotherapy model.

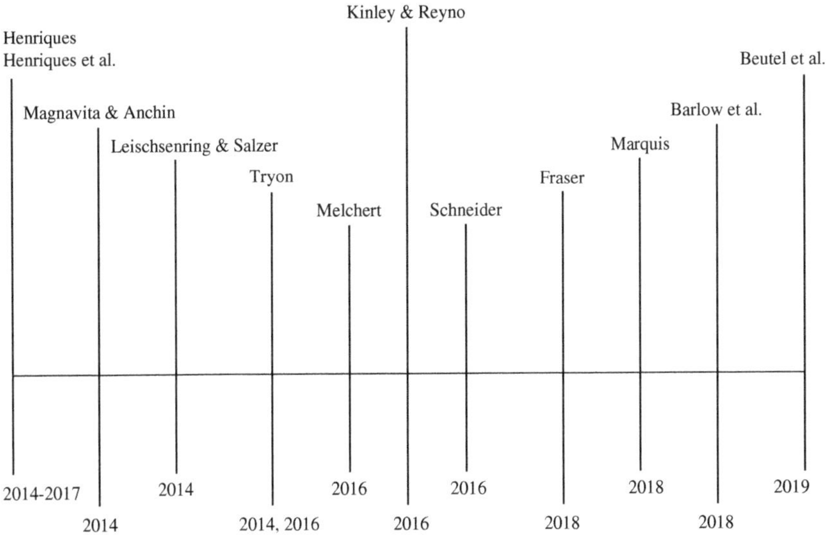

Figure 3.3 Contemporary integrated and unified models of psychotherapy. This figure illustrates a timeline that represents a brief history of contemporary integrated and unified treatment models from the time of DSM-5 (American Psychiatric Association, 2013) to the present.

Magnavita and Anchin's Unified Psychotherapy Model (2014)

In 2014, Magnavita and Anchin presented a unified psychotherapy framework, with its focus on holism, as a complex, all-inclusive, wide-ranging, framework of psychotherapy where therapists view patients' clinical presentation through several lenses. Chapters 1, 2, and 3 discuss the unified psychotherapy model of Magnavita and Anchin (2014). What is the unifying concept? The relational matrix (Mitchell, 1988) which contains the four subsystems or levels of a client's entire ecological system, intrapsychic-biological, interpersonal-dyadic, relational-dyadic, and sociocultural-familial, is a unifying, metatheoretical concept in which the biopsychosocial system is rooted (Magnavita & Anchin, 2014). Individuals are relational, and their personalities are further developed by their relationships with other people, commencing with attachments to caregivers (Magnavita & Anchin, 2014). The relational matrix facilitates an awareness of a sense of agency (distinctiveness or differentiation) and communion (relationship with others), contemporary ideas based on Sullivan's (1953) interpersonal theory of psychotherapy (Magnavita & Anchin, 2014). Whereas the emphasis of Freud's (1917, 1933) classical psychoanalytic model is on drives, a relational psychoanalytic approach, on the other hand, focuses on relationships, e.g., interpersonal psychoanalysis, object relations, self-psychology (Magnavita & Anchin, 2014). Later chapters of this book discuss the way in which attachment theory, a relational concept, plays a critical role in the development of the emotional disorders, e.g., anxiety.

The Nested Model (NM) of Henriques, Kleinman, and Asselin (2014) Based on Unified Theory

See Chapter 2 for the unified model developed by Henriques and colleagues (2014), the Nested Model (NM) of well-being.

The Unifying Approach of Tryon (2014, 2016)

What is the nature of a unified, neuroscience framework that views psychological material from a physical rather than from a mental perspective? Chapter 2 briefly described Tryon's (2014) Bio Psychology Network framework. Chapter 3 expands on Tryon's (2014, 2016) unifying approach. What comprises Tryon's (2014, 2016) unifying approach? Researchers assert that conflict among psychotherapy theories prevents integration based on theoretical unification (Castonguay, 2011; Goldfried, 1980); however, Tryon (2014, 2016) suggests that integration take place at the level of the concept or at the level of psychological principles rather than at the level of methodology, thereby facilitating a greater degree of comprehensiveness. Tryon (2014) proposed that psychological integration and theoretical unification can emerge when clinicians, theorists, and researchers develop physical rather than mental concepts, and he offered a bio psychology framework that integrates neuroscience and views psychological material from a physical rather than from a mental perspective. In 2016, he offered a cognitive neuroscience foundation that theoretically unifies several orientations, facilitates integration with meaning, and he showed how an applied psychological science (APS) clinical orientation facilitates theoretical unification across behavioral, pharmacologic, psychodynamic, cognitive, and cognitive-behavioral clinical orientations.

A similar position is taken by Melchert (2016), who, like Tryon (2016), suggested a unified approach that incorporates a neuroscience foundation; however, it is argued that the aforementioned unifying paradigms are but a flight to reductionism (Fraser, 2018). Tryon (2014), on the other hand, asserts that he introduces ideas that represent the opposite of reductionism, and he underscores the concept of emergence, the way in which complexity emerges from modest elements, the way and why psychology exists. Just as chemists are not afraid of reductionism in that they are not concerned that physicists will replace them and biologists are not afraid of physicists and chemists, so too psychologists do not need to feel concerned about neuroscience if the concept of emergence exists for them (Tryon, 2014). For Tryon (2014), cognitive neuroscience emphasizes biological explanations and how neural networks can explain cognition.

What are the core concepts of Tryon's (2014, 2016) unified approach? Tryon (2016) puts forth core concepts that identify the essence of the aforementioned clinical orientations. He defines key concepts that are related to the clinical orientations, and highlights mechanisms that are important to natural science renditions. The following comprise Tryon's (2014) core principles: Processing that is unconscious, memory and learning, transformation, and activation/reactivation.

What is a core concept? A core concept is central to a particular clinical orientation when individuals cannot hold a particular clinical orientation without agreeing with that specific concept (Tryon, 2016). For example, individuals need to agree with the concept of unconscious processing in order to hold a psychodynamic clinical perspective (Summers & Barber, 2010; Tryon, 2016). According to Tryon (2016), the unifying APS orientation is congruent with a psychodynamic approach in its emphasis on unconscious processing in that that the flow of activations through neural networks occurs unconsciously. More specifically, a natural science approach seeks to use mechanisms that pertain to a particular phenomenon to explain the cause of that phenomenon (Pennington, 2014; Tryon, 2016). The resolution of unconscious motives can be explained by an understanding of the mechanisms of neural network models that identify causal patterns beginning with unconscious activations prior to presenting as conscious (McClleland, 2010; O'Reilly & Munakat, 2000, Tryon, 2018). Tryon's (2014) unified theory offers mechanism conceptualizations that can explain different psychological ideas as well as the reason that interventions with empirical support work, and his theory is consistent with five different orientations, e.g., psychodynamic, pharmacologic, and others.

According to Tryon's (2014) unified theory of psychological science, which is based on core and corollary network concepts or principles, if a clinician were to adopt his network approach, the therapist would identify with concepts or principles rather than with eminent psychologists or with clinical orientations because the Bio Psychology Network Theory includes these orientations. Tryon (2014) explains that his model guides a clinician to view a client's issues as physical rather than mental and to view therapy as involving brain changes, thereby removing the stigma related to seeking psychotherapy. His unified theory can help reconcile the disharmonies among mental health professionals and can promote the study of a mature psychological science. This approach can allow the behavioral clinician to more easily include psychological mindedness and the psychodynamic clinician to include, with greater ease, the goal of decreasing symptoms (Tryon, 2014).

What are other examples of core concepts? With respect to a behavioral clinical orientation, Tryon (2016) views the operant as a core concept. He asserts that a unifying APS clinical orientation that includes neural networks that are trained rather than automated supports the notion of an applied behavior analysis (ABA) form of a behavioral clinical orientation. In short, the features of neural networks of the APS clinical orientation, similar to the operant conditioning of ABA, rely on learning (Tryon, 2016). The core concepts of Wolpe's (1958) systematic desensitization and exposure and response prevention are learning and memory. Tryon (2016) explains that the APS orientation supports Wolpe's (1958) behavioral perspective because it derives from natural science's mechanisms (Bear, Connors, & Paradiso, 2007) that view learning as an outcome of memory formation.

In addition to describing core concepts that pinpoint the conceptual essence of a few of the major clinical orientations and showing how a unifying APS orientation is consistent with these clinical orientations, Tryon (2016) identifies key concepts that are related to the major clinical orientations and shows how the key concepts that are related to these approaches correspond to the unifying APS orientation. Unlike core concepts, which are critical for a particular clinical approach, key concepts are related, but not critical to the particular clinical orientation (Tryon, 2016). For example, the notion of schema is a key rather than a core or critical concept of the cognitive approach (Young, Kosko, & Weishaar, 2006), and the unifying APS orientation relies upon the neural network models to recognize schema thought information (Rumelhart, Smolensky, McClelland, & Hinton, 1986).

What are the advantages of Tryon's (2016) unifying perspective? By relying on core concepts, key concepts, and principles, Tryon (2016) demonstrates that the APS clinical orientation, based on cognitive neuroscience, facilitates theoretical psychotherapy unification that is meaningful across several major clinical orientations. Rather than relying on manuals and methods, Tryon's (2016) innovative approach allows therapists to comprehensively customize therapy according to the specific needs of their patients. The aforementioned transtheoretical clinical approach of the APS offers a unifying coherent theoretical foundation that facilitates the use of a variety of methods from different orientations without confining psychotherapists to only one theoretical treatment approach (Tryon, 2016).

Schneider's (2016) Existential-Integrative Psychotherapy Model (ET)

In 2016, Schneider designed an existential-integrative (EI) psychotherapy model which relies on Rollo May's (1958) (e.g., May, Angel, & Ellenberger, 1958; Schneider & May, 1995) and James Bugental's (1987) existential-humanistic research. Existential-integrative therapy facilitates the integration of several treatment approaches within an existential or experiential perspective, e.g., existential and CBT (Schneider, 2016). EI, an example of assimilative integration, is the most advanced integrative treatment that has existential psychotherapy as its base (Wolfe, 2016).

Schneider (2016) explains that an EI therapist aims to facilitate the concept of choice or freedom for clients within the client's limits. Chapter 10 includes a discussion of how existential-integrative psychotherapy models can be applied to treat individuals with PTSD.

Kinley and Reyno's (2016) Integrated Neurobiological Model

How does an integrated neurobiological model relate to patients' emotional disorders? Recently, Kinley and Reyno (2016) developed a model of psychotherapy integration that relies on the relationship between mind and body, an approach that is based on the connection between neurobiological and psychological concepts. A focus of Kinley and Reyno's (2016) integrated neurobiological psychotherapy model is on the integration of poorly regulated circuitry, interventions, at every phase of the disorder, which depend upon neuronal impairments, and on neurological change mechanisms that underlie patients' emotional disorders. Chapter 5 discusses how Kinley & Reyno's (2016) integration of neuroscience and psychotherapy treatment applies to generalized anxiety disorder (GAD).

Fraser's (2018) Unifying Approach

What is a key concept of Fraser's (2018) unifying approach? In 2018, Fraser, in his exploration of the shared content of different psychotherapy approaches, proposed a unifying approach that explains patients' problems and integrates interventions that are effective for their problems, and he suggested a paradigm that focuses on the process of change to assist in the integration of different psychotherapy perspectives. He proposed that an alternate paradigm or metatheory, a view of process that integrates change along with the notion of systems that are based on process and the effect of context, underlies psychotherapy treatments that work.

The Character Adaptation Systems Theory (CAST) of Henriques (2017)

The CAST or character adaptation systems theory of Henriques (2017) is described in Chapters 1 and 2.

The Metatheoretical Integral or Unifying Model of Marquis (2018)

An all-inclusive metatheoretical quadratic framework is the unifying or integral model of Marquis (2018). From a metatheoretical rather than a theoretical view, the integral model of Marquis (2018) offers principles rather than practice directives. Integral therapy has an experiential feel with a focus on the developmental needs of individual patients (Marquis, 2018). Chapter 1 includes a brief discussion of the unified approach to psychotherapy of Marquis (2018), and Chapter 5 demonstrates how the integral, metatheoretical model of Marquis (2018) can be applied in clinical practice, within the context of a case study of a patient with generalized anxiety disorder (GAD).

The Emotion-Focused Psychodynamic Therapy (EFPP) of Beutel, Greenberg, Lane, and Subic-Wrana (2019)

How can emotion-focused therapy be integrated with psychodynamic therapy? Recently, Beutel and colleagues (2019) developed emotion-focused psychodynamic therapy (EFPP) along with a transdiagnostic manual to treat individuals with anxiety disorders. EFPP considers both psychodynamic tensions of an intrapsychic and interpersonal nature as well as the transformation of emotions (Beutel et al., 2019).

Summary

This chapter provided a brief history of some of the integrated and unified models of psychotherapy from the 1930s until the present (see Table 3.) The next chapter discusses the integrated and unified theoretical approaches as they relate to the etiology of the anxiety disorders. Although integrated treatment is practiced around the world today, and it is the wave of the future, there continues to be a deficit of empirically supported education that focuses on psychotherapy integration (Aafjes-van Doorn, Klinar Alfaro, Fialová, & Kamsteeg, 2018; Wachtel, 2010).

References

Aafjes-van Doorn, K., Klinar Alfaro, D., Fialová, M., & Kamsteeg, C. (2018). Psychotherapy integration training around the globe: A personal and empirical perspective. *Journal of Psychotherapy Integration, 28*(4), 505–520. doi: 10.1037/int0000135

Alexander, F., & French, T. (1946). *Psychoanalytic psychotherapy*. New York: Ronald Press.

Allen, D. (1993). Unified psychotherapy. In G. Striker & J. Gold (Eds.), *Comprehensive handbook of psychotherapy integration* (pp. 125–137). New York, NY: Plenum Press.

American Psychiatric Association. (2013). *Diagnostic and statistical manual of mental disorders* (5th ed.). Washington, DC: Author.

Angyal, A. (1941). *Foundations for a science of personality*. Oxford, England: Commonwealth Fund.

Angyal, A. (1982). *Neurosis and treatment: A holistic theory*. New York, NY: Da Capo Press.

Barlow, D. H., Allen, L. B., & Choate, M. L. (2004). Toward a unified treatment for emotional disorders. *Behavior Therapy, 35*(2), 205–230. doi: 10.1016/S0005-7894(04)80036-4

Barlow, D. H., Farchione, T. J., Bullis, J. R., Gallagher, M. W., Murray-Latin, H., Sauer-Zavala, S., … Cassiello-Robbins, C. (2017). The unified protocol for transdiagnostic treatment of emotional disorders compared with diagnosis-specific protocols for anxiety disorders: A randomized clinical trial. *JAMA Psychiatry, 74*(9), 875–884. doi: 10.1001/jamapsychiatry.2017.2164.

Barlow, D. H., Farchione, T. J., Fairholme, C. P., Ellard, K. K., Boisseau, C. L., Allen, L. B., & Ehrenreich-May, J. T. (2011). *Unified protocol for transdiagnostic treatment of emotional disorders: Therapist guide*. New York, NY: Oxford University Press.

Barlow, D. H., Farchione, T. J., Sauer-Zavala, S., Murray-Latin, H., Ellard, K. K., Bullis, J. R., … Cassiello-Robbins, C. (2018). *Unified protocol for transdiagnostic treatment of emotional disorders: Therapist guide* (2nd ed.). New York: Oxford University Press.

Bear, M. F., Connors, B. W., & Paradiso, M. A. (2007). *Neuroscience: Exploring the brain* (3rd ed.). Baltimore, MD: Lippincott, Williams & Wilkins.

Beutel, M. E., Greenberg, L., Lane, R. D., & Subic-Wrana, C. (2019). Treating anxiety disorders by emotion-focused psychodynamic psychotherapy (EFPP)—An integrative, transdiagnostic approach. *Clinical Psychology and Psychotherapy, 26*(1), 1–13. doi: 10.1002/cpp.2325

Bohart, A. (1982). Similarities between cognitive and humanistic approaches to psychotherapy. *Cognitive Therapy and Research, 6*(3), 24–249.

Bowen, M. (1976). Theory and practice of family therapy. In P. J. Guerin, Jr. (Ed.), *Family therapy: Theory and practice* (pp. 42–90). New York, NY: Gardner Press.

Bowlby, J. (1973). *Attachment and loss, Vol. 2. Separation*. New York, NY: Basic Books.

Bowlby, J. (1977). The making and breaking of affectional bonds. I. Aetiology and psychopathology in the light of attachment theory. *British Journal of Psychiatry, 130*(3), 201–210. doi: 10.1192/bjp.130.3.201

Bowlby, J. (1988). *A secure base: Parent-child attachment and healthy human development*. New York, NY: Basic Books.

Bugental, J. (1987). *The art of the psychotherapist*. New York, NY: Norton.

Castonguay, L. (2011). Psychotherapy, psychopathology, research, and practice: Pathways of connections and integration. *Psychotherapy Research, 21*(2), 125–140. doi: 10.1080/10503307.2011.563250

Castonguay, L. G., Eubanks, C. F., Goldfried, M. R., Muran, J. C., & Lutz, W. (2015). Research on psychotherapy integration: Building on the past, looking to the future. *Psychotherapy Research, 25*(3), 365–382. doi: 10.1080/10503307.2015.1014010

Dawkins, R. (1982). *The extended phenotype*. Oxford, UK: Oxford University Press. doi: 10.1016/j.jad.2017.11.036

Dollard, J., & Miller, N. E. (1950). *Personality and psychotherapy: An analysis in terms of learning, thinking and culture*. New York, NY: McGraw-Hill.

Engel, G. L. (1980). The clinical application of the biopsychosocial model. *The American Journal of Psychiatry, 137*(5), 535–544.

Fernández-Álvarez, H., Consoli, A. J., & Gómez, B. (2016). Integration in psychotherapy: Reasons and challenges. *American Psychologist, 71*(8), 820–830.

Frank, J. D. (1961). *Persuasion and healing: A comparative study of psychotherapy*. Oxford, UK: Johns Hopkins University Press.

Fraser, J. (2018). *Unifying effective psychotherapies: Tracing the process of change*. Washington, DC: American Psychological Association.

French, T. M. (1933). Interrelations between psychoanalysis and the experimental work of Pavlov. *American Journal of Psychiatry, 89*(6), 1165–1203.

Freud, S. (1917). *A general introduction to psychoanalysis* (J. Riviere, Trans.). New York, NY: Liveright (Work republished in 1963).

Freud, S. (1933). *New introductory lectures on psychoanalysis*. New York, NY: Norton.

Gilbert, M., & Shmukler, D. (1996). *Brief therapy with couples: An integrative approach*. New York: John Wiley & Sons.

Goldfried, M. R. (1980). Toward the delineation of therapeutic change principles. *American Psychologist, 35*(11), 991–999. doi: 10.1037/0003-066X.35.11.991

Goldfried, M. R., Pachankis, J. E., & Bell, A. C. (2005). A history of psychotherapy integration. In J. C. Norcross & M. R. Goldfried (Eds.), *Handbook of psychotherapy integration* (2nd ed., pp. 24–60). New York, NY: Oxford University Press. doi: 10.1093/med:psych/9780195165791.003.0002

Greben, D. H. (2004). Integrative dimensions of psychotherapy training. *The Canadian Journal of Psychiatry, 49*(4), 238–248. doi: 10.1177/070674370404900404

Greenberg, L. S., & Johnson, S. M. (1988). *Emotionally focused therapy for couples*. New York, NY: Guilford Press.

Hassin, R. R., Uleman, J. S., & Bargh, J. A. (Eds.). (2005). *The new unconscious*. New York, NY: Oxford University Press.

Henriques, G. (2011). *A new unified theory of psychology*. New York, NY: Springer Press. doi: 10.1007/978-1-4614-0058-5

Henriques, G. (2017). Character adaptation systems theory: A new big five for personality and psychotherapy. *Review of General Psychology, 21*(1), 9–22. doi: 10.1037/gpr0000097

Henriques, G., Kleinman, K., & Asselin, C. (2014). The nested model of well-being: A unified approach. *Review of General Psychology, 18*(1), 7–18. doi: 10.1037/a0036288

Jensen, J. P., Bergin, A. E., & Greaves, D. W. (1990). The meaning of eclecticism: New survey and analysis of components. *Professional Psychology: Research and Practice, 21*(2), 124–130.

Jones-Smith, E. (2006). The strength-based counseling model. *Counseling Psychologist, 34*(1), 13–79. doi: 10.1177/0011000005277018.

Jones-Smith, E. (2012). *Theories of counseling and psychotherapy: An integrative approach*. Thousand Oaks, CA: Sage.

Kinley, J. L., & Reyno, S. M. (2016). Project for a scientific psychiatry: A neurobiologically informed, phasic, brain-based model of integrated psychotherapy. *Journal of Psychotherapy Integration, 26*(1), 61–73. doi: 10.1037/a0039636

Kubie, L. S. (1934). Relation of the conditioned reflex to psychoanalytic technic. *Archives of Neurology and Psychiatry, 32*(6), 1137–1142. doi: 10.1001/archneurpsyc.1934.02250120014002

Lazarus, A. A. (1967). In support of technical eclecticism. *Psychological Reports, 21*(2), 415–416.

Lazarus, A. A. (2005). Multimodal therapy. In J. C. Norcross & M. R. Goldfried (Eds.), *Handbook of psychotherapy integration* (2nd ed., pp. 105–120). New York, NY: Oxford University Press.

Lebow, J. L. (1987). Integrative family therapy: An overview of major issues. *Psychotherapy: Theory, Research, Practice, Training, 24*(3S), 584–594.

Lebow, J. L. (1997). The integrative revolution in couple and family therapy. *Family Process, 36*(1), 1–17. doi: 10.1111/j.1545-5300.1997.00001.x

Leichsenring, F., & Salzer, S. (2014). A unified protocol for the transdiagnostic psychodynamic treatment of anxiety disorders: An evidence-based approach. *Psychotherapy, 51*(2), 224–245. doi: 10.1037/a0033815

Leichsenring, F., & Steinert, C. (2018). Towards an evidence-based unified psychodynamic protocol for emotional disorders. *Journal of Affective Disorders, 232*, 400–416.

Magnavita, J. J. (2006). In the search of the unifying principles of psychotherapy: Conceptual, empirical, and clinical convergence. *American Psychologist, 61*, 882–892. doi: 10.1037/0003-066X.61.8.882

Magnavita, J. J. (2008). Psychoanalytic psychotherapy. In J. L. Lebow (Ed.), *Twenty-first century psychotherapies: Contemporary approaches to theory and practice* (pp. 206–236). Hoboken, NJ: John Wiley & Sons.

Magnavita, J. J. (2012). Advancing clinical science using system theory as the framework for expanding family psychology with unified psychotherapy. *Couple and Family Psychology: Research and Practice, 1*(1), 3–13. doi: 10.1037/a0027492

Magnavita, J. J., & Anchin, J. C. (2014). *Unifying psychotherapy: Principles, methods, and evidence from clinical science*. New York, NY: Springer.

Marquis, A. (2018). *Integral psychotherapy: A unifying approach*. New York, NY: Routledge.

May, R. (1958). Contributions of existential psychotherapy. In R. May, E. Angel & H. F. Ellenberger (Eds.), *Existence: A new dimension in psychiatry and psychology* (pp. 37–91). New York, NY: Basic Books.

May, R., Angel, E., & Ellenberger, H. F. (Eds.). (1958). *Existence: A new dimension in psychiatry and psychology*. New York, NY: Basic Books. doi: 10.1037/11321-000

McClelland, J. L. (2010). Emergence in cognitive science. *Topics in Cognitive Science*, *2*(4), 751–770. doi: 10.1111/j.1756-8765.2010.01116.x

McWilliams, N. (2017). Integrative research for integrative practice: A plea for respectful collaboration across clinician and researcher roles. *Journal of Psychotherapy Integration*, *27*(3), 283–295. doi: 10.1037/int0000054

Melchert, T. P. (2016). Leaving behind our preparadigmatic past: Professional psychology as a unified clinical science. *American Psychologist*, *71*(6), 486–496. doi: 10.1037/a0040227

Messer, S. (1992). A critical examination of belief structures in integrative and eclectic psychotherapy. In J. C. Norcross & M. R. Goldfried (Eds.), *Handbook of psychotherapy integration* (2nd ed., pp. 130–168). New York: Basic Books.

Minuchin, S., & Fishman, H. C. (1981). *Family therapy techniques*. Cambridge, MA: Harvard University Press.

Mitchell, S. A. (1988). *Relational concepts in psychoanalysis: An integration*. Cambridge, MA: Harvard University Press.

Muse, M. D., Moore, B. A., & Stahl, S. M. (2013). Benefits and challenges of integrative treatment. In S. M. Stahl & B. A. Moore (Eds.), *Anxiety disorders: A guide for integrating psychopharmacology and psychotherapy* (pp. 3–24). New York, NY: Routledge.

Newman, C. F. (1989). Cognitive therapy, countertransference, and the borderline patient (Unpublished manuscript). Philadelphia, PA: Center for Cognitive Therapy.

Norcross, J. C. (Ed.). (1986). *Handbook of eclectic psychotherapy*. New York, NY: Brunner/Mazel.

Norcross, J. C. (Ed.). (1987). *Casebook of eclectic psychotherapy*. New York, NY: Brunner/Mazel.

Norcross, J. C. (2005). A primer on psychotherapy integration. In J. C. Norcross & M. R. Goldfried (Eds.), *Handbook of psychotherapy integration* (2nd ed., pp. 3–23). New York, NY: Oxford University Press.

Norcross, J. C., & Goldfried, M. R. (2005). The future of psychotherapy integration: A roundtable. *Journal of Psychotherapy Integration*, *15*(4), 392–471. doi: 10.1037/1053-0479.15.4.392

Norcross, J. C., & Halgin, R. P. (2005). Training in psychotherapy integration. In J. C. Norcross & M. R. Goldfried (Eds.), *Handbook of psychotherapy integration* (2nd ed., pp. 439–458). New York, NY: Oxford University Press.

Norcross, J. C., & Popple, L. M. (2017). *Supervision essentials for integrative psychotherapy*. Washington, DC: American Psychological Association.

O'Reilly, R. C., & Munakata, Y. (2000). *Computational explorations in cognitive neuroscience: Understanding the mind by simulating the brain*. Cambridge, MA: The MIT Press.

Patterson, T. (1997). Theoretical unity and eclecticism: Pathways to coherence in family therapy. *American Journal of Family Therapy*, *25*, 97–109.

Pennington, B. F. (2014). *Explaining abnormal behavior: A cognitive neuroscience perspective*. New York, NY: Guilford Press.

Pinsof, W. M. (1995). *Integrative IPCT: A synthesis of biological, individual, and family therapies*. New York, NY: Basic Books.

Prochaska, J. O. (1979). *Systems of psychotherapy: A transtheoretical analysis*. Oxford, England: Dorsey.

Quinn, N. (2003). Cultural selves. In J. LeDoux, J. Debiec & H. Moss (Eds.), *The self: From soul to brain. Annals of the New York Academy of Science, Vol. 1001* (pp. 145–176). New York, NY: Academy of Sciences.

Rogers, C. R. (1951). *Client-centered therapy*. Boston, MA: Houghton-Mifflin.
Rosenzweig, S. (1936). Some implicit common factors in diverse methods of psychotherapy. *American Journal of Orthopsychiatry, 6*(3), 412–415. doi: 10.1111/j.1939-0025.1936.tb05248.x
Rumelhart, D. E., Smolensky, P., McClelland, J. L., & Hinton, G. E. (1986). Schemata and sequential thought processes in PDP models. In J. L. McClelland, D. E. Rumelhart & The PDP Research Group, *Parallel distributed processing: Explorations in the microstructure of cognition*, (Vol. 2, pp. 7–57). Cambridge, MA: MIT Press.
Safran, J. D., & Segal, Z. V. (1990). *Interpersonal process in cognitive therapy*. Northvale, NJ: Jason Aronson.
Schneider, K. J. (2008). *Existential-integrative psychotherapy: Guideposts to the core of practice*. New York, NY: Routledge.
Schneider, K. J. (2016). Existential-integrative therapy: Foundational implications for integrative practice. *Journal of Psychotherapy Integration, 26*(1), 49–55.
Schneider, K. J., & May, R. (1995). *The psychology of existence: An integrative, clinical perspective*. New York, NY: McGraw-Hill.
Schore, A. N. (2009). Relational trauma and the developing right brain: An interface of psychoanalytic self psychology and neuroscience. *Annals of the New York Academy of Sciences, 1159*, 189–203. doi: 10.1111/j.1749-6632.2009
Simon, G. M. (2004). An examination of the integrative nature of emotionally focused therapy. *The Family Journal, 12*(3), 254–262. doi: 10.1177/1066480704264348
Staats, A. W. (1983). *Psychology's crisis of disunity: Philosophy and method for a unified science*. New York, NY: Praeger.
Sternberg, R. J., & Grigorenko, E. L. (2001). Unified psychology. *American Psychologist, 56*(12), 1069–1079. doi: 10.1037//0003-066X.56.12.1069
Stricker, G. (2010). A second look at psychotherapy integration. *Journal of Psychotherapy Integration, 20*(4), 397. doi: 10.1037/a0022037
Stricker, G., & Gold, J. (2006). *Introduction: An overview of psychotherapy integration*. In G. Stricker & J. Gold (Eds.), *A casebook of psychotherapy integration* (pp. 3–16). Washington, DC: American Psychological Association.
Sullivan, H. S. (1953). *The interpersonal theory of psychiatry*. New York, NY: Norton.
Summers, R. F., & Barber, J. P. (2010). *Psychodynamic therapy: A guide to evidence-based practice*. New York, NY: Guilford.
Tryon, W. W. (2014). *Cognitive neuroscience and psychotherapy: Network principles for a unified theory*. New York: Academic Press.
Tryon, W. W. (2016). Transtheoretic transdiagnostic psychotherapy. *Journal of Psychotherapy Integration, 26*(3), 273–287. doi: 10.1037/a0040041
Tryon, W. W. (2018). Unconscious processing: Comment on Hornsey and Fielding (2017). *American Psychologist, 73*(5), 685–686. doi: 10.1037/amp0000311
Ventura, R., & Stavrianopoulos, K. (2014). Being a person-centered therapist and the challenge of working with the emotionally focused therapy model: A case study. *Person-Centered and Experiential Psychotherapies, 13*(2), 169–183. doi: 10.1080/14779757.2013.871575
Wachtel, P. L. (1977). *Psychoanalysis and behaviorism: Toward an integration*. New York, NY: Basic Books.
Wachtel, P. L. (1997). *Psychoanalysis, behavior therapy, and the relational world*. Washington, DC: American Psychological Association. doi:10.1037/10383-000
Wachtel, P. L. (2010). Psychotherapy integration and integrative psychotherapy: Process or product?. *Journal of Psychotherapy Integration, 20*(4), 406–416. doi: 10.1037/a0022032

Wilber, K. (2000). *Integral psychology: Consciousness, spirit, psychology, therapy*. Boston, MA: Shambhala Publications.

Wolfe, B. E. (2005). *Understanding and treating anxiety disorders: An integrative approach to healing the wounded self.* Washington, DC: American Psychological Association.

Wolfe, B. E. (2016). Existential-humanistic therapy and psychotherapy integration: A commentary. *Journal of Psychotherapy Integration, 26*(1), 56–60. doi: 10.1037/int0000023

Wolpe, J. (1958). *Psychotherapy by reciprocal inhibition*. Stanford, CA: Stanford University Press.

Young, J. E., Klosko, J. S., & Weishaar, M. E. (2006). *Schema therapy: A practitioner's guide.* New York, NY: Guilford.

Zarbo, C., Tasca, G. A., Cattafi, F., & Compare, A. (2015). Integrative psychotherapy works. *Frontiers in Psychology, 6*, 2021. doi: 10.3389/fpsyg.2015.02021

Zarbo, C., Tasca, G. A., Cattafi, F., & Compare, A. (2016). Integrative psychotherapy works. *Frontiers in Psychology, 6*, 2021. doi: 10.3389/fpsyg.2015.02021

Ziv-Beiman, S., & Shahar, G. (2015). Psychotherapy Integration. In R. L. Cautin & S. O. Lilienfeld (Eds.), *The encyclopedia of clinical psychology* (pp. 1–6). New York, NY: Wiley. Advanced online publication. doi: 10.1002/9781118625392 .wbecp189

Part II

Integrated and Unified Psychotherapy Approaches for the Anxiety Disorders

Whereas the first part of the book prepared the groundwork for integrated and unified approaches, the second part, "Integrated and Unified Psychotherapy Approaches for the Anxiety Disorders," discusses the integrated and unified etiological and psychotherapy models as they apply to specific anxiety disorders. Part II consists of Chapter 4, "The Etiology of the Anxiety Disorders: Themes that Underlie Integrated Psychotherapy Models of the Anxiety Disorders," Chapter 5, "Generalized Anxiety Disorder (GAD)," Chapter 6, "Panic Disorder (PD)," Chapter 7, "Phobias: Social Anxiety Disorder (SAD) (Social Phobia) and Specific Phobia (SP)," and Chapter 8, "Separation Anxiety Disorder (SAD) and Adult Separation Anxiety Disorder (ASAD)." Part II begins with Chapter 4 which explores the etiology of the anxiety disorders, the concepts, themes, and thoughts that underlie integrated psychotherapy models for the anxiety disorders. Chapter 5 describes the etiology and the clinical practice applications of integrated and unified psychotherapy treatment models for generalized anxiety disorder (GAD). Chapter 6 discusses the etiology and clinical practice applications of integrated and unified psychotherapy treatment models for panic disorder (PD). Chapters 7 discusses the etiology and clinical practice applications of integrated and unified psychotherapy treatment models for phobias such as social anxiety disorder (SAD) (social phobia) and specific phobia (SP). Chapter 8 explores the etiology and integrated and unified psychotherapy approaches for separation anxiety disorder (SAD) and adult separation anxiety disorder (ASAD).

4 The Etiology of the Anxiety Disorders

Themes that Underlie Integrated Psychotherapy Models of the Anxiety Disorders

Introduction

Various themes underlie integrated etiological models for the anxiety disorders, and these concepts may interact across the different biological, psychological, cultural, and social aspects of an individual's life (Ingersoll & Marquis, 2014). This chapter describes themes that underlie the integrated and unified psychotherapy models of the anxiety disorders. It explores the development and maintenance of the anxiety disorders within the context of integrated and unified perspectives.

The Theme of Self-Wounds (Wolfe, 2005)

There are key themes or concepts that underlie integrated and unified psychotherapy models for the anxiety disorders. For example, Wolfe (2005) developed an integrative etiological perspective of self-wounds aimed at offering an integrative view of the nature, formulation, and continuance of the anxiety disorders. He selected both common and unique characteristics of cognitive-behavioral, existential, biomedical, and psychodynamic approaches to the anxiety disorders as a basis for developing his model.

According to Wolfe's model (2005), the anxiety disorders derive from an experience of a troubled self or a sense of a disaster or a catastrophe which is linked to a distressing emotion. Indeed, Wolfe's (2005) model set forth an etiological approach to the anxiety disorders that recognizes an existential basis of anxiety (Schneider, 2008). Chapter 3 described Schneider's (2008) existential-integrative psychology framework.

There are common factors that comprise the etiology of the anxiety disorders. Wolfe (2005) posits the following common factors: Genetics, a threatening experience, and a perception of self as ineffective.

Genetics

Some individuals have genetic vulnerabilities that act as catalysts for an anxiety disorder to emerge (Buckholtz & Lindenbergh, 2012; Wolfe, 2003). For example, the serotonin transporter 5-HTT gene variant has been shown to be related to anxiety disorders and correlated with neuroticism as well as with elevated stress (Buckholtz & Lindenbergh, 2012).

Threat

There are common elements (i.e., fear, avoidance, negative emotion) and distinctive aspects (i.e., threat object and scope of perceived danger) that comprise the etiology of the anxiety disorders (Craske & Waters, 2005; Watson & Clark, 1984). With respect to common elements, the conditioning of fear, a type of classical conditioning where individuals learn associations between stimuli and negative experiences, shapes much of today's research on the anxiety disorders (Greene, Bailey, & Neumeister, 2013). The common aspect of trauma plays a key role in the development and maintenance of the anxiety disorders (Barlow, 2004; Davanloo, 2005; Marquis, 2018). With respect to unique elements such as the threat object and the breadth of the perceived danger, the threat object for generalized anxiety disorder is broader than that for panic disorder; however, the threat scenario for social anxiety disorder is much less broad (i.e., performance), and the scope for specific phobia is the least broadly defined (i.e., specific objects) (Craske & Waters, 2005).

The Perception of an Ineffective Self

The third common factor that comprises the etiology of the anxiety disorders is the perception of self as ineffective (Wolfe, 2005). Wolfe's (2005, 2006) integrated etiological approach to anxiety consists of a conscious layer where a patient foresees a threat as well as an unconscious layer that reflects the notion of self-wounds, the unresolved emotional damage from the past, and the fear of exposing intensely painful self perceptions (Alladin, 2014). The implicit and explicit levels of Wolfe's (2005, 2006) etiological model of anxiety comprise the patient's story about the meaning of symptoms or the way in which the patient suffers with internally painful experiences (Alladin, 2014). The notion of self-wounds or painful perceptions of the self that underlies Wolfe's (2005, 2006) integrated model of the etiology of anxiety can explain the shame against which individuals with anxiety disorders attempt to defend (Alladin, 2014). The concept of self-wounds and an impaired perception of self underlie Wolfe's (2005, 2006) integrated etiological perspective in that it helps to explain the meaning of symptoms and fears of exposure that individuals with anxiety perceive to be shameful (Alladin, 2014). Anxiety denotes an unconscious fear of injury to a self that is wounded and protected by maladaptive defenses, e.g., avoidance (Alladin, 2014).

According to Wolfe (2005), the following are types of self-wounds that produce anxiety: A self that is vulnerable on a physiological level, a self that is not capable, that feels shame, that feels alone, and a self that feels conflicted.

Wolfe (2005) proposed the following sources of self-wounds: Betrayals, concerns about expressing affect, trauma, embarrassment, and ineffective reactions to existential issues.

The concept of self-wounds or emotional damage to the self is a key focus of Wolfe's (2005) integrated psychotherapy approach for the anxiety disorders, a perspective that integrates psychodynamic, behavioral, cognitive, and experiential therapies (Alladin, 2014). When patients experience a high level of anxiety, they begin, at a conscious level, to anticipate disasters, which reflect, unconsciously, their worry about exposing self-wounds or deeply painful emotions that they do not wish to reveal (Alladin, 2014; Wolfe, 2005, 2006). The aforementioned explicit and implicit layers comprise the etiology of anxiety symptoms and their meaning (Alladin, 2014; Wolfe, 2005, 2006).

Patients with anxiety disorders frequently feel powerless, a feeling similar to the helplessness experienced by infants (Freud, 1926/1959; Ingersoll & Marquis, 2014; Wolfe, 2003). Anxiety disorders develop as a consequence of past painful events, emotional tensions, and the suppression of facing pain again, and the wounded self may generate unconscious conflicts (Alladin 2014; Wolfe, 2005). Individuals who are anxious may possess unconscious fears of insults to the self that is already wounded, and the self employs distorted defenses, e.g., avoidance, to cope with the existing wounds (Alladin, 2014). The finding that psychodynamic treatment for the anxiety disorders can have a positive outcome (e.g., Leichsenring, 2005) may indirectly provide evidence for the idea that patients' anxieties are lessened when they work out their unconscious conflicts. Each specific anxiety disorder, i.e., panic disorder, generalized anxiety disorder, contains different content matter related to a painful self-experience, and each employs a different way to ward off the pain (Wolfe, 2005; Alladin, 2014). Although interventions that focus on patients' symptoms are needed, deeper and more lasting interventions focus on resolving unconscious conflicts that cause the anxiety (Alladin, 2014).

A Neuroscience Theme

Neural Circuitry

The etiology of the anxiety disorders can be viewed from a neuroscience perspective. Chapter 3 discussed the integrated neurobiological psychotherapy model of Kinley and Reyno (2016). A focus of Kinley and Reyno's (2016) model is on the integration of poorly regulated circuitry. The identification of common and distinct maladaptive neural circuitry can shed light on change processes (Kinley & Reyno, 2016). For example, the amygdalocentric model of anxiety, with its theory on the dysfunctional processing of fear, specifies that the areas of the brain involved in the anxiety disorders include the amygdala, the prefrontal cortex, and the hippocampus, and the model underscores how the amygdala generates an adaptive response to a fearful event through its association with the hippocampus and the prefrontal cortex, both participants in the processing of fear (Greene et al., 2013; Rauch, Shin, & Phelps, 2006; Ray, 2018). There is greater activation of the amygdala and weaker activation of the prefrontal cortex in individuals with anxiety disorders than in individuals who do not have anxiety disorders (Greene et al., 2013; Rauch et al., 2006; National Institute of Mental Health (NIMH), 2008). Stresses and relational trauma can negatively influence the neural networks that comprise emotional regulation (how patients have an effect on the timing and perception of their emotions), resulting in the development of emotional disorders such as anxiety (Gross, 1998; Kinley & Reyno, 2016; Puetz et al., 2014). In general, individuals with an anxiety disorder tend to have patterns of brain activity that are more asymmetrical along with consistently higher than normal sympathetic functioning (Barlow, 2004; Ingersoll & Marquis, 2014).

Neurotransmitters

Which neurotransmitters are involved in the anxiety disorders? Gamma-aminobutyric acid has been shown to be a key neurotransmitter involved in anxiety (Ray, 2018). Anxiety conditions are associated with dysfunction in the serotonergic system, a neurotransmitter system involving serotonin in the amygdala, and with impairment in the noradrenergic system, a neurotransmitter system involving norepinephrine in the locus coeruleus (Pelligrino, Pierce, & Walkup, 2011).

The Relationship Between a Transdiagnostic Approach and the Brain's Neural Circuitry

Is there a relationship between a transdiagnostic approach and the brain's neural circuitry? The etiology of the anxiety disorders can be considered from a transdiagnostic perspective based on the notion of the brain's neural networks. The attempt to explain psychological ideas from a physical perspective dates back to Freud, a neurologist, who was subject to the scientific constraints of his time (Tryon, 2014). Tryon (2016) showed how natural science mechanisms can explain psychological ideas. His transdiagnostic applied psychological science (APS) approach (described in Chapter 3), which is based on a biopsychology network (BPN), relies on the concept of the brain's neural networks, can explain how psychotherapy results in changes in the brain, and is consistent with findings such as Del Casale et al.'s (2011), where imaging demonstrated changes to the structure of the brain of clients with obsessive-compulsive disorder who received cognitive-behavioral therapy.

Patients with similar susceptibilities can be vulnerable to developing anxiety and depression (Kennedy & Barlow, 2018). For example, a patient's tendency to ruminate may be associated with both anxiety and depression (Nolen-Hoeksema, 2000). The doubtful feelings that are characteristic of individuals who ruminate produce anxiety, and the more frequent the rumination, the higher the risk for depression (Nolen-Hoeksema, 2000). Consistent with the transdiagnostic unified protocol (UP), factors such as temperament have been shown to account for the co-occurrence of mental disorders such as generalized anxiety disorder, social anxiety disorder, panic disorder, depressive disorder, and posttraumatic stress disorder (Boettcher & Conklin, 2018; Brown & Barlow, 2009; Ruscio, Borkovec, & Ruscio, 2001). For example, a patient with a high tendency to ruminate in relation to negative emotions may develop a feeling of hopelessness, which can result in either depression and/or anxiety (Alloy, Kelly, Mineka, & Clements, 1990; Lyubomirsky, Tucker, Caldwell, & Berg, 1999; Nolen-Hoeksema, 2000).

The following vignette illustrates how a client with depressive symptoms begins to feels a bit hopeful, but then becomes consumed with anxiety. Her tendency towards rumination leads her down the path of mixed symptoms of depression and anxiety.

Vignette

Therapist: How have you been this week?

Patient: [With head hung low] At the beginning of the week, I thought a lot about whether I'll be able to afford my rent this month. My boss told me that he needs to reduce the number of hours he can offer me, and I felt kind of hopeless and I don't know what to do. Nothing seems to work out for me.

Therapist: You're thinking a lot about making ends meet.

Patient: Yeah … At the beginning of the week, my thinking over and over about how I might not make the rent was interfering with my concentration on my present job. I don't know why this was occurring. At the beginning of the week, I felt kind of down because I didn't know what to do. Couldn't concentrate on my tasks at work even though I'm waking up in the early morning hours.

Therapist: How were you towards mid and end of week?

Patient: Then, in the middle of the week, I heard about another possible job, and I started thinking about what that means, and wasn't certain about whether I should apply. I kept mulling the idea back and forth in my mind, weighing the expense and time about taking off from my present job to see if I can interview for a better one. I went over it a lot in my mind, and, then, towards the end of the week [pace of speech speeds up], I called the new job several times during one day because I felt so distressed, was worried about getting the new job, and then I was up all night thinking it over last night. I keep thinking about how to proceed. Then today, I was worried that I might not get an interview for the new job, and I called a few more times, and, finally, got an appointment, and now I'm worried about whether I'll do well at the interview for the new

> job. I keep worrying about whether I would do well on the interview, and I feel a little like it may work, but still feel edgy and nervous about the whole situation …

In this vignette, the patient, who generally presents as depressed, continues to ruminate. By the end of the week, she has figured out a possible solution to her problem. Whereas she begins to feel a bit more hopeful, she continues to ruminate, and, at the same time, her depression and hopelessness revert to incessant worry and symptoms of anxiety as she continues to ruminate about whether she may be able to salvage the situation.

The Theme of Insecure Attachments

What is the relationship between the relational concept of attachment and the etiology of the anxiety disorders? The theme of insecure attachment is present for many individuals with anxiety disorders in that insecure attachments tend to increase vulnerability to anxiety (Bowlby, 1988; Johnson, 2019; Leichsenring & Salzer, 2014). Bowlby (1973, 1977, 1988) asserted that the infants of caregivers who failed to take care of infants reliably and with sensitivity would have difficulty seeking emotional support from caregivers when distressed and exploring their environs, in general. Further, infant patterns of attachment have been found to be related to adult attachment patterns (Fraley, 2002). An attachment theory model with its robust and comprehensive base of developmental evidence can encourage therapists to think in an integrative way across a variety of clinical perspectives (Levy, Wesley, Temes, & Clouthier, 2015). For example, the attachment subtypes of anxious and fearful are related to vulnerability to generalized anxiety disorder (GAD), obsessive-compulsive disorder (OCD), and posttraumatic stress disorder (PTSD) (Ein-Dor & Doron, 2015; Johnson, 2019).

Impaired Attachment, the Regulation of Emotions, and a Transtheoretical Framework

What is the relationship between a transtheoretical model, the regulation of emotion, and dysfunctional attachment? Research has demonstrated that the regulation of emotions plays an important part in mental health (Aldao, Nolen-Hoeksema, & Schweizer, 2010; Fredrickson, Messina, & Grecucci, 2018; Hu, Zhang, Wang, Mistry, Ran, & Wang, 2014). A combination of emotions, conditioned anxiety, and the defenses can generate and maintain emotions that are not regulated (Fredrickson, Messina, & Grecucci, 2018). To understand an emotion and its accompanying anxiety, a Dysregulated Affective State (DAS; Grecucci, Theuninck, Frederickson, & Job, 2015), Fredrickson and colleagues (2018) proposed an integration of emotional neuroscience and Experiential-Dynamic Emotion Regulation (EDER), a framework of concepts that seeks to treat Dysregulated Affective States. The gist of EDER methodology is the synthesis of affect regulation scientific concepts and psychodynamic therapy (Fredrickson et al. 2018). According to Fredrickson and colleagues (2018), there is a distinction between the initial emotion itself and dysregulated states. The EDER methodology proposes that dysregulated emotions require regulation by the therapist because they impede healthy adaptation; however, patients need to express the initial physiological emotions without regulation by therapists (Fredrickson et al., 2018). According to Fredrickson and colleagues (2018), individuals can become overwhelmed by anxiety to the point that they may not recognize the emotion masked by the anxiety, and in this case, the anxiety, rather than the emotion, needs to be regulated. They suggest that EDER conceptualizations be used as a transtheoretical framework for promoting a patient's ability to regulate anxiety and that EDER's techniques can be incorporated within other perspectives.

The Theme of Vulnerability: A Vulnerability–Stress Model

What is the relationship between a vulnerability–stress model and the etiology of anxiety in the elderly? To understand the etiology of anxiety in the elderly, Beekman and colleagues (1998) suggested the use of a vulnerability–stress framework. For the elderly with anxiety disorders, vulnerability variables (e.g., female, low education level) are primary in the etiology, with stressors (e.g., deaths in the family) contributing secondarily (Beekman et al., 1998). For example, the vulnerability factor, being female, was related to several anxiety disorders in the elderly, but only showed statistical significance in phobic disorders (Beekman et al., 1998). With respect to an association between network factors and the etiology of anxiety in the elderly, the size of the contact network was found to contribute (Beekman et al., 1998). Different factors contributed to particular types of anxiety disorders (e.g., panic, phobias, obsessive-compulsive disorder), but loneliness was found to be related to the entire gamut of anxiety disorders in the elderly (Beekman et al., 1998).

An Integral Approach to the Etiology of the Anxiety Disorders

What is the relationship between the etiology of an emotional disorder and the intervention? The etiology or sources of a disorder and treatment are connected as it is easier to devise effective treatments if the etiology or sources of the disorder are understood (Ingersoll & Marquis, 2014). There is a myriad of causes of anxiety across physical, psychological, cultural, and social aspects of an individual's life (Ingersoll & Marquis, 2014). Integral psychotherapists recognize that anxiety is triggered by a complex interaction of biological, affective, cognitive, existential, interpersonal, cultural, and social aspects rather than by a linear cause (Ingersoll & Marquis, 2014).

If one views the anxiety disorders through the lens of an integral psychotherapy model (described in Chapter 2), the worry and fear that accompany the anxiety can be included in the upper-left individual interior quadrant (psychological), accompanying physical symptoms such as dizziness or hyperventilation and the genetic and biological parts may be represented within the upper-right individual exterior quadrant (medical), the effect of the frenetic pace of today's culture, within the lower-left group interior quadrant (cultural), and the societal pressures of global issues, e.g., terrorism, within the lower-right group exterior quadrant (social) (Ingersoll & Marquis, 2014).

A Unified Approach to the Etiology of the Anxiety Disorders

How does Magnavita's (2008) unified approach (discussed in Chapter 3) relate to the etiology of the anxiety disorders? Magnavita (2008) devised a unified psychotherapy approach that includes four subsystems of restructuring. The third subsystem, the relational-triadic, focuses on relationships that consist of more than two individuals. An example of a theme related to the etiology of the anxiety disorders that corresponds to the third subsystem, the relational-triadic, is illustrated in Magnavita and Anchin's (2014) unifying approach to psychotherapy. The notion of the relational-triadic, Magnavita and Anchin's (2014) third level of the total ecological system (TES) of their unifying approach to psychotherapy, can be considered an anxiety-regulating system beyond the dyad. When anxiety is not manageable in a dyad, a triangulated relationship manifests as a diathesis or point of vulnerability in order to regulate the anxiety (Magnavita & Anchin, 2014). A unifying approach to the anxiety disorders encourages mental health professionals to recognize triangulated relationships in the family and to facilitate differentiation within the triangular configuration, e.g., symptoms of anxiety that develop within the mother, father, child triangle (Magnavita & Anchin, 2014).

Summary

This chapter described themes, e.g., self-wounds, neuroscience, insecure attachments, transtheoretical, transdiagnostic, vulnerability–stress, that underlie integrated and unified etiological models for the anxiety disorders, and showed how these concepts can interact across the different physiological, psychological, and sociocultural aspects of the lifespan (Ingersoll & Marquis, 2014) (see Table 4.1). It explored the development and maintenance of the anxiety disorders within the context of integrated and unified perspectives. The next chapter discusses the integrated and unified etiological and psychotherapy models as they apply specifically to generalized anxiety disorder (GAD). Common dimensions of the anxiety disorders include the conditioning of fear (Greene, Bailey, & Neumeister, 2013) and the emergence of traumata as they evolve in

Table 4.1 The Etiology of the Anxiety Disorders: Themes

Self-Wounds	*Neuroscience*	*Transdiagnostic*	*Attachment*	*Vulnerability*	*Integral/Unified*
Genetics[a] Threat[a]	Neural Circuitry[b]	Trans-diagnostic and Neural Circuitry[c]	Insecure Attachments[d,e,f]	Vulner-ability–Stress Model[g]	Integral Psychotherapy: Psychological, Medical, Cultural, Social[h]
Perception of Ineffective Self[i,a]	Amygda-locentric Model of Anxiety[j,k,l]	Consistent with the transdiagnostic UP, temperament had been shown to account for the co-occurrence of mental disorders such as GAD, SAD, PD, depressive disorder, and PTSD.[m,n,o]	Dysregulated Affective State (DAS)[p] To understand and treat a DAS, the integration of emotional neuroscience and Experiential-Dynamic Emotion Regulation (EDER) was proposed.[q]		Unified Approach Four Subsystems of Restructuring[r] Total Ecological System (TES): Relational-Triadic[s]

[a]Wolfe (2005, 2006). [b]Kinley and Reyno (2016). [c]Tryon (2014, 2016). [d]Bowlby (1988). [e]Johnson (2019). [f]Leichsenring and Salzer (2014). [g]Beekman and colleagues (1998). [h]Ingersoll and Marquis (2014). [i]Alladin (2014). [j]Greene, Bailey, and Neumeister, (2013). [k]Rauch, Shin, and Phelps (2006). [l]Ray (2018). [m]Boettcher and Conklin (2018). [n]Brown and Barlow (2009). [o]Ruscio, Borkovec, and Ruscio (2001). [p]Grecucci, Theuninck, Frederickson, and Job (2015). [q]Fredrickson, Messina, and Grecucci (2018). [r]Magnavita(2008). [s]Magnavita and Anchin (2014).

the development and maintenance of the anxiety disorders for integrated and unified frameworks (Barlow, 2004; Davanloo, 2005; Marquis, 2018).

References

Aldao, A., Nolen-Hoeksema, S., & Schweizer, S. (2010). Emotion-regulation strategies across psychopathology: A meta-analytic review. *Clinical Psychology Review, 30*(2), 217–237. doi: 10.1016/j.cpr.2009.11.004

Alladin, A. (2014). The wounded self: New approach to understanding and treating anxiety disorders. *American Journal of Clinical Hypnosis, 56*(4), 368–388. doi: 10.1080/00029157.2014.880045

Alloy, L., Kelly, K., Mineka, S., & Clements, C. (1990). Comorbidity in anxiety and depressive disorders: A helplessness/hopelessness perspective. In J. D. Maser & C. R. Cloninger (Eds.), *Comorbidity of mood and anxiety disorders* (pp. 3–12). Washington, DC: American Psychiatric Association Press.

Barlow, D. H. (2004). *Anxiety and its disorders: The nature and treatment of anxiety and panic* (2nd ed.). New York, NY: Guilford.

Beekman, A. T., Bremmer, M. A., Deeg, D. J., Van Balkom, A. J., Smit, J. H., De Beurs, E., … van Tilburg, W. (1998). Anxiety disorders in later life: A report from the Longitudinal Aging Study Amsterdam. *International Journal of Geriatric Psychiatry, 13*(10), 717–726. doi: 10.1002/(sici)1099-1166(1998100)13:10<717::aid-gps857>3.0.co;2-m

Boettcher, H., & Conklin, L. R. (2018). Transdiagnostic assessment and case formulation: Rationale and application with the unified protocol. In D. H. Barlow & T. J. Farchione (Eds.), *Applications of the unified protocol for transdiagnostic treatment of emotional disorders* (pp. 17–37). New York, NY: Oxford University Press.

Bowlby, J. (1973). *Attachment and loss, Vol. 2. Separation.* New York, NY: Basic Books.

Bowlby, J. (1977). The making and breaking of affectional bonds. I. Aetiology and psychopathology in the light of attachment theory. *British Journal of Psychiatry, 130*(3), 201–210. doi: 10.1192/bjp.130.3.201

Bowlby, J. (1988). *A secure base: Parent-child attachment and healthy human development.* New York, NY: Basic Books.

Brown, T. A., & Barlow, D. H. (2009). A proposal for a dimensional classification system based on the shared features of the DSM-IV anxiety and mood disorders: Implications for assessment and treatment. *Psychological Assessment, 21*(3), 256–271. doi: 10.1037/a0016608

Buckholtz, J. W., & Meyer-Lindenberg, A. (2012). Psychopathology and the human connectome: Toward a transdiagnostic model of risk for mental illness. *Neuron, 74*(6), 990–1004. doi: 10.1016/j.neuron.2012.06.002

Craske, M. G., & Waters, A. M. (2005). Panic disorder, phobias, and generalized anxiety disorder. *Annual Review of Clinical Psychology, 1*, 197–225. doi: 10.1146/annurev.clinpsy.1.102803.143857

Davanloo, H. (2005). *Intensive short-term dynamic psychotherapy: Selected papers of Habib Davanloo.* New York, NY: Wiley.

Del Casale, A., Kotzalidis, G. D., Rapinesi, C., Serata, D., Ambrosi, E., Simonetti, A., … Girardi, P. (2011). Functional neuroimaging in obsessive-compulsive disorder. *Neuropsychobiology, 64*(2), 61–85. doi: 10.1159/000325223

Ein-Dor, T., & Doron, G. (2015). Psychopathology and attachment. In J. Simpson & S. Rholes (Eds.), *Attachment theory and research: New directions and emerging themes* (pp. 346–373). New York, NY: Guilford Press.

Fraley, R. C. (2002). Attachment stability from infancy to adulthood. Meta-analysis and dynamic modeling of developmental mechanisms. *Personality and Social Psychology Review*, *6*(2), 123–151. doi: 10.1207/S15327957PSPR0602_03

Frederickson, J. J., Messina, I., & Grecucci, A. (2018). Dysregulated anxiety and dysregulating defenses: Toward an emotion regulation informed dynamic psychotherapy. *Frontiers in Psychology*, *9*, 2054. doi: 10.3389/fpsyg.2018.02054

Freud, S. (1959). Inhibitions, symptoms and anxiety. In J. Strachey (Ed. and trans.), *The standard edition of the complete works of Sigmund Freud*, (Vol. 20, pp. 87–172). London: Hogarth Press. (original work published 1926).

Grecucci, A., Theuninck, A., Frederickson, J., & Job, R. (2015). Mechanisms of social emotion regulation: From neuroscience to psychotherapy. In M. L. Bryant (Ed.), *Emotion regulation: Processes, cognitive effects and social consequences* (pp. 57–84). New York, NY: Nova Science Publishers.

Greene, A. M., Bailey, C. R., & Neumeister, A. (2013). A biopsychosocial approach to anxiety. In S. M. Stahl & B. A. Moore (Eds.), *Anxiety disorders: A guide for integrating psychopharmacology and psychotherapy* (pp. 25–50). New York, NY: Routledge.

Gross, J. J. (1998). The emerging field of emotion regulation: An integrative review. *Review of General Psychology*, *2*(3), 271–299. doi: 10.1037/1089-2680.2.3.271

Hu, T., Zhang, D., Wang, J., Mistry, R., Ran, G., & Wang, X. (2014). Relation between emotion regulation and mental health: A meta-analysis review. *Psychological Reports*, *114*(2), 341–362. doi: 10.2466/03.20.PR0.114k22w4

Ingersoll, R. E., & Marquis, A. (2014). *Understanding psychopathology: An integral exploration.* Upper Saddle River, NJ: Pearson Education.

Johnson, S. M. (2019). *Attachment theory in practice: Emotionally focused therapy (EFT) with individuals, couples, and families*. New York, NY: Guilford.

Kennedy, K. A., & Barlow, D. (2018). The unified treatment for transdiagnostic treatment of emotional disorders: An introduction. In D. H. Barlow & T. J. Farchione (Eds.), *Applications of the unified protocol for transdiagnostic treatment of emotional disorders* (pp. 1–16). New York, NY: Oxford University Press.

Kinley, J. L., & Reyno, S. M. (2016). Project for a scientific psychiatry: A neurobiologically informed, phasic, brain-based model of integrated psychotherapy. *Journal of Psychotherapy Integration*, *26*(1), 61–73. doi: 10.1037/a0039636

Leichsenring, F. (2005). Are psychodynamic and psychoanalytic therapies effective? A Review of empirical data. *International Journal of Psycho-Analysis*, *86*(3), 841–868. doi: 10.1516/RFEE-LKPN-B7TF-KPDU

Leichsenring, F., & Salzer, S. (2014). A unified protocol for the transdiagnostic psychodynamic treatment of anxiety disorders: An evidence-based approach. *Psychotherapy*, *51*(2), 224–245. doi: 10.1037/a0033815

Levy, K. N., Wesley, S., Temes, C. M., & Clouthier, T. L. (2015). An integrative attachment theory framework of personality disorders. In S. K. Huprich (Ed.), *Personality disorders: Toward theoretical and empirical integration in diagnosis and assessment* (pp. 315–343). Washington, DC: American Psychological Association.

Lyubomirsky, S., Tucker, K., Caldwell, N. D., & Berg, K. (1999). Why ruminators are poor problem solvers: Clues from the phenomenology of dysphoric rumination. *Journal of Personality and Social Psychology*, 77(5), 1041–1060. doi: 10.1037/0022-3514.77.5.1041

Magnavita, J. J. (2008). Psychoanalytic psychotherapy. In J. L. Lebow (Ed.), *Twenty-first century psychotherapies: Contemporary approaches to theory and practice* (pp. 206–236). Hoboken, NJ: John Wiley & Sons.

Magnavita, J. J., & Anchin, J. C. (2014). *Unifying psychotherapy: Principles, methods, and evidence from clinical science.* New York, NY: Springer.
Marquis, A. (2018). *Integral psychotherapy: A unifying approach.* New York, NY: Routledge.
National Institute of Mental Health. (2008). *Posttraumatic stress disorder.* DHHS Publication No. ADM 08-3561. Washington, DC: US Government Printing Office.
Nolen-Hoeksema, S. (2000). The role of rumination in depressive disorders and mixed anxiety/depressive symptoms. *Journal of Abnormal Psychology, 109*(3), 504–511. doi: 10.1037/0021-843X.109.3.504
Pelligrino, L., Pierce, C., & Walkup, J. T. (2011). Pharmacological management of childhood and adolescent anxiety disorders. In W. K. Silverman & A. P. Field (Eds.), *Anxiety disorders in children and adolescents* (2nd ed., pp. 367–391). New York, NY: Cambridge University Press.
Puetz, V. B., Kohn, N., Dahmen, B., Zvyagintsev, M., Schüppen, A., Schultz, R. T., … Konrad, K. (2014). Neural response to social rejection in children with early separation experiences. *Journal of the American Academy of Child and Adolescent Psychiatry, 53*(12), 1328–1337. doi: 10.1016/j.jaac.2014.09.004
Rauch, S. L., Shin, L. M., & Phelps, E. A. (2006). Neurocircuitry models of posttraumatic stress disorder and extinction: Human neuroimaging research—Past, present, and future. *Biological Psychiatry, 60*(4), 376–382. doi: 10.1016/j.biopsych.2006.06.004
Ray, W. J. (2018). *Abnormal psychology.* Thousand Oaks, CA: Sage.
Ruscio, A. M., Borkovec, T. D., & Ruscio, J. (2001). A taxometric investigation of the latent structure of worry. *Journal of Abnormal Psychology, 110*(3), 413–422. doi: 10.1037//0021-843X.130.3.413
Schneider, K. J. (2008). *Existential-integrative psychotherapy: Guideposts to the core of practice.* New York, NY: Routledge.
Tryon, W. (2014). *Cognitive neuroscience and psychotherapy: Network principles for a unified theory.* Cambridge: Academic Press.
Tryon, W. W. (2016). Transtheoretic transdiagnostic psychotherapy. *Journal of Psychotherapy Integration, 26*(3), 273–287. doi: 10.1037/a0040041
Watson, D., & Clark, L. A. (1984). Negative affectivity: The disposition to experience aversive emotional states. *Psychological Bulletin, 96*(3), 465–490. doi: 10.1037/0033-2909.96.3.465
Wolfe, B. E. (2003). Integrative psychotherapy of the anxiety disorders. In J. C. Norcross &M. R. Goldfried (Eds.), *Handbook of psychotherapy integration* (2nd ed., pp. 263–280). New York, NY: Oxford University Press.
Wolfe, B. E. (2005). *Understanding and treating anxiety disorders: An integrative approach to healing the wounded self.* Washington, DC: American Psychological Association.
Wolfe, B. E. (2006). An integrative perspective on the anxiety disorders. In G. Stricker & J. Gold (Ed.). *A casebook of psychotherapy integration* (pp. 65–77). Washington, DC: American Psychological Association.

5 Generalized Anxiety Disorder (GAD)

Introduction

How common is generalized anxiety disorder (GAD)? In a survey on the use of outpatient therapy services, it was found that 63% of clients reported anxiety symptoms as their reason for beginning treatment (Albani, Blaser, Geyer, Schmutzer, & Brähler, 2010). Of all the anxiety disorders, generalized anxiety disorder (GAD) is the most common; however, GAD can be resistant to treatment, and those patients who receive sufficient treatment range only from 20% to 32% (Porensky et al., 2009; Revicki et al., 2012; Watson & Greenberg, 2017). Costs for health care and lost work output for patients with generalized anxiety disorders are greater than for patients with other disorders, and there is an effect of intergenerational spread of chronic worry and anxiety from parents with generalized anxiety to the next generation (Watson & Greenberg, 2017).

This chapter focuses on integrated and unified etiology approaches and psychotherapy treatment models for generalized anxiety disorder. At the end of the chapter, a case study is presented to demonstrate the implementation of a unified psychotherapy approach for generalized anxiety disorder (GAD). For this case study, the therapist treated a patient with generalized anxiety disorder by using Marquis' (2018) Integral or unified, four quadrant psychotherapy approach (Upper Right, Upper Left, Lower Right, and Lower Left).

Symptoms of Generalized Anxiety Disorder (GAD)

What are the symptoms of generalized anxiety disorder (GAD)? According to the *Diagnostic and Statistical Manual of Mental Disorders, 5th edition (*DSM-5) (American Psychiatric Association, 2013), individuals who have the common disorder, generalized anxiety disorder (GAD), worry incessantly about a broad range of incidents that can happen, expect negative events to occur, seem to be irritable, have a lot of muscle tension, may have difficulty sleeping and concentrating, and can experience a high degree of psychosocial impairment (American Psychiatric Association, 2013; Comer, 2015; Orsillo, Roemer, & Barlow, 2003). What are the distinctions between the symptoms of GAD and the symptoms of other anxiety disorders, e.g., specific phobia (SP)? Chapter

4 discussed the distinctive aspects that comprise the etiology of the anxiety disorders (Craske & Waters, 2005; Watson & Clark 1984). With respect to distinctive elements such as the threat object and the scope of the perceived harm, it was explained in Chapter 4 that the threat object for generalized anxiety disorder is broader than for panic disorder and that the scope for specific phobia is the least broadly defined (i.e., specific objects) (Craske & Waters, 2005). Whereas individuals with specific phobia (SP) have anxiety about one particular item and their worry tends to be specific, individuals with GAD worry about a variety of issues and tend to perceive worry as overwhelming and broad (American Psychiatric Association, 2013; Fredette et al., 2013).

Individuals with GAD tend to have difficulty regulating their emotions. They experience affect intensely, tend to catastrophize, may have difficulty discerning their emotions (alexithymia), and have difficulty calming their negative affect (Mennin & Fresco 2010; Mennin, Heimberg, Turk, & Fresco, 2005; Tryon, 2014). A sense of danger is overblown in the minds of individuals who have generalized anxiety disorder. Examples of thoughts that prevail in the minds of adults with GAD include chronic worries such as "What if I get sick while traveling?" or "What if I don't get the promotion on the job?" The fears and worries of individuals with GAD tend to interfere with their daily performance. The worry of individuals with GAD results in brief relief from physiological stress (Ray, 2018).

Diagnosis of Generalized Anxiety Disorder (GAD)

In the U.S., generalized anxiety disorder (GAD) and depression are diagnosed more often than other emotional disorders (Ray, 2018). An adult who experiences extreme worry and anxiety for six months can be said to have a generalized anxiety disorder (GAD) (American Psychiatric Association, 2013). Generally, individuals with a generalized anxiety disorder have worries that are hard to control, avoid risk, and seek reassurance (APA, 2013; Ray, 2018). To receive a diagnosis of GAD, an individual needs to have a physiological symptom such as elevated muscle tension that accompanies the chronic worries (APA, 2013; Ray, 2018). Patients with GAD share the interpersonal characteristics of low agency (the extent of persuasion that one has, e.g., low persuasion) and high communion (the extent that an individual pursues a connection with others, e.g., caring that is problematic) (Gómez Penedo, Constantino, Coyne, Westra, & Antony, 2017).

Prevalence of Generalized Anxiety Disorder (GAD)

Prevalence

What is the prevalence of generalized anxiety disorder (GAD)? Anxiety disorders, given their prevalence and related economic effects, are considered an important public health issue (Kessler, Petukhova, Sampson, Zaslavsky, & Wittchen, 2012; Wittchen et al., 2011). The rates of lifetime prevalence for GAD vary between approximately 4% and 7% (Bolognesi, Baldwin, & Ruini, 2014; Witchen et al., 2002). Kessler and colleagues (2005) report the lifetime prevalence to be almost 6%. More recent rates of lifetime prevalence vary between approximately 2% and 6% (Watson & Greenberg, 2017). The estimate for the 12-month in the U.S. is approximately 3% for adults (APA, 2013).

According to Angst et al. (2016), 21% of adults have generalized anxiety disorder at some point in their lives. More than twice the number of women have GAD than do men (Ray, 2018). The most frequent anxiety disorder in the elderly is GAD (Porensky et al., 2009); however, after age 74, GAD will develop in fewer than 1% of people (Kessler et al., 2005; Wolitzky-Taylor, Castriotta, Lenze, Stanley, & Craske, 2010). Although anxiety symptoms and disorders occur frequently in the elderly, they occur less frequently than in adults who are younger (Bryant, Jackson, Ames, 2008; Wolitzky-Taylor et al., 2010). According to Beekman and colleagues (1998), the risk variables for anxiety disorders in the elderly either begin in early life or they are comprised of stressors that tend to occur frequently as individuals age; however, it is, generally, not possible to prevent or cure most of them. Whereas the incidence of GAD does not decrease in the elderly, the rates for the other anxiety disorders tend to decrease in the aged (Beekman et al., 1998).

Onset

When in the life cycle does generalized anxiety disorder (GAD) emerge? GAD's onset is in contrast to the onset of the other anxiety disorders. Whereas some anxiety disorders emerge in childhood, generalized anxiety disorder tends to begin later, with uncommon occurrences before early adolescence; however, in contrast to the finding that GAD begins later in life, others assert that since individuals with GAD relate that they have felt anxious throughout the course of their lives, it is likely that GAD's onset occurs when individuals are children or adolescents (Andlin-Sobocki & Wittchen, 2005; Paus, Keshavan, & Giedd, 2008; Watson, Timulak, & Greenberg 2019). The finding that GAD's onset can emerge subtly for individuals, with symptoms of general anxiety experienced from the time that they were children, is supported by many (Anderson, Noyes, & Crowe, 1984). GAD tends to reach its highest level in middle age, and it wanes after middle age (Ray, 2018).

Comorbidity

Does generalized anxiety disorder (GAD) occur with other emotional disorders, and which emotional disorders are likely to occur with GAD? GAD is highly comorbid with other emotional disorders (Carter, Wittchen, Pfister &

Kessler, 2001; Timulak & McElvaney, 2018). Generally, individuals with one anxiety disorder tend to encounter another anxiety disorder either at the same time or at another time in their lives (Comer, 2015; Rodriguez et al., 2004). The anxiety disorder that is most likely to occur with GAD is social anxiety disorder (Borkovec, Abel, & Newman, 1995). There is quite a bit of overlap between the mood and anxiety disorders (Barlow, Allen, & Choate, 2004), and depression tends to occur with high frequency in both younger adults and the elderly with anxiety disorders (Wolitzky-Taylor et al., 2010).

Heritability

Are there genetic links to generalized anxiety disorder (GAD)? For generalized anxiety disorder, heritability ranges from 15% to 30% (Kendler & Baker, 2007; Ray, 2018).

An Integrative Etiology of Generalized Anxiety Disorder (GAD): Focus, Underpinnings, and Causes of GAD

This section discusses the etiology of generalized anxiety disorder (GAD) from an integrative point of view and lays out the implicit and explicit causes implicated in the development and maintenance of generalized anxiety disorder (GAD). The factors in common as well as the factors that are unique to the etiology and maintenance of generalized anxiety disorder are presented. There is an extensive range of etiological theories (e.g., Freud's [1917, 1933] overwhelming neurotic or moral anxiety, Lang, McTeague and Bradley's [2014] genetic and biological predispositions and brain circuits) that include themes that contribute to the development and maintenance of generalized anxiety (Comer, 2015).

Psychodynamic Themes and Generalized Anxiety Disorder (GAD)

How do psychodynamic theorists conceptualize generalized anxiety disorder (GAD)? The current way that we view generalized anxiety disorder as excessive worrying is consistent with Freud's (1894) notion of "fearful expectation" in his description of anxiety neurosis (Leichsenring & Salzer, 2014). What function does the worrying of patients with GAD fulfill? The excessive worrying of individuals with generalized anxiety disorder may be viewed as a defense mechanism that serves to ward off a deeper threat such as trauma (Borkovec, 1994; Leichsenring and Salzer, 2014). Comer (2015) contrasts Freud's earlier view of the development of generalized anxiety disorder with later psychodynamic theorists. For example, whereas Freud (1917, 1933) holds that generalized anxiety disorder occurs when neurotic and moral anxiety overtake the defenses of an individual, other psychodynamic therapists (e.g., Sharf, 2012) assert that generalized anxiety disorder derives from deficiencies in the early child–parent relationship (Comer, 2015).

The Developmental Theory of Attachment and Generalized Anxiety Disorder (GAD)

What is the relationship between attachment theory and the development of generalized anxiety disorder (GAD)? A common theme that emerges for individuals with generalized anxiety is the developmental notion of attachments that are not secure or impaired child–parent relationships (Crits-Christoph, Connolly, Azarian, Crits-Christoph, & Shappell, 1996; Lichtenstein & Cassidy, 1991). Anxiety may have become part of the attachment pattern of children who perceive the world as unsafe and insecure (Ray, 2018). Children with an attachment pattern that is not secure worry that others will not take care of them, and, thus, nothing will work out for them (Ray, 2018). Whereas a sociocultural perspective of the etiology of anxiety disorders posits that societal threats and cultural stresses may give rise to an environment in which individuals are prone to develop generalized anxiety disorder, a humanistic approach (e.g., Rogers, 1951) asserts that individuals with GAD have not received positive regard that is unconditional from caregivers, which leads to them being highly critical of themselves (Comer, 2015).

An interpersonal/psychodynamic approach to generalized anxiety disorder underscores cognitive/emotional treatment of patients' traumatic experiences and attachment issues. For example, the psychodynamic works of Manfredi et al. (2011) and Jenkins (1968) show a relationship between an overprotective style of parenting and offspring who are anxious (Comer, 2015). Barlow's (2004) assertion that an individual's cognitive predisposition to anxiety can be traced to a style of parenting that is controlling is not inconsistent with the aforementioned psychodynamic approach. The common theme of attachment is present as a concept for several theories that explain the etiology of GAD.

Cognitive, Metacognitive, and Emotion-Focused Themes and Generalized Anxiety Disorder (GAD)

What are the cognitive and metacognitive themes that are related to generalized anxiety disorder (GAD)? The metacognitive framework of generalized anxiety disorder asserts that patients with GAD cope with perceived harm by worrying (Haseth et al., 2019; Wells, 1995). Cognitive researchers have suggested that anxiety derives from schemas of fear that include stimulus connections that are inaccurate representations of relationships (Foa & Kozak, 1986).

According to emotion-focused theory, the etiology of GAD originates in a set of dysfunctional emotion schemes where patients feel fearful and vulnerable when they access memories replete with threatening experiences that they suffered at a time when they did not receive adequate soothing and support (Watson et al., 2019). Maladaptive functioning in individuals with GAD derives from dysfunctional affect schemes of dread and shame along with a difficulty in regulating emotion (Goldman, 2019; Timulak & McElvaney, 2018; Watson & Greenberg, 2017). Generally, patients with GAD cannot adequately address their needs because they have not been validated (Watson & Greenberg, 2017). In order to protect themselves from being overwhelmed by painful affect when their feelings are dismissed, individuals with generalized anxiety worry and become anxious (Watson & Greenberg, 2017). A primary contributor to GAD is the lack of capacity of individuals with this disorder to bring themselves to a place of soothing (Watson & Greenberg, 2017, Watson et al., 2019).

The Theme of Self-Wounds and Generalized Anxiety Disorder (GAD)

How does an integrative perspective of self-wounds relate to generalized anxiety disorder (GAD)? Wolfe (2003) developed an integrative approach to the anxiety disorders that views patients with anxiety disorders as having a disturbed self-perception, and that the source of an anxiety disorder is based on a patient's expectation of "self-endangerment" or harm to the self. (Chapter 1 described the link between the aforementioned conceptualization of anxiety and Roger's [1951] notion of self-concept and Kohut's [1971] conceptualization of self-object theory which underlie the etiology of the anxiety disorders.) Wolfe's (2003) model recognizes that whereas some individuals have genetic vulnerabilities that act as catalysts for an anxiety disorder to emerge, the cause for GAD is heavily weighted towards clients' hurtful life experiences, the self-wounds that individuals' damaging life experiences produce, and the defenses that individuals with GAD use to avoid their past wounds. Individuals with anxiety disorders continuously suffer with their unconscious, feared catastrophes about which they worry excessively, and their emotions are fraught with pain (Wolfe, 2003).

Processes that contribute to the development of GAD include an individual's difficulty with social proficiencies, an individual's incorporation of the toxic opinions of others about one's value, and the formation of underlying conflicts about the verbalization of feelings (Wolfe, 2005). Processes that contribute to the maintenance of GAD include worrying, the chronicity of unconscious conflicts, avoidance, and the management of impressions (Wolfe, 2005).

The Theme of Death Anxiety and Generalized Anxiety Disorder (GAD)

How does death anxiety contribute to the development and maintenance of generalized anxiety disorder? According to Wolfe (2008), the etiology of the anxiety disorders needs to take death anxiety into consideration because it is the most common source for patients with anxiety disorders. Wolfe (2003, 2008) suggests that patients with GAD use several defenses to cope with their self-wounds and anxiety. They may be self-preoccupied with their anxiety, they may avoid the objects and settings that are connected to the anxiety, and/or they may become enmeshed in interpersonal behavior patterns of negativity (Wolfe, 2003, 2008).

To develop a psychodynamic understanding of the psychological defenses that individuals use against death anxiety, Bassett (2007) integrated two theories: Terror Management Theory (TMT) (Greenberg, Pyszczynski, & Solomon, 1986) and Separation Theory (Firestone, 1994). Both theories underscore the effect of past experiences on the development of psychological defenses and recognize that adult defenses develop as a reaction to anxiety over abandonment by parents (Bassett, 2007). Death anxiety emerges as an existential worry about one's extinction that takes the place of concerns about neglect experienced from parents, and the integration of the two theories offers a more complete understanding of adult defenses by broadening the number and type of psychological defenses against death anxiety (Bassett, 2007; Firestone, 1984).

Neuroscience and Generalized Anxiety Disorder (GAD)

How does neuroscience contribute to the causes of generalized anxiety disorder (GAD)? According to Comer (2015), certain brain circuits, or a network of associated brain formations, are linked to particular emotional reactions. Whereas several research studies implicate the amygdala, the prefrontal cortex, and anterior cingulate cortex in the development of generalized anxiety disorder (e.g., Lang, McTeague, & Bradley, 2014; McClure al., 2007; Schienle, Hettema, Cáceda, & Nemeroff, 2011), it is suggested that a different circuit is involved in the development of panic disorder (Comer, 2015). Chapter 6 discusses the brain circuits and neurotransmitters involved in panic disorder. Neuroscience investigations propose that patients with GAD seem predisposed to neural overactivity and emotional overarousal, and it is hard for these individuals to regulate their emotions (Newman, Llera, Erickson, Przeworski, & Castonguay, 2013; Stevens, Jendrusina, Sarapas, & Behar, 2014; Timulak & McElvaney, 2018).

Generalized Anxiety Disorder (GAD) and Other Anxiety Disorders

What is the relationship between generalized anxiety disorder and the other anxiety disorders? It has been proposed that the different anxiety disorders have developed from generalized anxiety disorder (Brown, Barlow, & Liebowitz, 1994; May, 1979; Wolfe, 2005). In their discussion of common and distinct variables that contribute to the etiology of the anxiety disorders, Craske and Waters (2005) point out that GAD shares characteristics of threat-related patient behaviors such as avoidance and fear with other anxiety disorders (i.e., specific phobia and panic disorder); however, the anxiety disorders vary according to the scope and object of the danger, with the broadest threat-reaction taking place in GAD. Their model that aims to predict the beginning of an anxiety disorder entails issues related to a patient's vulnerability towards anxiety and a patient's history with vulnerability pertaining more to GAD, and history more to specific phobia. Compared to other anxiety disorders, GAD's fear stimuli are the least constricted, and GAD is associated with the highest level of neuroticism (Craske & Waters, 2005; Mineka, Watson, & Clark, 1998). Thus, the associative link for acquiring anxiety pertains less to GAD than to the other anxiety disorders, e.g., phobias (Craske & Waters, 2005).

Characteristic of individuals with GAD and some of the other anxiety disorders is a propensity to suffer negative affect across a broad range of situations without the presence of an external stressful event (Craske & Waters, 2005; Watson & Clark, 1984). Whereas negative affect is shared among the anxiety disorders, distinctive variables can discern among them (Craske & Waters, 2005; Zinbarg & Barlow, 1996). Cognitive theory posits variables of risk and associative learning variables that account for the etiology and maintenance of the anxiety disorders (Craske & Waters, 2005). For example, there are different kinds of distinct learning experiences (e.g., traumatic conditioning, the observation of a traumatized model, and the relating of potentially dangerous information) that account for less of the variance for GAD than for panic disorder and the phobias (Craske & Waters, 2005; Rachman, 1978). More specifically, the fear cues are less defined for GAD than for the other anxiety disorders, and when compared to the other anxiety disorders, GAD is the disorder that is highest on negative emotions, but unique effects for GAD contribute to less variance than for the other anxiety disorders (Craske & Waters, 2005; Mineka et al., 1998). Craske and Waters (2005) explain that the associative learning variables play more of an active role for the phobias and panic disorder than they do for GAD, and, therefore, it is understandable that when negative incidents take place, individuals with GAD experience connections of threat that pertain to an extensive range of adjacent stimuli rather than perceptions of direct cues of threat as experienced by individuals with specific phobia.

Summary

Various psychological theories, frameworks, and models, e.g., the cognitive avoidance theory of worry of Borkovec, Alcaine, & Behar (2004), the metacognitive orientation of Wells (1999), have been proposed to conceptualize generalized anxiety disorder and to explain the excessive worry about future outcomes manifested by individuals with GAD (Ingersoll & Marquis, 2014; Timulak & McElvaney, 2018). This portion described the etiology of generalized anxiety disorder (GAD) from an integrative point of view and delineated the causes implicated in the development and maintenance of generalized anxiety disorder (GAD). Which features are characteristic of individuals with generalized anxiety disorder? Emotional avoidance and interpersonal difficulties are involved in the etiology of GAD (Newman, Castonguay, Borkovec, Fisher, & Nordberg, 2008). The shared focus is on the patient's avoidance of emotional experiences (Alladin, 2014; Lee, Orsillo, Roemer, & Allen 2010).

Clinical Practice Applications of Single-School, Integrated, and Unified Psychotherapy Treatment Models for Generalized Anxiety Disorder (GAD)

Do individuals with generalized anxiety disorder (GAD) tend to seek treatment, and if so, when? The symptoms of GAD can wax and wane, and often clients experience symptoms for approximately 10 years prior to seeking therapy (Comaty & Advokat, 2013). It has been found that GAD can be resistant to treatment, that only about half of clients with GAD benefit from brief interventions, and that several clients who receive treatment will show symptoms later in time (Borkovec, Newman, Pincus, & Lytle, 2002; Hanrahan, Field, Jones, & Davey, 2013; Watson et al., 2019). On the other hand, what clinicians view as resistance to treatment, in fact may not turn out to be resistance. Much of what is concluded to be patient resistance during psychotherapy may be ambivalence about behavior change (Arkowitz, 2002).

The Problem With Single School Cognitive-Behavioral Approaches for Generalized Anxiety Disorder (GAD)

How effective is cognitive-behavioral therapy for generalized anxiety disorder (GAD)?

Examples of single-school cognitive-behavioral approaches for GAD include relaxation, exposure, and problem-solving (Borkovec et al., 2004; Dugas & Robichaud, 2007; Murphy et al., 2017). The previous section on the etiology of GAD emphasized the need to address the issue of worry for patients with GAD. Murphy et al. (2017) explain that to target worry in patients with GAD, cognitive-behavioral models use psychoeducation, shaping, and belief restructuring (e.g., Behar, DiMarco, Hekler, Mohlman, & Staples, 2009). Cognitive-behavioral therapists such as Zinbarg, Craske, and Barlow (2006) have treated GAD by employing imagery exposure. Relaxation treatment along with desensitization or relaxation treatment alone has been demonstrated to be beneficial for patients with GAD (Goldfried, 1971; Muse, Moore, & Stahl, 2013; Öst, 1987). Applied relaxation (AR) has been shown to be as beneficial as CBT post treatment, but after 12 months, 58% showed gains with CBT, and 33%, with AR (Bolognesi et al., 2014, Borkovec & Costello, 1993). The rates of remission for CBT and applied relaxation are 60% and 51%, respectively (Bolognesi et al., 2014). Treatment for an anxiety disorder can work at any age (King & Barrowclough, 1991). For example, therapy that includes relaxation training is suggested for elderly individuals who have anxiety (Ayers, Sorrell, Thorp, & Wetherell, 2007).

In what ways have CBT treatments fallen short in the treatment of GAD? Cognitive-behavioral exposure may be difficult to enact for patients with GAD because of the broad range and chronic characteristics of the feared stimuli of patients with GAD (Murphy et al., 2017). When the object or situation that is feared can be easily identified (e.g., specific phobia), CBT methods seem to be more effective than psychodynamic therapy; however, when it is more difficult to identify the feared object or situation (e.g., generalized anxiety disorder, panic disorder), it is preferable to use exploratory methods, as in psychodynamic therapy, in order to uncover an individual's conflicts, defenses, and sources of anxiety (Marquis, 2018). Furthermore, cognitive-behavioral therapy for generalized anxiety disorder has not included interventions for either interpersonal difficulties or emotional avoidance (Newman, Castonguay, Borkovec, & Molnar, 2004). Research has shown that cognitive-behavioral therapy reduces the feelings of worry that clients with anxiety disorders experience; however, at termination more than 35% of patients are not functioning well (Covin, Ouimet, Seeds, & Dozois, 2008; Ladouceur et al., 2000; Newman & Llera, 2011).

Nevertheless, it appears that CBT continues to dominate because it is an evidence-based treatment (Jones-Smith, 2012). Cognitive-behavioral therapy (CBT) has been shown to be a well-recognized and effective intervention for GAD; however, the rates of recovery for CBT are only approximately 50% (Hanrahan et al., 2013; Timulak et al., 2018). There are patients who do not prefer CBT for their psychotherapy for GAD, and high premature termination rates for individuals with anxiety disorders who have received CBT are not unusual (Taylor, Abramowitz, & McKay, 2012; Timulak et al., 2018). Although it has been shown that CBT is used as a preferred approach for GAD, many individuals, particularly the elderly, do not hold on to long term positive effects that are lasting (Bolognesi et al., 2014).

Whereas cognitive-behavioral treatments have been somewhat helpful in treating GAD, GAD is the least effectively treated of the anxiety disorders (Brown et al. 1994; Newman, Castonguay, Borkovec, Fisher, & Nordberg, 2008; Orsillo et al., 2003). In fact, it is suggested that fewer than 50% of patients respond to cognitive-behavioral treatments for GAD (Cuijpers et al., 2014). It is possible that a cognitive-behavioral psychotherapist who persists with a CBT treatment approach for patients with GAD who resist CBT may be contributing to the repetition of these patients original interpersonal difficulties, e.g., their tendency to relent by employing a nonassertive position when confronted by a dominant other (Constantino & Westra, 2012). The nonassertive position that patients with GAD tend to employ in their interpersonal relationships might be contributing to their disorder and interpersonal problems, and the traditional CBT techniques may be exacerbating the interpersonal difficulties characteristic of patients with GAD (Gómez Penedo et al., 2017).

Although cognitive-behavioral treatment (e.g., relaxation training) has been effective in decreasing the symptoms of GAD, many individuals who have received cognitive-behavioral treatment do not reach satisfying levels of "end-state" behaviors (Orsillo et al., 2003, p. 222; Ray, 2018). A comprehensive psychotherapy treatment approach needs to include different formulations that comprise the etiology of the anxiety disorders (Zerbe, 1990). Integrated treatments are needed, specifically those targeting the interpersonal and emotional difficulties of individuals with GAD.

Integrated Psychotherapy Treatment Models for Generalized Anxiety Disorder (GAD)

Cognitive-Behavioral Therapy (CBT) and Interpersonal and Emotional Processing Therapy (IEP) for Generalized Anxiety Disorder (GAD)

How can an integration of cognitive-behavioral therapy (CBT) and other treatments help patients with generalized anxiety disorder (GAD) who do not profit from a single-school therapy such as CBT by itself? Can an integration of cognitive-behavioral therapy (CBT) and interpersonal and emotional processing therapy (IEP) help patients who do not benefit much from a monotherapy such as CBT by itself? The next section highlights the interpersonal difficulties of individuals with generalized anxiety disorder and illustrates how the integration of cognitive-behavioral therapy (CBT) with interpersonal processing therapy (IEP) can help patients with GAD.

Although cognitive-behavioral therapy (CBT) is effective for GAD, it does not help all patients with GAD, and it does not adequately target the emotional avoidance and interpersonal problems that make up the etiology of GAD (Hanrahan et al., 2013; Newman, Castonguay, Borkovec, Fisher, & Nordberg, 2008). To meet the needs of patients with generalized anxiety disorder who have not progressed with traditional cognitive-behavior therapy, Newman et al. (2004) proposed an integrated psychotherapy approach that integrates interpersonal therapy with standard CBT. Schottenbauer, Glass, and Arnkoff (2005) point out that the aforementioned integrated approach is an example of parallel-concurrent integration where two or more kinds of therapy are offered during distinct sessions or during different parts of a session. The interpersonal-emotional part of the therapy is kept distinct from the cognitive-behavioral part (Newman et al., 2004; Schottenbauer et al, 2005). The psychotherapy integrative approach of Newman et al. (2004) is particularly useful for patients with GAD who have problems with processing their emotions (Schottenbauer et al., 2005).

How can interpersonal therapy help patients with generalized anxiety face their emotions? Newman, Castonguay, Borkovec, Fisher, and Nordberg (2008) developed an integrative psychotherapy approach that includes cognitive-behavioral therapy (CBT) and interpersonal and emotional processing therapy (IEP) to treat the emotional avoidance and interpersonal difficulties of patients with GAD. They showed that the symptoms of patients with GAD were reduced post treatment, and the reduction of symptoms endured upon follow-up, one year later. The findings support therapists who assist patients to shift from CBT to IEP during therapy sessions and are consistent with results that show that therapists who facilitate a corrective relationship during therapy make it possible for patients to attain improved relationship experiences outside of therapy (Henry & Strupp, 1994; Newman, Castonguay, Borkovec, Fisher, & Nordberg, 2008; Wachtel, 1977). It is suggested that the effect size for the integrated treatment, IEP, for GAD is greater than the average effect size for a monotherapy such as CBT (Bolognesi et al., 2014; Borkovec & Ruscio, 2001; Newman, Castonguay, Borkovec, Fisher, & Nordberg, 2008).

CBT Integrated With Motivational Interviewing (MI) for Generalized Anxiety Disorder (GAD)

How can an integration of cognitive-behavioral therapy (CBT) and motivational interviewing (MI) help patients who do not benefit much from a monotherapy by itself? This section highlights an integrated psychotherapy treatment approach that is personalized for the patient and shows the benefits of the integration of cognitive-behavioral therapy (CBT) with motivational interviewing (MI) for patients with GAD.

When cognitive-behavioral therapy for patients with GAD who tend to worry a lot was compared to an integrated treatment of both cognitive-behavioral therapy and motivational interviewing (MI), it was found that after treatment, both groups equally decreased the tendency to worry; however, the patients who received the integrated treatment showed significantly less worry from the time of treatment completion through a year follow-up than did patients who received only CBT (Westra, Constantino, and Antony, 2016). Arkowitz and Westra (2004) suggest that whereas CBT assists patients to enact change, MI focuses on motivation and on the resolution of ambivalence linked to change. MI, initially developed by Miller and Rollnick (1991, 2002) as a person-centered framework that is directive, aims at encouraging client self-exploration associated with change (Westra & Dozois, 2006). A therapist treating with CBT facilitates client change; however, a practitioner using MI encourages patients to be their own advocates (Westra & Dozois, 2006). Whereas MI has a portion that is directive, aimed at encouraging patients to make behavioral changes themselves, it is first and foremost involved with change motivation rather than with the establishment of a plan for behavioral change (Westra & Dozois, 2006). MI was initially used for clients' difficulties with substance use (Miller, 1983); however, it has been expanded to include a broad scope of behavioral issues (Miller & Rose, 2009). Rollnick, Miller, and Butler (2008) call for therapists to allow patients to voice their own behavior changes, to work to understand the rationale of patients for wanting change, to employ quality and empathic listening, and to empower patients to discover how they can facilitate their own change.

The research of Gómez Penedo et al. (2017) supports the findings of Westra and colleagues (2016) that patients with GAD who are nonassertive were found to have a continued decrease in worry during follow-up only with the integrated treatment, MI-CBT, rather than with CBT. Furthermore, it has been shown that patients treated with MI-CBT were found to have fewer interpersonal difficulties than patients treated with only CBT (Constantino, Westra, Antony, & Coyne, 2016). A context-responsive psychotherapy integration approach outlines a perspective where markers or contexts guide treatment adaptations (Constantino, Bernecker, Boswell, & Castonguay, 2013; Gómez Penedo et al., 2017). For example, if patients have interpersonal difficulties such as nonassertiveness, then an integrated psychotherapy approach whereby MI methods are integrated with CBT could generate a better outcome and a longer period of improvement (Constantino et al., 2013; Gómez Penedo et al., 2017).

These findings encourage therapists to carefully assess their patients interpersonal problems prior to treatment as they can assist both in treatment selection and during treatment so that patients with GAD have the opportunity to revise their interpersonal problems (e.g., by taking a position that is different from the psychotherapist rather than displaying submissive behaviors) (Gómez Penedo et al., 2017). A therapist's willingness to recognize the interpersonal problems of patients with GAD and to tailor interventions based on these patients' issues suggests a responsiveness that moves beyond a diagnosis that is strictly by category (Gómez Penedo et al., 2017).

Metacognitive Therapy (MCT) and the Integration of Mindfulness and CBT for Generalized Anxiety (GAD)

How can metacognitive therapy offer a benefit for patients with generalized anxiety disorder (GAD)? Metacognitive therapy (MCT) is a recommended intervention for GAD, and aims to modify thought processes rather than the content (Haseth et al., 2019; National Institute for Health and Clinical Excellence [NICE], 2011; Wells, 1995). It has been suggested that Group MCT (g-MCT), a cost-effective intervention, could be as efficacious a treatment as individual MCT and CBT (Haseth et al., 2019).

How can the integration of mindfulness and CBT benefit patients with generalized anxiety disorder (GAD)? Whereas mindfulness techniques have been used in religion, they can be applied to secular scenarios as well. For example, Creswell (2017) discusses the neurobiological processes of mindfulness treatments and how they have been applied using evidence-based research to a variety of settings, e.g., military, workplace. Bolognesi and colleagues (2014) offer examples of psychotherapy approaches for generalized anxiety disorder (GAD) that include mindfulness perspectives, e.g., acceptance-based behavior therapy (ABBT; Roemer & Orsillo, 2005, 2007), an integrated treatment approach that includes components of acceptance and commitment therapy (ACT; Hayes, Strosahl, & Wilson, 1999), and mindfulness CBT (Segal, Williams, & Teasdale, 2002). The integration of mindfulness methods, e.g., acceptance and commitment therapy (ACT), into existing cognitive-behavioral interventions may increase the quality of life for those with GAD (Hayes, 2004; Hayes, Strosahl, & Wilson, 2011; Orsillo et al., 2003). Some researchers, however, found that CBT was superior to mindfulness/ acceptance interventions in decreasing anxiety (Newby, McKinnon, Kuyken, Gilbody, & Dalgleish, 2015).

See the section of this chapter, "Unified Treatment Approaches for Anxiety," which explains that mindfulness is incorporated as a module into the transdiagnostic unified protocol (UP) of Barlow, Farchione, and colleagues (2011). The UP was published as a therapist guide and patient workbook to help patients with emotional states that are characterized by negativity (Barlow,

Ellard et al., 2011; Barlow, Farchione et al., 2011, 2018; Kennedy & Barlow, 2018).

The Integration of Neuroscience and Psychotherapy Treatment for Generalized Anxiety Disorder (GAD)

How can the relationship between neurobiological and psychological concepts help with generalized anxiety disorder (GAD)? Kinley and Reyno (2016), in their integrated neurobiological approach, propose that several psychotherapy treatments e.g., mindfulness, emotion-focused, and others, can help with impaired affect regulation. Chapter 3 described their model of psychotherapy integration, a transdiagnostic framework with a neurobiological rationale for clinical issues, which underscores a link between mind and body, an association between neurobiological and psychological ideas, the self-regulation of emotions, and the integration of impaired brain circuitry. Theirs is a brain-based and phasic approach with a well-delineated therapeutic intervention that is suggested at each phase of an emotional disorder depending on the key neuronal impairments. Kinley and Reyno (2016) suggest that some individuals need greater amounts of care at an earlier phase of psychotherapy and move more slowly through the phasic intervention hierarchy because of their more impaired or disrupted neural network, which may have been affected earlier in life.

Integrating Psychodynamic, Humanistic, Behavioral, and Cognitive Approaches in the Treatment of Generalized Anxiety Disorder (GAD)

The finding that patients with an attachment style that is dismissive had a better outcome with integrative treatment than with cognitive-behavioral therapy (CBT) tends to suggest that incorporating psychodynamic, humanistic, and interpersonal treatments into a CBT framework offers a greater openness to the needs and impairments of certain types of patients with GAD (Castonguay, Eubanks, Goldfried, Muran, & Lutz, 2015; Newman, Castonguay, Fisher, & Borkovec, 2008). In his article, "An Integrated Approach to the Treatment of Anxiety Disorders and Phobias," Gold (1993) described a model that integrates psychodynamic, behavioral, humanistic, and cognitive ideas and techniques while relying on the attachment theory of Bowlby (1980) and Guidano (1987). His integrated therapy model of the anxiety disorders and phobias consists of three phases, which include assessment, the resolution of symptoms, and the exploration of a client's past experiences of attachment along with the correction of maladaptive attachments.

How can integrative approaches that focus on psychodynamic and interpersonal themes benefit clients with generalized anxiety disorder (GAD)? The integrative approaches, cyclical psychodynamic theory and integrative relational therapy, have frequently been used as a treatment for anxiety and interpersonal problems (Wachtel, 1977; Wachtel, 1997; Wachtel, Kruk, &

McKinney, 2005). A focus of the aforementioned interventions is on vicious circles or the manner in which patients' intrapsychic states or patterns from the past emerge on a daily basis and elicit reactions from other individuals that mimic earlier patterns (Wachtel et al., 2005). (The cyclical psychodynamic perspective and the concept of vicious circles are discussed in the section on "Theoretical Integration" in Chapter 2.) Cyclical psychodynamics is derived from a psychoanalytic relational approach and a synthesis of psychodynamic, systemic, and cognitive-behavioral perspectives (Wachtel, 2014; Wachtel et al., 2005; Wachtel & Wachtel, 1986). A goal of the cyclical psychodynamic perspective along with integrative relational psychotherapy is to promote a corrective affective experience within the working alliance so that the patient can establish productive ways to interact with other individuals outside of therapy (Wachtel et al., 2005).

How can an integrated psychotherapy approach that focuses on self-wounds benefit patients with GAD? (Chapter 4 and the section on "The Theme of Self-Wounds and Generalized Anxiety Disorder (GAD)" presented in this chapter discussed the theme of self-wounds promoted in Wolfe's [2003, 2005, 2006] integrative model.) Wolfe's (2003, 2005, 2006) and Alladin's (2014) conceptualizations of self-wounds and clients' persistent conflicts based on their subjective perceptions lend themselves to integrated etiological and treatment approaches to anxiety that address both symptom reduction as well as the need to help patients reveal the undiscoverable along with their unconscious conflicts related to their anxieties. When a patient perceives the self to be in danger, feelings of powerlessness and helplessness emerge, and a loss of control ensues (Wolfe, 2003). A therapist who adheres to an integrative approach needs both to aim at symptom reduction and to help the patient with GAD recognize the unconscious meaning of the felt anxiety, worry, and painful emotions that are associated with the perceived harm (Wolfe, 2003). Wolfe's (2003) integrative intervention model for the anxiety disorders includes both the reduction of symptoms and an exploration of underlying conflicts that set off the anxiety. His integrative four-stage approach to the anxiety disorders includes forming a working relationship, offering instruction about relevant methods to reduce the anxiety, discovering the patient's conflicts or self-wounds, and assisting patients to resolve their conflicts or heal their self-wounds. By making use of Wolfe's (2003) integrative model that draws on aspects of cognitive-behavioral, psychodynamic, and experiential orientations of psychotherapy, therapists can help patients with anxiety disorders decrease their symptoms, and they can employ an emotion-focused treatment that helps patients to explore their existential urgencies. Wolfe (2008) proposed an integrated psychotherapy treatment for the anxiety disorders within the setting of a therapeutic relationship that blends a treatment that focuses on symptoms, e.g., tools that help patients reduce their anxiety, with a deeper phase of treatment, the modification of patients' strategies, e.g., avoidance, that prevent them from facing their self-wounds and existential issues. Wolfe's (2005, 2013) integrated psychotherapy approach underscores insight into a client's self and interpersonal issues, generates changes in behavior, and can have an effect upon the cognitive and emotional sources of a client's impaired view of the self.

Alladin (2014) relies on Wolfe's (2005, 2006) integrated etiological theory and psychotherapy approach along with his conceptualization of self-wounds in his development of an integrated model, cognitive hypnotherapy, that combines psychodynamic, behavioral, cognitive, and experiential treatment approaches for the management of anxiety. Alladin's (2014) integrated psychotherapy treatment model employs conscious and unconscious methods along with hypnotic and cognitive techniques in the treatment of anxiety disorders. His approach utilizes hypnotherapy to achieve a relaxation response which is important for patients with anxiety disorders. Whereas clients diagnosed with an anxiety disorder tend to ruminate about threats on a chronic basis and their psychological and physiological repertoire is one of constriction, hypnosis can help them to enhance their expression, broaden their awareness, increase positive feelings, and heighten their emotional experience (Alladin, 2014; Brown & Fromm, 1990).

Although treatment that is focused on anxiety symptoms is necessary (e.g., imaginal or in vivo exposure), it is not sufficient, for it may be more in-depth treatment that helps patients to resolve unconscious conflicts that underlie their anxiety disorders (Alladin, 2014; Wolfe, 2003, 2005, 2006). It is important to assess the first therapeutic entry point correctly because failure to do so can interfere with the patient's therapy process (Wolfe, 2006). For example, consider the situation where a therapist assesses that a patient has an anxiety disorder and begins with cognitive-behavioral strategies upon noting Wolfe's (2006) assertion that the change of behavior is the first entry point for most individuals. Wolfe's (2006) call for assessment is well taken as patients, indeed, may want to change their behavior, but may wish for a corrective relationship in therapy prior to engaging in cognitive-behavioral exercises, and a therapist who attempts to begin with cognitive-behavioral strategies without first assessing a patient's level of comfort with that procedure can interfere with the process of therapy.

How can assimilative integration models of psychotherapy assist in the treatment of patients with anxiety disorders? Chapter 2 discussed how the fourth type of integration, assimilative integration, differs from the other three types in that it anchors itself to a unitary therapy framework while integrating tenets from other psychotherapy frameworks (Castonguay et al., 2015; Norcross, 2005). Recently, Glock, Hilsenroth, and Curtis (2018) showed that an integrative psychotherapy perspective can be effective for the anxiety disorders. The findings of Glock and colleagues (2018) support an assimilative integration approach such as Gold and Stricker's (2012) where methods are derived from already established psychotherapy models that are tailored to the needs of each particular patient. Glock et al.'s (2018) study of integrative psychotherapy for anxiety, the first investigation of client ratings of particular psychotherapy interventions linked to outcome, showed that clients viewed several kinds of treatment approaches to be beneficial for their difficulties with anxiety. It was suggested that certain kinds of psychodynamic-interpersonal and cognitive-behavioral methods are critical for change for patients with anxiety (Glock et al., 2018). Specifically, patients rated the item where a psychotherapist offers different ways to understand situations as most helpful for the psychodynamic-interventional portion and the item where a psychotherapist offers explicit directions for resolving difficulties as the most helpful for the cognitive-behavioral part (Glock et al., 2018).

With respect to assimilative integration therapies that are psychodynamic, Sell, Möller, and Taubner (2018) integrated imagery and hypnotic trances into their guided imagery psychotherapy (GIP) and hypnopsychotherapy and found improvements in patients' well-being, quality of relationships, and psychological mindedness post treatment. It has been shown that the improvements that can be attributed to psychodynamic interventions are lasting and seem to reach beyond the remission of symptoms (Shedler, 2010).

Are there integrated humanistic treatments for GAD? Barekati, Bahmani, Naghiyaaee, Afrasiabi, and Mars (2017) showed how an integrated cognitive-existential approach to group psychotherapy can decrease cognitive distortions and existential anxieties in the elderly. Using an integrated cognitive-existential framework, they addressed Yalom's (1980) notion of existential anxiety and its application during group therapy for older individuals. Alternative integrated psychodynamic, humanistic, behavioral, and cognitive interventions to the monotherapies include the integrative treatment, cognitive-behavioral hypnotherapy, which has been shown to be beneficial for individuals with GAD (e.g., Baker, 2001) and the integrative psychotherapy approach based on the work of Gilbert and Orlans (2011) which employs both humanistic and psychodynamic orientations and has been effective in the treatment of both anxiety and depression (van Rijn & Wild, 2013).

Emotion-Focused Therapy (EFT) (Johnson, 1996, 2019): An Integrated Treatment for Generalized Anxiety Disorder (GAD)

Comprehensive integrated treatments need to target the emotional difficulties of individuals with generalized anxiety disorder (GAD). What does an emotion-focused therapy (EFT) orientation mean for a therapist? Emotion-focused therapy is an exploration into the world of another while holding that person's experience and world, and it is a quest to understand what it takes to be human (Johnson, 2019). What does EFT mean for a client? It is to live in a safe and benign place where growth can take place on an internal and interpersonal level (Johnson, 2019).

How does emotion-focused therapy integrate treatment for generalized anxiety disorder (GAD)? An integrated treatment for GAD, emotion-focused therapy (EFT), incorporates elements from person-centered, Gestalt, and other humanistic or existential therapies (Greenberg, Rice & Elliott, 1993). Therapists have developed EFT in order to help patients decrease the symptoms of generalized anxiety disorder on a long-term basis by transforming patients' hurtful emotions and damaging organizations of the self (Greenberg, 2011; Timulak & McElvaney, 2016; Watson & Greenberg, 2017). EFT, initially, integrated the gestalt therapy of Fritz Perls (1969) and the client-centered therapy of Carl Rogers (1951), both of which derive from a humanistic-existential approach, and, then, emerged to integrate a theory that shows the way in which affect changes throughout psychotherapy (Goldman, 2019). Originally, EFT was used in relation to depression, trauma, and couples who have difficulties in their relationships (Greenberg & Johnson, 1988; Greenberg & Watson, 2006; Paivio & Pascual-Leone, 2010). Recently, EFT has been used in relation to GAD (Timulak & McElvaney, 2016; Timulak & McElvaney, 2018; Watson & Greenberg, 2017). It is hard for patients with GAD to process emotions (Behar et al., 2009; Newman & Llera, 2011). Thus, EFT with its focus on the transformation of hurtful affect is a suitable treatment for individuals with GAD (Timulak et al., 2018; Timulak & McElvaney, 2016). Although most interventions for GAD highlight work with anxiety and worry, emotion-focused therapy (Greenberg, 2011; Greenberg et al. 1993) focuses primarily on heightening awareness of emotions, on the recognition of the underlying experiences of emotion and what sets them off, on improving the regulation of emotions, on transforming dysfunctional emotions, and on reflecting on affect that works (Greenberg, 2006, Timulak et al., 2018; Timulak & McElvaney, 2018).

What is the difference between the emotion-focused therapy (EFT) and cognitive-behavioral approaches with respect to worry? Emotion-focused therapy (EFT) is a complex type of psychotherapy that focuses on emotional building (Timulak & McElvaney, 2018). In contrast to cognitive-behavioral approaches to worry, emotion-focused therapy (EFT) targets the level of affective activation, the level of emotional awareness of the worry process (Murphy et al., 2017). The goal of EFT is to develop access to emotions that are healthy, e.g., anger that is assertive, and to promote self-soothing rather than to focus on restructuring of beliefs about worry or on methods of problem-solving (Murphy et al., 2017). The purpose of EFT is to alter the way in which emotion is processed so that the client can discover novel meaning (Johnson, 2019).

What are some of the tasks of EFT? The primary tasks of EFT include imaginary chair conversations, e.g., two-chair conversation for conflict or criticism of the self and for interruption of the self, empty chair conversation for business that has not been completed (Elliott, Watson, Goldman, & Greenberg, 2004; Murphy et al., 2017). Murphy and colleagues (2017) explain that EFT encourages the client to engage in the task of chair dialogue, to feel the effect of worry, and to experience healthy affect in order to cultivate resilience to the worry process. For example, the two-chair conversation for worry encourages a patient to become more aware with regard to worry, to experience its effect, and to confront the worry (Timulak & McElvaney, 2018). EFT that targets worry is more active than imaginal exposure in that individuals can combat worry by using transformative affect, altering one emotion by initiating another emotion (Greenberg, 2011; Murphy et al., 2017).

How do emotion-focused therapists (EFT) work with individuals with GAD? The emotion-focused psychotherapy approach relies on developing a caring working relationship and promotes experiential assignments (Greenberg et al., 1993). In some ways, treating anxiety may be more complex than treating depression as GAD can emerge after a long history of patients' experiences being invalidated (Watson et al., 2019). During emotion-focused therapy, the emotion schemes of fear and worry experienced by individuals with GAD need to be evoked, experienced as tolerable, and altered by compassion and assertiveness (Goldman, 2019). EFT therapists who focus on building an attuned relationship and facilitating experiential assignments such as worry chair conversations (Murphy et al., 2017) can help patients who have received little or no support to reorganize their self-structures while working towards emotion processing, painful affective transformation, and building patient confidence (Watson et al., 2019). The primary therapeutic work with individuals with GAD focuses on helping them to transform their distress by adopting new, adaptive ways of coping such as developing anger that is assertive and encouraging the capacity for self-soothing (Watson et al., 2019). Primary processes that result in change include the integration of meaning and emotion, key concepts that are promoted in emotion-focused therapy, an integrated experiential emotion-focused treatment (Goldman, 2019).

Pharmacotherapy, Combined Medication and Therapy, and Generalized Anxiety Disorder

How do patients with generalized anxiety disorder (GAD) fare with monotherapy, pharmacotherapy, and a combination of monotherapy and pharmacotherapy? Since the 1950s benzodiazepines such as alprazolam (Xanax) or clonazepam (Klonopin) have been used in the treatment of anxiety (Gorman, 2016; Julien, 2013). Today, benzodiazepines, given their side effects, are classified as sedative-hypnotic medications rather than as anxiolytics (Julien, 2013). Although benzodiazepines have been found to be beneficial for adults, they have not been demonstrated to be significantly effective for children and adolescents (Pelligrino, Pierce, & Walkup, 2011). Given that the GABA activity of patients with anxiety is decreased, which results in a lower inhibition of portions of the brain responsible for threat reaction, benzodiazepines tend to affect GABA activity and decrease anxiety in approximately 65% to 70% of patients with GAD (Ray, 2018; Roemer, Orsillo, & Barlow, 2002).

In the 1990s, azapirones, e.g., buspirone, were introduced, and these had an effect on the brain's serotonin receptors (Ray, 2018). Buspirone (Buspiron, Wellbutrin) may be effective for adult patients who have not tried benzodiazepines, tends to be focused on the cognitive concerns of generalized anxiety disorder, and has fewer side effects than the benzodiazepines; however its usefulness is limited as a unitary therapy (Comaty & Advokat, 2013; Ray, 2018).

A window for the integration of psychological treatments with pharmacotherapy for GAD involves a view of neuroscience. Gorman (2016) suggests that researchers use neuroscience to discover ways in which antidepressants and psychodynamic therapy may be combined for patients with anxiety disorders. Psychopharmacology, e.g., serotonin-specific reuptake inhibitors (SSRIs) and serotonin-norepinephrine reuptake inhibitors (SNRIs) frequently have been shown to help patients with anxiety (Julien, 2013; Katzman et al., 2011). Paroxetine (Paxil) was the initial SSRI that was recommended for GAD (Comaty & Advokat, 2013). In the late 1980s, fluoexetine (Prozac), was introduced as the first SSRI to work both as an antidepressant and as an anxiolytic, and other SSRIs were introduced in the 1990s (Julien, 2013). The SNRIs that can benefit patients with GAD include venlefaxine (Effexor) and duloxetine (Cymbalta) (Julien, 2013).

For children with anxiety disorders, the SSRIs are preferred because of safety and effectiveness (Pelligrino, Pierce, & Walkup, 2011). Benzodiazepines are generally contraindicated in the elderly with generalized anxiety disorder, and the SSRIs are preferred (Julien, 2013).The following example of psychotherapy treatments provides a comparison of monotherapy to combination therapy (therapy with medication) in the treatment of GAD. Brief therapy such as brief Adlerian psychodynamic psychotherapy (B-APP), derived from the individual psychology of Adler (Mosak, 1979), and supportive-expressive psychodynamic therapy (Crits-Christoph et al., 1996), an interpersonal intervention, have been shown to be effective for GAD. Approximately 40% to 60% of patients with GAD show full improvement with either pharmacotherapy or psychological interventions (Ray, 2018). Some studies find that monotherapy (Adlerian psychodynamic, the brief kind) and combination therapy (B-APP with pharmacological intervention) are effective for GAD (Ferrero et al., 2007). Others show that therapy is more advantageous than only medication (Borkovec & Ruscio, 2001; Comaty & Advokat, 2013; Otto, Smits, & Reese, 2004). In general, recent studies demonstrate that only infrequently is combination therapy more effective over time than monotherapy or medication alone for patients with anxiety disorders (Gorman, 2016; Aaronson, Katzman, & Moster, 2015). The small amount of research that shows the superiority of combination therapy (psychotropics and psychodynamic therapy) for clients with anxiety includes brief interventions and reports results for research samples that are small (Gorman, 2016).

Anderson and Palm (2006) found that although medications decrease the anxiety symptoms of patients with GAD, pharmacotherapy does not alter the primary feature of GAD, the chronic worry that patients with GAD experience. It has been shown that psychotherapy is as effective as medication in the treatment of GAD, and it is the intervention of choice given a lesser number of side effects and improved rates of remission (Muse et al., 2013). Whereas individuals with panic disorder were almost three times more likely to refuse medication over therapy as an intervention, no differences were found in rates of refusal between pharmacotherapy and psychotherapy for individuals with GAD (Swift, Greenberg, Tompkins, & Parkin, 2017). GAD has a more chronic course than panic disorder post pharmacotherapy (Orsillo et al., 2003; Woodman, Noyes, Black, Schlosser, & Yagia, 1999).

Unified Treatment Approaches for Anxiety

Unified therapy treatments that are transdiagnostic and that emphasize the similarities among disorders have been developed both for psychodynamic therapy and for cognitive-behavioral therapy (Barlow, Farchione et al., 2011, 2018; Leichsenring & Steinert, 2018). The next section discusses two unified treatments, Barlow et al.'s (2004, 2018) and Barlow, Farchione et al.'s (2011) cognitive-behavioral unified protocol (UP) and the unified psychodynamic psychotherapy (UPP-ANXIETY) model of Leichsenring and Salzer (2014). Both Leichsenring and Salzer's (2014) unified psychodynamic psychotherapy for anxiety (UPP-ANXIETY), an effective transdiagnostic treatment for the anxiety disorders, and Barlow et al.'s (2004) unified CBT treatment protocol share several common characteristics (Leichsenring and Salzer, 2014).

Barlow et al.'s (2004, 2017, 2018) and Barlow, Farchione et al.'s (2011) Cognitive-Behavioral Unified Protocol (UP)

Are emotional disorders more similar than different? Some have suggested that transdiagnostic CBT treatments for anxiety reflect a shift towards a dimensional rather than a disorder-specific framework and are more efficient for clients and clinicians (Bullis et al., 2015; Clark, 2009; García-Escalera, Chorot, Valiente, Reales, & Sandín, 2016). A rationale for developing a transdiagnostic perspective that is unified is that similar propensities seem to render patients vulnerable to developing a broad range of disorders including anxiety, depression, stress, panic, and obsessions (Kennedy & Barlow, 2018). Mental disorders are more similar than different, and a common feature is the negative response to intense affective experiences (Kennedy and Barlow, 2018). Anxiety and mood disorders share common elements such as emotional regulation, e.g., Barlow, Farchione et al.'s (2011, 2018) unified protocol (UP). The UP demonstrates the way in which anxiety and depression can be combined into a common overarching concept – negative affect disorder.

What is the nature of transdiagnostic treatments? The transdiagnostic unified protocol (UP), published as a workbook for clients and a guide for therapists, can assist clients with a shared temperament of neuroticism to cope more adaptively with their negative affective states (Barlow, Ellard et al., 2011; Barlow, Farchione et al., 2011, 2018; Kennedy & Barlow, 2018). The UP consists of various modules, e.g., motivation, psychoeducation, in vivo exposure, mindfulness, and others, that teach affect regulation skills (Cassiello-Robins, Murray-Latin, & Sauer-Zavala, 2018; Ellard et al., 2010). When the UP was compared with single-disorder protocols (SDPs) for generalized anxiety disorder (GAD), it was found that the UP was as effective a treatment as the SDPs; however, the dropout rate for UP was lower than for the SDPs (Barlow et al., 2017; Kennedy and Barlow, 2018). Employing the UP, Boettcher and Conklin (2018) developed a functional treatment model for the transdiagnostic assessment of emotional disorders with an emphasis on patients' neurotic traits that comprise the etiology of these disorders, a model that highlights how patients' connections with their emotions have an effect upon their problems. In an effort to decrease obstacles to engaging in empirically based interventions, researchers have recently broadened the UP's range to include a web-based intervention program (Cassiello-Robins et al. 2018).

Both the UP and EFT posit aspects that are common in depression and anxiety, e.g., perceived threat, and emphasize graded exposure whereby patients can perceive threat by feeling and processing it in varied ways (Johnson, 2019). Whereas the UP with its cognitive-behavioral emphasis is not suited to the theory of attachment as it emphasizes that the common element in the development of anxiety and depression is neuroticism and temperament (Barlow, Farchione et al. (2011), there are those who suggest that the theory of attachment offers a model that is more explanatory (Johnson, 2019).

Unified Psychodynamic Psychotherapy (UPP-ANXIETY)

Leichsenring and Salzer (2014) compared Barlow et al.'s (2004) unified treatment model for emotional disorders to their own unified psychodynamic psychotherapy (UPP-ANXIETY) and noted that Barlow et al.'s (2004) model covered a broader range of disorders (depressive and anxiety) than the UPP-ANXIETY (anxiety disorders). Barlow et al.'s (2004) unified model as well as other unified CBT treatment protocols (e.g., Erickson, Janeck, & Tallman, 2007; McEvoy & Nathan, 2007; Schmidt et al., 2012) share common aspects with UPP-ANXIETY (Leichsenring and Salzer, 2014). These common treatment principles include how to begin and end psychotherapy, important for both proponents of CBT as well as psychodynamic treatment (PDT) (Leichsenring and Salzer, 2014). A primary difference between Barlow et al.'s (2004) unified model and the UPP-ANXIETY of Leichsenring and Salzer, 2014 is that UPP-ANXIETY does not include the use of exposure in the way that it is applied by the unified CBT treatment models (Leichsenring and Salzer, 2014).

Recently, Leichsenring and Steinert (2018) recommended integrating the principles for anxiety and depression into one unified psychodynamic treatment protocol (UPP-EMO) that is comprised of seven modules, and they point out similarities and differences between their model and Barlow et al.'s (2004) unified treatment for emotional disorders. The following vignette focuses on Leichsenring and Steinert's (2018) Module 6 of the unified psychodynamic protocol for "emotional disorders" (UPP-EMO), a vignette that includes the notion of defining and working on the core conflict.

Vignette

Therapist: Can you tell me what happens when you try to sleep?
Patient: Before bed, I check my phone, then read a little.
Therapist: What seems to be your concern?
Patient: I start to worry about details. Like, um … , what if I get sick for my presentation tomorrow. Then my mind wonders and I begin to worry about my daughter who is not doing that well with her friends. I finally fall asleep after about two hours, but then I get up early in the morning and start to worry again.
Therapist: It sounds like when you try to go to sleep, it's one worry after another.
Patient: Yeah. I worry a lot during the day too. I worry so much that it's getting me down. And now I'm having trouble functioning and getting through the day.
Therapist: It appears that you're getting anxious about being anxious, and it's beginning to paralyze you.

In this vignette, the therapist begins to facilitate the identification of the core conflict for a patient with mixed anxiety and depression. In the next portion of Module 6, the therapist may focus on the isolated emotion that the patient avoids, work through the patients' defenses that maintain the underlying conflict, and facilitate a more adaptive plan.

Summary

The results of psychotherapy treatments differ depending upon which anxiety disorder is targeted. Compared to other anxiety disorders, GAD is the least effectively treated of the anxiety disorders (Brown et al., 1994; Orsillo et al., 2003).

To manage anxiety means to encourage patients to accept the anxiety without employing defenses that involve avoidance or escape and without blowing the anxiety out of proportion (Muse et al., 2013). This section discussed integrated and unified psychotherapy treatment approaches for generalized anxiety disorder (GAD). An integrative approach underscores the need for therapists to include their patients in the process of integrating theories and treatments rather than to adhere to a prior preexisting intervention plan (Oddli and McLeod, 2017). Empathy, an essential integrative ingredient of therapy, characterizes different therapeutic approaches, and encourages psychotherapists joining with their clients at the outset (Bohart & Greenberg, 1997; Wolfe, 2013). There is a need for integrated approaches that target patients' interpersonal and emotional needs, and the rationale for an integrated focus on the interpersonal and emotional is discussed. Therapists need to target the interpersonal and emotional aspects of GAD as well as clients' difficulties tolerating events that are not guaranteed, and change has been found to be dependent upon the goodness of fit of the therapeutic alliance between therapist and client (Constantino, Castonguay, and Schut, 2001; Dugas et al., 2010; Newman & Llera, 2011).

How to Implement Integral Psychotherapy in Clinical Practice for Generalized Anxiety Disorder (GAD)

An integral or unified psychotherapy model, with its focus on deepening affect, can assist patients to experience anxiety within the safe setting of a therapeutic relationship (Ingersoll & Marquis, 2014). Chapter 3 described the metatheoretical quadratic framework of the integral or unifying model of Marquis (2018). The following case study relies on this approach to treat a patient with generalized anxiety disorder (GAD).

The therapist, for this case study, treated a patient with generalized anxiety disorder by employing Marquis' (2018) Integral, four quadrant psychotherapy approach (Upper Right quadrant, Upper Left quadrant, Lower Right quadrant, and Lower Left quadrant). According to Marquis (2018), The Upper Left (UL) quadrant represents the experiential, intrapsychic portion of the individual, the Upper Right (UR) quadrant corresponds to the behavioral, external dimension of the individual, the Lower Left (LL) quadrant represents the cultural, internal portion of the interpersonal, intersubjective, or collective, and the Lower Right (LR) quadrant corresponds to the social system, which involves the external dimension of the collective. In this case study, rather than maintaining a linear quadratic approach, the therapist shifted dynamically and fluidly among quadrants to suit the patient's developmental and minute-to-minute needs.

Ricardo, a 36-year-old Hispanic graduate student in the art department at a major university, sought therapy for his feelings of chronic worry about his ability to support his wife and his daughter's physical disabilities and her recent outbursts of anger. Ricardo was referred by the chair of his department after Ricardo's art professors informed the chair that they had noticed that Ricardo seemed to be without sleep and more nervous than usual. Although he has experienced symptoms of anxiety on a daily basis for over four years, only recently has Ricardo suffered sleepless nights. Generally, he feels overwhelmed by his attempts to keep up with paying the bills, work at school, and his part-time job as a waiter at a fine-dining restaurant in the city. More than once during the past few weeks, Ricardo has called friends late into the night to express his worries, and, more recently, woke his wife in the middle of the night to express his endless fears and worries about his upcoming exams, his concern, despite doing well in his program, that he would lose his scholarship and be compelled to drop out of his program, his fears that the restaurant supervisor would fire him, or that he would become ill and not be able to work. His wife and his friends dismissed his fears as silly and unwarranted. Initially, Ricardo refused to contact a therapist and preferred to talk to his friends about his difficulties even though they minimized his troubles, but his wife and a friend from his high school years recently persuaded Ricardo to seek assistance from the university's counseling center for his uncontrollable worrying and his tendency to wake his wife almost every night to discuss his problems.

The clinical psychologist at the university found that although Ricardo expressed concern about his fears, about his constant worry and nerves that once he started to worry he had difficulty stopping, about his stress at home when his wife complained daily about his small paycheck, about his stress at school related to keeping up with his graduate studies, and his somatic symptoms such as headaches, nausea, frequent muscle tension, palpitations, and sleepless nights, he did not speak much about having anxiety.

Ricardo reported that his father died when he was a young boy, his mother had a difficult time supporting Ricardo, and his siblings, Diego, and Julia, and his mother frequently asked him when he came home from school to accept part-time jobs to help to support the family. Ricardo reported that he was often ashamed that he did not have a father to accompany him to sports events. Ricardo reported that more recently he felt as if he could not get enough breath in, and his worries seemed to be increasing to the point that he had difficulty concentrating on his art work and presentations.

The therapist used a unified psychotherapy approach (Marquis, 2018) to treat Ricardo's generalized anxiety disorder. Generalized anxiety warrants treatment that addresses more than one or two quadrants.

Upper Right (UR) quadrant: Intervening from the Upper Right (UR) means targeting the physiological, behavioral, and genetic. For Ricardo's behavioral symptoms of anxiety, the clinical psychologist used imagery exposure (Zinbarg, Craske, & Barlow, 2006). More specifically, imaginal exposure, e.g., worry exposure (Hoyer et al., 2009), along with applied relaxation techniques, muscle relaxation, and breathing exercises, were used to target Ricardo's symptoms of anxiety. Along with the aforementioned behavioral interventions, the clinical psychologist encouraged Ricardo to engage in an aerobic exercise program offered at his local gym. Ricardo requested medication for his anxiety, and the therapist referred him to a psychiatrist who prescribed Xanax (alprazolam) for his anxiety and insomnia. With respect to the genetic component of the Upper Right, Ricardo has a family history of anxiety, and his brother, Diego, was recently hospitalized for posttraumatic stress disorder after multiple deployments in Afghanistan. Ricardo related that his mother tends to worry about everything and has a difficulty time sleeping. Although his mother did not seek help for her anxiety, it seems likely that she suffered from symptoms of anxiety for a major portion of her life. It seems that Ricardo may have inherited his tendency towards anxiety from his mother. Recently, Ricardo's sister, Julia, was diagnosed with panic disorder.

Upper Left (UL) quadrant: Whereas psychotherapy treatments that correspond to the Upper Right (UR) quadrant of an integral model include behavioral and pharmacological as well as exercise, psychotherapy interventions that correspond to the Upper Left (UL) can include a psychodynamic view of a patient from an intrapsychic perspective (Ingersoll & Marquis, 2014; Marquis, 2018). By intervening with brief psychodynamic therapy from the Upper Left (UL), the therapist was able to help Ricardo address the intrapsychic aspects of his condition. In order to protect himself from becoming overwhelmed by painful affect when his feelings are not recognized, Ricardo tends to worry and display symptoms of anxiety. Within the UL quadrant, the therapist was able to help Ricardo explore the underpinnings of his anxiety, e.g., his unconscious and conflictual feelings and the worry defense that he employs in order to protect himself from further pain. To help Ricardo understand how his dysfunction derives from maladaptive emotional schemes related to shame and his difficulty in regulating affect, the therapist used an integrated experiential/ humanistic emotion-focused therapy. The ability to internalize compassion for the self and to maintain a position of self-soothing are key components promoted by an emotion-focused treatment (Watson & Greenberg, 2017). The emotion-focused therapy facilitated Ricardo's ability to understand how his early feelings of pain had been dismissed and how attuning to his emotions and needs by using worry chair conversations help him to process his emotions, elevate his self-esteem, build a stronger self-concept, and transform the worry defense and shame to self-compassion and comfort.

Lower Left (LL) quadrant: Emotion-focused therapy for generalized anxiety disorder includes the formation of a strong therapeutic alliance (Greenberg et al., 1993). By intervening from the Lower Left (LL), the therapist addressed interpersonal elements rather than the intrapsychic aspects of the Upper Left (UL) quadrant. From the start, the therapist worked on building a strong therapeutic relationship with Ricardo that underscored authenticity and attunement. A relational healing alliance that is accompanied by acceptance, empathy, attunement, and warmth has been demonstrated to help patients with anxiety (Levy Berg, Sandell, & Sandahl, 2009; Timulak & McElvaney, 2018). In line with attachment research (Fosha, 2000), it has been established that anxiety can impede a patient's development, particularly when a caregiver is not available. The therapist was careful to create a safe environment and was emotionally available for Ricardo. Within the LL quadrant, work was focused on the interpersonal rather than on the intrapsychic, with an emphasis on helping Ricardo model and extend the therapeutic dyad by building quality relationships with friends and members of his own family. Ricardo has a sister, Julia, who seems to be sympathetic to his tensions and conflicts, and Ricardo began meeting her once a month for lunch. The therapist emphasized the building of positive social relationships at school, and encouraged Ricardo to seek assistance with his projects by reaching out to colleagues in the art department.

Lower Right (LR) quadrant: Treatments that correspond to the Lower Right (LR) quadrant include assisting patients to connect with support services, e.g., financial aid (Ingersoll & Marquis, 2014). Working from the context of the Lower Right (LR) quadrant, the therapist referred Ricardo, his wife, and his daughter to a family therapist. By intervening from the LR with

Table 5.1 Generalized Anxiety Disorder (GAD)

Etiology	*Integrated*	*Unified*
Psychodynamic Themes Excessive worrying as a defense mechanism that serves to ward off a deeper threat such as trauma (Borkovec, 1994; Leichsenring & Salzer, 2014). Developmental Theory of Attachment (Crits-Christoph, Connolly, Azarian, Crits-Christoph, & Shappell, 1996; Lichtenstein & Cassidy, 1991)	Integration of CBT and Interpersonal therapy (Newman, Castonguay, Borkovec, & Molnar, 2004) CBT and Interpersonal and Emotional Processing Therapy (IEP) (Newman, Castonguay, Borkovec, Fisher, & Nordberg, 2008) CBT Integrated with Motivational Interviewing (MI) (Gómez Penedo, Constantino, Coyne, Westra, & Antony, 2017; Miller and Rollnick, 1991, 2002; Gómez Penedo, Constantino, Coyne, Westra, & Antony, 2016; Westra & Dozois, 2006) Metacognitive Therapy (MCT) (Haseth et al., 2019; Wells, 1995;) Mindfulness CBT (Segal, Williams, & Teasdale 2002)	A Unified Psychodynamic Psychotherapy for Anxiety (UPP-ANXIETY) Leichsenring and Salzer (2014) A transdiagnostic unified psychotherapy treatment for the anxiety disorders
Cognitive (Foa & Kozak, 1986) Metacognitive (Haseth et al., 2019; Wells, 1995) Emotion-Focused themes or emotion schemes (Watson, Timulak, & Greenberg, 2019)	Integration of Neuroscience and Psychotherapy (Kinley & Reyno, 2016)	A Cognitive-Behavioral Unified Protocol (UP) Barlow et al. (2004, 2017, 2018) and Barlow, Farchione et al. (2011)
Self-Wounds (Wolfe, 2003, 2005) Death Anxiety (Wolfe, 2008)	Integrating Psychodynamic, Humanistic, Interpersonal and CBT (Castonguay, Eubanks, Goldfried, Muran, & Lutz, 2015; Newman, Castonguay, Fisher, & Borkovec, 2008)	Leichsenring and Salzer (2014) noted that Barlow et al.'s (2004) model covered a broader range of disorders (depressive and anxiety) than the UPP- ANXIETY (anxiety disorders).
Neuroscience Although research implicates the amygdala, the prefrontal cortex, and anterior cingulate cortex in the development of generalized anxiety disorder (e.g., Lang, McTeague, & Bradley, 2014; McClure al., 2007; Schienle, Hettema, Cáceda, & Nemeroff, 2011), a different circuit is involved in the development of panic disorder (Comer, 2015).	Emotion-focused Therapy (EFT) Greenberg (2011) Johnson (1996, 2019) Timulak & McElvaney (2016) Watson & Greenberg (2017) Watson, Timulak, & Greenberg (2019)	Leichsenring and Steinert (2018) recommended integrating the principles for anxiety and depression into one unified psychodynamic treatment protocol (UPP-EMO) that is comprised of seven modules, and they point out similarities and differences between their model and Barlow et al.'s (2004) unified treatment for emotional disorders.

its focus on the systemic, the therapist referred Ricardo to a counselor who helped him procure a small grant for an art history project. Ricardo's therapist suggested several free social-service and after-school programs that were available for his daughter.

Summary

Symptoms of generalized anxiety disorder (GAD) tend to increase during stressful periods, and patients with GAD tend to report that their symptoms of anxiety, worry, and nervousness have been present throughout most of their lives, suggesting the effect of early-life influences in the etiology of GAD (Watson & Greenberg, 2017). Unlike the phobias, GAD does not have a distinct precipitant (Watson & Greenberg, 2017).

This chapter described the etiology of GAD, its development and maintenance, and discussed integrated and unified etiology approaches and psychotherapy treatment models for GAD (see Table 5.1). Towards the end of the chapter, a brief case study was presented to demonstrate how a therapist employed the unified psychotherapy approach of Marquis (2018), an integral, four quadrant psychotherapy approach, to treat a patient with GAD.

References

Aaronson, C. J., Katzman, G., & Moster, R. L. (2015). Combination pharmacotherapy and psychotherapy for the treatment of major depressive and anxiety disorders. In P. E. Nathan & J. M. Gorman (Eds.), *A guide to treatments that work* (4th ed., pp. 507–543). New York, NY: Oxord University Press.

Albani, C., Blaser, G., Geyer, M., Schmutzer, G., & Brähler, E. (2010). Outpatient psychotherapy in Germany from the patient perspective: Part 1: Health care situation. *Psychotherapeut*, *55*(6), 503–514.

Alladin, A. (2014). The wounded self: New approach to understanding and treating anxiety disorders. *American Journal of Clinical Hypnosis*, *56*(4), 368–388. doi: 10.1080/00029157.2014.880045

American Psychiatric Association. (2013). *Diagnostic and statistical manual of mental disorders* (5th ed.). Washington, DC: Author.

Anderson, I. M., & Palm, M. E. (2006). Pharmacological treatments for worry: Focus on generalized anxiety disorder. In G. C. L. Davey & A. Wells (Eds.), *Worry and its psychological disorders: Theory, assessment and treatment* (pp. 305–334). West Sussex, England: John Wiley & Sons.

Anderson, J. C., Noyes, R., & Crowe, R. R. (1984). A comparison of PD and generalized anxiety disorder. *American Journal of Psychiatry*, *141*(4), 572–575. doi: 10.1176/ajp.141.4.572

Andlin-Sobocki, P., & Wittchen, H.-U. (2005). Cost of anxiety disorders in Europe. *European Journal of Neurology*, *12* (Suppl. 1), 39–44. doi: 10.1111/ j.1468-1331.2005.01195.x

Angst, J., Paksarian, D., Cui, L., Merikangas, K. R., Hengartner, M. P., Ajdacic-Gross, V., … Rössler, W. (2016). The epidemiology of common mental disorders from age 20 to 50: Results from the prospective Zurich cohort study. *Epidemiology of Psychiatric Sciences*, *25*(1), 24–32. doi: 10.1017/S204579601500027X

Arkowitz, H. (2002). Toward an integrative perspective on resistance to change in psychotherapy. *Journal of Clinical Psychology, 58*(2), 219–227. doi: 10.1002/jclp.1145

Arkowitz, H., & Westra, H. A. (2004). Integrating motivational interviewing and cognitive behavioral therapy in the treatment of depression and anxiety. *Journal of Cognitive Psychotherapy, 18*(4), 337–350.

Ayers, C. R., Sorrell, J. T., Thorp, S. R., & Wetherell, J. L. (2007). Evidence-based psychological treatments for late-life anxiety. *Psychology and Aging, 22*(1), 8–17. doi: 10.1037/0882-7974.22.1.8

Baker, H. (2001). Hypnosis for anxiety reduction and ego-enhancement. *Australian Journal of Clinical and Experimental Hypnosis, 29*(2), 147–151.

Barekati, S., Bahmani, B., Naghiyaaee, M., Afrasiabi, M., & Marsa, R. (2017). The effectiveness of cognitive-existential group therapy on reducing existential anxiety in the elderly. *World Family Medicine, 15*(8), 75–83. doi: 10.5742/MEWFM.2017.93059

Barlow, D. H. (2004). *Anxiety and its disorders: The nature and treatment of anxiety and panic* (2nd ed.). New York, NY: Guilford Press.

Barlow, D. H., Allen, L. B., & Choate, M. L. (2004). Toward a unified treatment for emotional disorders. *Behavior Therapy, 35*(2), 205–230. doi: 10.1016/S0005-7894(04)80036-4

Barlow, D. H., Ellard, K. K., Fairholme, C. P., Farchione, T. J., Boisseau, C. L., Allen, L. B., & Ehrenreich-May, J. T. (2011). *Unified protocol for transdiagnostic treatment of emotional disorders: Client workbook.* New York, NY: Oxford University Press.

Barlow, D. H., Farchione, T. J., Bullis, J. R., Gallagher, M. W., Murray-Latin, H., Sauer-Zavala, S., … Cassiello-Robbins, C. (2017). The unified protocol for transdiagnostic treatment of emotional disorders compared with diagnosis-specific protocols for anxiety disorders: A randomized clinical trial. *JAMA Psychiatry, 74*(9), 875–884. doi: 10.1001/jamapsychiatry.2017.2164

Barlow, D. H., Farchione, T. J., Fairholme, C. P., Ellard, K. K., Boisseau, C. L., Allen, L. B., & Ehrenreich-May, J. T. (2011). *Unified protocol for transdiagnostic treatment of emotional disorders: Therapist guide.* New York, NY: Oxford University Press.

Barlow, D. H., Farchione, T. J., Sauer-Zavala, S., Murray-Latin, H., Ellard, K. K., Bullis, J. R., … Cassiello-Robbins, C. (2018). *Unified protocol for transdiagnostic treatment of emotional disorders: Therapist guide* (2nd ed.). New York, NY: Oxford University Press.

Bassett, J. F. (2007). Psychological defenses against death anxiety: Integrating terror management theory and Firestone's separation theory. *Death Studies, 31*(8), 727–750. doi: 10.1080/07481180701490628

Beekman, A. T., Bremmer, M. A., Deeg, D. J., van Balkom, A. J., Smit, J. H., de Beurs, E., … van Tilburg, W. (1998). Anxiety disorders in later life: A report from the Longitudinal Aging Study Amsterdam. International Journal of Geriatric Psychiatry, 13(10), 717–726. doi: 10.1002/(SICI)1099-1166(1998100)13:10<717::AID-GPS857>3.0.CO;2

Behar, E., DiMarco, I. D., Hekler, E. B., Mohlman, J., & Staples, A. M. (2009). Current theoretical models of generalized anxiety disorder (GAD): Conceptual review and treatment implications. *Journal of Anxiety Disorders, 23*(8), 1011–1023. doi: 10.1016/j.janxdis.2009.07.006

Boettcher, H., & Conklin, L. R. (2018). Transdiagnostic assessment and case formulation: Rationale and application with the unified protocol. In D. H. Barlow & T. J. Farchione (Eds.), *Applications of the unified protocol for transdiagnostic treatment of emotional disorders* (pp. 17–37). New York, NY: Oxford University Press.

Bohart, A. C., & Greenberg, L. S. (1997). *Empathy reconsidered: New directions in psychotherapy.* Washington, DC: American Psychological Association. doi: 10.1037/10226-000

Bolognesi, F., Baldwin, D. S., & Ruini, C. (2014). Psychological interventions in the treatment of generalized anxiety disorder: A structured review. *Journal of Psychopathology, 20*, 111–126.

Borkovec, T. D. (1994). The nature, function and origin of worry. In G. C. L. Davey & F. Tallis (Eds.), *Worrying: Perspectives on theory, assessment and treatment.* New York, NY: Wiley.

Borkovec, T. D., Abel, J. L., & Newman, H. (1995). Effects of psychotherapy on comorbid conditions in generalized anxiety disorder. *Journal of Consulting and Clinical Psychology, 63*(3), 479–483. doi: 10.1037/0022-006X.63.3.479

Borkovec, T. D., Alcaine, O., & Behar, E. (2004). Avoidance theory of worry and generalized anxiety disorder. In R. G. Heimberg, C. L. Turk & D. S. Mennin (Eds.), *Generalized anxiety disorder: Advances in research and practice* (pp. 77–108). New York, NY: Guilford Press.

Borkovec, T. D., & Costello, E. (1993). Efficacy of applied relaxation and cognitive-behavioral therapy in the treatment of generalized anxiety disorder. *Journal of Consulting and Clinical Psychology, 61*(4), 611–619.

Borkovec, T. D., Newman, M. G., Pincus, A. L., & Lytle, R. (2002). A component analysis of cognitive-behavioral therapy for generalized anxiety disorder and the role of interpersonal problems. *Journal of Consulting and Clinical Psychology, 70*(2), 288–298. doi: 10.1037/0022-006x.70.2.288

Borkovec, T. D., & Ruscio, A. M. (2001). Psychotherapy for generalized anxiety disorder. *The Journal of Clinical Psychiatry, 62* (Suppl. 11), 37–42.

Bowlby, J. (1980). *Attachment and loss: Vol. 3. Loss.* New York, NY: Basic Books.

Brown, D. P., & Fromm, E. (1990). Enhancing affective experience and its expression. In D. C. Bryant, C., Jackson, H., & Ames, D. (2008). The prevalence of anxiety in older adults: Methodological issues and a review of the literature. *Journal of Affective Disorders, 109*(3), 233–250. doi: 10.1016/j.jad.2007.11.008

Brown, T. A., Barlow, D. H., & Liebowitz, M. R. (1994). The empirical basis of generalized anxiety disorder. *The American Journal of Psychiatry, 151*(9), 1272–1280. doi: 10.1176/ajp.151.9.1272

Bullis, J. R., Sauer-Zavala, S., Bentley, K. H., Thompson- Hollands, J., Carl, J. R., & Barlow, D. H. (2015). The unified protocol for transdiagnostic treatment of emotional disorders: Preliminary exploration of effectiveness for group delivery. *Behavior Modification, 39*(2), 295–321..

Carter, R. M., Wittchen, H. U., Pfister, H., & Kessler, R. C. (2001). One-year prevalence of subthreshold and threshold DSM-IV generalized anxiety disorder in a nationally representative sample. *Depression and Anxiety, 13*(2), 78–88. doi: 10.1002/da.1020

Cassiello-Robins, C., Murray-Latin, H., & Sauer-Zavala, S. (2018). The unified protocol. In D. H. Barlow & T. J. Farchione (Eds.), *Applications of the unified protocol for transdiagnostic treatment of emotional disorders* (pp. 291–301). New York, NY: Oxford University Press.

Castonguay, L. G., Eubanks, C. F., Goldfried, M. R., Muran, J. C., & Lutz, W. (2015). Research on psychotherapy integration: Building on the past, looking to the future. *Psychotherapy Research, 25*(3), 365–382. doi: 10.1080/10503307.2015.1014010

Clark, D. A. (2009). Cognitive behavioral therapy for anxiety and depression: Possibilities and limitations of a transdiagnostic perspective. *Cognitive Behaviour Therapy, 38* (Suppl. 1), 29–34. doi: 10.1080/16506070902980745

Comaty, J. E., & Advokat, C. (2013). Generalized anxiety disorder. In S. M. Stahl & B. A. Moore (Eds.), *Anxiety disorders: A guide for integrating psychopharmacology and psychotherapy* (pp. 97–132). New York, NY: Routledge.

Comer, R. J. (2015). *Abnormal psychology*. New York, NY: Worth Publisher.

Constantino, M. J., Bernecker, S. L., Boswell, J. F., & Castonguay, L. G. (2013). Context-responsive psychotherapy integration as a framework for a unified clinical science: Conceptual and empirical considerations. *Journal of Unified Psychotherapy and Clinical Science, 2*(1), 1–20.

Constantino, M. J., Castonguay, L. G., & Schut, A. J. (2001). The working alliance: A flagship for the scientific-practitioner model in psychotherapy. In G. Shick Tryon (Ed.), *Counseling based on process research* (pp. 81–131). New York, NY: Allyn & Bacon.

Constantino, M. J., & Westra, H. A. (2012). An expectancy-based approach to facilitating corrective experiences in psychotherapy. In L. G. Castonguay & C. E. Hill (Eds.), *Transformation in psychotherapy: Corrective experiences across cognitive, behavioral, humanistic, and psychodynamic approaches* (pp. 121–139). Washington, DC: American Psychological Association. doi: 10.1037/13747-008

Constantino, M. J., Westra, H. A., Antony, M. M., & Coyne, A. E. (2016, June). Integrative motivational interviewing and cognitive-behavioral therapy for generalized anxiety disorder: Secondary outcomes of a randomized controlled trial. Paper presented at the Society for the Exploration of Psychotherapy Integration Society annual meeting, Dublin, Ireland.

Covin, R., Ouimet, A. J., Seeds, P. M., & Dozois, D. J. A. (2008). A meta-analysis of CBT for pathological worry among clients with GAD. *Journal of Anxiety Disorders, 22*(1), 108–116. doi: 10.1016/j.janxdis.2007.01.002

Craske, M. G., & Waters, A. M. (2005). Panic disorder, phobias, and generalized anxiety disorder. *Annual Review of Clinical Psychology, 1*, 197–225. doi: 10.1146/annurev.clinpsy.1.102803.143857

Creswell, J. D. (2017). Mindfulness interventions. *Annual Review of Psychology, 68*, 491–516. doi: 10.1146/annurev-psych-042716-051139

Crits-Christoph, P., Connolly, M. B., Azarian, K., Crits-Christoph, K., & Shappell, S. (1996). An open trial of brief supportive-expressive psychotherapy in the treatment of generalized anxiety disorder. *Psychotherapy: Theory, Research, Practice, Training, 33*(3), 418–430. doi: 10.1037/0033-3204.33.3.418

Cuijpers, P., Sijbrandij, M., Koole, S., Huibers, M., Berking, M., & Andersson, G. (2014). Psychological treatment of generalized anxiety disorder: A meta-analysis. *Clinical Psychology Review, 34*(2), 130–140. doi: 10.1016/j.cpr.2014.01.002

Dugas, M. J., Brillon, P., Savard, P., Turcotte, J., Gaudet, A., Ladouceur, R., ... & Gervais, N. J. (2010). A randomized clinical trial of cognitive-behavioral therapy and applied relaxation for adults with generalized anxiety disorder. *Behavior Therapy, 41*(1), 46–58. doi: 10.1016/j.beth.2008.12.004

Dugas, M. J., & Robichaud, M. (2007). *Cognitive- behavioral treatment for generalized anxiety disorder: From science to practice*. New York, NY: Routledge.

Ellard, K. K., Fairholme, C. P., Boisseau, C. L., Farchione, T. J., & Barlow, D. H. (2010). Unified protocol for the transdiagnostic treatment of emotional disorders: Protocol development and initial outcome data. *Cognitive and Behavioral Practice, 17*(1), 88–101. doi: 10.1016/j.cbpra.2009.06.002

Elliott, R., Watson, J., Goldman, R. N., & Greenberg, L. S. (2004). *Learning emotion-focused therapy: The process-experiential approach to change*. Washington, DC: American Psychological Association.

Erickson, D. H., Janeck, A., & Tallman, K. (2007). A cognitive-behavioral group for patients with various anxiety disorders. *Psychiatric Services, 58*(9), 1205–1211. doi: 10.1176/ps.2007.58.9.1205

Ferrero, A., Pierò, A., Fassina, S., Massola, T., Lanteri, A., Daga, G. A., & Fassino, S. (2007). A 12-month comparison of brief psychodynamic psychotherapy and pharmacotherapy treatment in subjects with generalized anxiety disorders in a community setting. *European Psychiatry, 22*(8), 530–539. doi: 10.1016/j.eurpsy.2007.07.004

Firestone, R. W. (1984). A concept of the primary fantasy bond: A developmental perspective. *Psychotherapy, 21*(2), 218–225. doi: 10.1037/h0085976

Firestone, R. W. (1994). Psychological defenses against death. In R. A. Neimeyer (Ed.), *Death anxiety handbook* (pp. 217–241). Washington, DC: Taylor Francis.

Foa, E. B., & Kozak, M. J. (1986). Treatment of anxiety disorders: Implications for psychopathology. In A. H. Tuma & J. D. Maser (Eds.), *Anxiety and the anxiety disorders* (pp. 421–452). Hillsdale, NJ: Erlbaum.

Fosha, D. (2000). *The transforming power of affect: A model for accelerated change.* New York, NY: Basic Books.

Fredette, C., El-Baalbaki, G., Neron, S., & Palardy, V. (2013). Using hypnosis in the treatment of anxiety disorders: Pros and cons. In F. Durbano (Ed.), *New insights into anxiety disorders* (pp. 343–377). InTech. doi: 10.5772/53768

Freud, S. (1894). On the grounds for detaching a particular syndrome from neurasthenia under the description anxiety neurosis. In J. Strachey (Ed.), *The standard ed. of the complete psychological works of Sigmund Freud* (Vol. 3, pp. 85–117). London, UK: Hogarth Press.

Freud, S. (1917). *A general introduction to psychoanalysis* (J. Riviere, Trans.). New York, NY: Liveright (Work republished in 1963).

Freud, S. (1933). *New introductory lectures on psychoanalysis.* New York, NY: Norton.

García-Escalera, J., Chorot, P., Valiente, R. M., Reales, J. M., & Sandín, B. (2016). Efficacy of transdiagnostic cognitive-behavioral therapy for anxiety and depression in adults, children and adolescents: A meta-analysis. *Revista de Psicopatología y Psicología Clínica, 21*(3), 147. doi: 10.5944/rppc.vol.21.num.3.2016.17811

Gilbert, M., & Orlans, V. (2011). *Integrative therapy, 100 key points and techniques.* London, England: Routledge.

Glock, G., Hilsenroth, M., & Curtis, R. (2018). Therapeutic interventions patients with anxiety problems find most helpful: A case for integration? *Journal of Psychotherapy Integration, 28*(2), 233–241. doi: 10.1037/int0000075

Gold, J., & Stricker, G. (2012). Psychotherapy integration and integrative psychotherapies. In G. Stricker & T. Widiger (Eds.), *Handbook of psychology*, (Vol. 8, pp. 345–366). New York, NY: Wiley.

Gold, J. R. (1993). An integrated approach to the treatment of anxiety disorders and phobias. In G. Stricker & J. R. Gold (Eds.), *Comprehensive handbook of psychotherapy integration* (pp. 293–301). New York, NY: Plenum Press.

Goldfried, M. R. (1971). Systematic desensitization as training in self-control. *Journal of Consulting and Clinical Psychology, 37*(2), 228–234. doi: 10.1037/h0031974

Goldman, R. N. (2019). History and overview of emotion-focused therapy. In L. S. Greenberg & R. N. Goldman (Eds.), *Clinical handbook of emotion-focused therapy* (pp. 3–35). Washington, DC: American Psychological Association.

Gómez Penedo, J. M., Constantino, M. J., Coyne, A. E., Westra, H. A., & Antony, M. M. (2017). Markers for context-responsiveness: Client baseline interpersonal problems moderate the efficacy of two psychotherapies for generalized anxiety disorder. *Journal of Consulting and Clinical Psychology, 85*(10), 1000–1011. doi: 10.1037/ccp0000233

Gorman, J. M. (2016). Combining psychodynamic psychotherapy and pharmacotherapy. *Psychodynamic Psychiatry, 44*(2), 183–209. doi: 10.1521/pdps.2016.44.2.183

Greenberg, J., Pyszczynski, T., & Solomon, S. (1986). The causes and consequences of a need for self-esteem: A terror management theory. In R. F. Baumeister (Ed.), *Public self and private self* (pp. 189–212). New York, NY: Springer-Verlag.

Greenberg, L. (2006). Emotion-focused therapy: A synopsis. *Journal of Contemporary Psychotherapy, 36*(2), 87–93. doi: 10.1007/s10879-006-9011-3

Greenberg, L., & Johnson, S. M. (1988). *Emotionally focused therapy for couples*. New York, NY: Guilford Press.

Greenberg, L. S. (2011). *Emotion-focused therapy*. Washington, DC: American Psychological Association.

Greenberg, L. S., Rice, L. N., & Elliott, R. (1993). *Facilitating emotional change: The moment-by-moment process*. New York, NY: Guilford Press.

Greenberg, L. S., & Watson, J. C. (2006). *Emotion-focused therapy for depression*. Washington, DC: American Psychological Association.

Guidano, V. (1987). *The development of the self*. New York, NY: Guilford Press.

Hanrahan, F., Field, A. P., Jones, F. W., & Davey, G. C. L. (2013). A meta-analysis of cognitive therapy for worry in generalized anxiety disorder. *Clinical Psychology Review, 33*(1), 120–132. doi: 10.1016/j.cpr.2012.10.008

Haseth, S., Solem, S., Sørø, G. B., Bjørnstad, E., Grøtte, T., & Fisher, P. (2019). Group metacognitive therapy for generalized anxiety disorder: A pilot feasibility trial. *Frontiers in Psychology, 10*, 290. doi: 10.3389/fpsyg.2019.00290

Hayes, S. C. (2004). Acceptance and commitment therapy, relational frame therapy, and the third wave of behavioral and cognitive therapies. *Behavior Therapy, 35*, 639–665. doi: 10.1016/j.beth.2016.11.006

Hayes, S. C., Strosahl, K., & Wilson, K. G. (1999). *Acceptance and commitment therapy: An experiential approach to behavior change*. New York, NY: The Guilford Press.

Hayes, S. C., Strosahl, K. D., & Wilson, K. G. (2011). *Acceptance and commitment therapy: The process and practice of mindful change* (2nd ed.). New York, NY: Guilford Press.

Henry, W. P., & Strupp, H. H. (1994). The therapeutic alliance as interpersonal process. In A. O. Horvath & L. S. Greenberg (Eds.), *The working alliance: Theory, research, and practice* (pp. 51–84). New York, NY: Wiley.

Hoyer, J., Beesdo, K., Gloster, A. T., Runge, J., Höfler, M., & Becker, E. S. (2009). Worry exposure versus applied relaxation in the treatment of generalized anxiety disorder. *Psychotherapy and Psychosomatics, 78*(2), 106–115. doi: 10.1159/000201936

Ingersoll, R. E., & Marquis, A. (2014). *Understanding psychopathology: An integral exploration*. Upper Saddle River, NJ: Pearson Education.

Jenkins, R. L. (1968). The varieties of children's behavioral problems and family dynamics. *American Journal of Psychiatry, 124*(10), 1440–1445. doi: 10.1176/ajp.124.10.1440

Johnson, S. M. (1996). *The practice of emotionally focused therapy: Creating connection*. New York, NY: Brunner/Mazel.

Johnson, S. M. (2019). *Attachment theory in practice: Emotionally focused therapy (EFT) with individuals, couples, and families*. New York, NY: Guilford Press.

Jones-Smith, E. (2012). *Theories of counseling and psychotherapy: An integrative approach*. Thousand Oaks, CA: Sage.

Julien, R. M. (2013). Pharmacological treatment of anxiety disorders across the lifespan. In S. M. Stahl & B. A. Moore (Eds.), *Anxiety disorders: A guide for integrating psychopharmacology and psychotherapy* (pp. 51–70). New York, NY: Routledge.

Katzman, M. A., Copeland, A., Klassen, L. J., Chokka, P., & Brawman-Mintzer, O. (2011). Pharmacotherapy for generalized anxiety disorder. *Psychiatric Annals, 41*(2), 95–103. doi: 10.3928/00485713-20110203-08

Kendler, K. S., & Baker, J. H. (2007). Genetic influences on measures of the environment: A systematic review. *Psychological Medicine, 37*(5), 615–626. doi: 10.1017/S0033291706009524

Kennedy, K. A., & Barlow, D. (2018). The unified treatment for transdiagnostic treatment of emotional disorders: An introduction. In D. H. Barlow & T. J. Farchione (Eds.), *Applications of the unified protocol for transdiagnostic treatment of emotional disorders* (pp. 1–16). New York, NY: Oxford University Press.

Kessler, R. C., Berglund, P., Demler, O., Jin, R., Merikangas, K. R., & Walters, E. E. (2005). Lifetime prevalence and age-of-onset distributions of DSM-IV disorders in the National Comorbidity Survey Replication. *Archives of General Psychiatry, 62*(6), 593–602. doi: 10.1001/archpsyc.62.6.593.

Kessler, R. C., Petukhova, M., Sampson, N. A., Zaslavsky, A. M., & Wittchen, H. U. (2012). Twelve-month and lifetime prevalence and lifetime morbid risk of anxiety and mood disorders in the United States. *International Journal of Methods in Psychiatric Research, 21*(3), 169–184. doi: 10.1002/mpr.1359

King, P., & Barrowclough, C. (1991). A clinical pilot study of cognitive behavioural therapy for anxiety disorders in the elderly. *Behavioral and Cognitive Psychotherapy, 19*(4), 337–345. doi: 10.1017/S0141347300014038

Kinley, J. L., & Reyno, S. M. (2016). Project for a scientific psychiatry: A neurobiologically informed, phasic, brain-based model of integrated psychotherapy. *Journal of Psychotherapy Integration, 26*(1), 61–73. doi: 10.1037/a0039636

Kohut, H. (1971). *The analysis of the self.* New York, NY: International Universities Press.

Ladouceur, R., Dugas, M. J., Freeston, M. H., Léger, E., Gagnon, F., & Thibodeau, N. (2000). Efficacy of a cognitive–behavioral treatment for generalized anxiety disorder: Evaluation in a controlled clinical trial. *Journal of Consulting and Clinical Psychology, 68*(6), 957–964. doi: 10.1037/0022-006X.68.6.957

Lang, P. J., McTeague, L. M., & Bradley, M. M. (2014). Pathological anxiety and function/dysfunction in the brain's fear/defense circuitry. *Restorative Neurology and Neuroscience, 32*(1), 63–77. doi: 10.3233/RNN-139012

Lee, J. K., Orsillo, S. M., Roemer, L., & Allen, L. B. (2010). Distress and avoidance in generalized anxiety disorder: Exploring the relationships with intolerance of uncertainty and worry. *Cognitive Behavior Therapy, 39*(2), 126–136. doi: 10.1080/16506070902966918

Leichsenring, F., & Salzer, S. (2014). A unified protocol for the transdiagnostic psychodynamic treatment of anxiety disorders: An evidence-based approach. *Psychotherapy, 51*(2), 224–245. doi: 10.1037/a0033815

Leichsenring, F., & Steinert, C. (2018). Towards an evidence-based unified psychodynamic protocol for emotional disorders. *Journal of Affective Disorders, 232*, 400–416. doi: 10.1016/j.jad.2017.11.036

Levy Berg, A., Sandell, R., & Sandahl, C. (2009). Affect-focused body psychotherapy in patients with generalized anxiety disorder: Evaluation of an integrative method. *Journal of Psychotherapy Integration, 19*(1), 67–85. doi: 0.1037/a0015324

Lichtenstein, J., & Cassidy, J. (1991, April). *The inventory of adult attachment (INVAA): Validation of a new measure.* Paper presented at the Society for Research in Child Development. Seattle, WA.

Manfredi, C., Caselli, G., Rovetto, F., Rebecchi, D., Ruggiero, G. M., Sassaroli, S., & Spada, M. M. (2011). Temperament and parental styles as predictors of ruminative brooding and worry. *Personality and Individual Differences, 50*(2), 186–191. doi: 10.1016/j.paid.2010.09.023

Marquis, A. (2018). *Integral psychotherapy: A unifying approach.* New York, NY: Routledge.

May, R. (1979). *The meaning of anxiety*. New York, NY: Washington Square Press.

McClure, E. B., Monk, C. S., Nelson, E. E., Parrish, J. M., Adler, A., Blair, R. J., ... Pine, D. S. (2007). Abnormal attention modulation of fear circuit function in pediatric generalized anxiety disorder. *Archives of General Psychiatry, 64*(1), 97–106. doi: 10.1001/archpsyc.64.1.97

McEvoy, P. M., & Nathan, P. (2007). Effectiveness of cognitive behavior therapy for diagnostically heterogeneous groups: A benchmarking study. *Journal of Consulting and Clinical Psychology, 75*(2), 344–350. doi: 10.1037/0022-006X.75.2.344

Mennin, D. S., & Fresco, D. M. (2010). Emotion regulation as an integrative framework for understanding and treating psychopathology. In A. M. Kring & D. M. Sloan (Eds.), *Emotion regulation and psychopathology: A transdiagnostic approach to etiology and treatment* (pp. 356–379). New York, NY: Guilford Press.

Mennin, D. S., Heimberg, R. G., Turk, C. L., & Fresco, D. M. (2005). Preliminary evidence for an emotion dysregulation model of generalized anxiety disorder. *Behaviour Research and Therapy, 43*(10), 1281–1310. doi: 10.1016/j.brat.2004.08.008

Miller, W. R. (1983). Motivational interviewing with problem drinkers. *Behavioural Psychotherapy, 11*(2), 147–172. doi: 10.1017/S0141347300006583

Miller, W. R., & Rollnick, S. (1991). *Motivational interviewing: Preparing people to change addictive behavior*. New York, NY: The Guilford Press

Miller, W. R., & Rollnick, S. (2002). *Motivational interviewing: Preparing people for change* (2nd ed.). New York, NY: Guilford Press.

Miller, W. R., & Rose, G. S. (2009). Toward a theory of motivational interviewing. *American Psychologist, 64*(6), 527–537. doi: 10.1037/a0016830

Mineka, S., Watson, D., & Clark, L. A. (1998). Comorbidity of anxiety and unipolar mood disorders. *Annual Review of Psychology, 49*, 377–412. doi: 10.1146/annurev.psych.49.1.377

Mosak, H. H. (1979). Adlerian psychotherapy. In R. J. Corsini (Ed.), *Current psychotherapies* (2nd ed., pp. 44–94). Itasca, IL: F.E. Peacock.

Murphy, J., Rowell, L., McQuaid, A., Timulak, L., O'Flynn, R., & McElvaney, J. (2017). Developing a model of working with worry in emotion–focused therapy: A discovery-phase task analytic study. *Counselling and Psychotherapy Research, 17*(1), 56–70. doi: 10.1002/capr.12089

Muse, M. D., Moore, B. A., & Stahl, S. M. (2013). Benefits and challenges of integrative treatment. In S. M. Stahl & B. A. Moore (Eds.), *Anxiety disorders: A guide for integrating psychopharmacology and psychotherapy* (pp. 3–24). New York, NY: Routledge.

National Institute for Health and Clinical Excellence [NICE]. (2011). *Generalised anxiety disorder in adults: Management in primary, secondary and community care (NICE clinical Guideline 113)*. London: The British Psychological Society.

Newby, J. M., McKinnon, A., Kuyken, W., Gilbody, S., & Dalgleish, T. (2015). Systematic review and meta-analysis of transdiagnostic psychological treatments for anxiety and depressive disorders in adulthood. *Clinical Psychology Review, 40*, 91–110. doi: 10.1016/j.cpr.2015.06.002

Newman, M. G., Castonguay, L. G., Borkovec, T. D., Fisher, A. J., & Nordberg, S. S. (2008). An open trial of integrative therapy for generalized anxiety disorder. *Psychotherapy: Theory, Research, Practice, Training, 45*(2), 135–147. doi: 10.1037/0033-3204.45.2.135

Newman, M. G., Castonguay, L. G., Borkovec, T. D., & Molnar, C. (2004). Integrative psychotherapy. In R. G. Heimberg, C. L., Turk & D. S. Mennin (Eds.), *Generalized anxiety disorders: Advances in research and practice* (pp. 320–350). New York, NY: Guilford Press.

Newman, M. G., Castonguay, L. G., Fisher, A. J., & Borkovec, T. B. (2008, November). The addition of interpersonal and emotional processing techniques to the treatment of generalized anxiety disorder. Paper presented at the Annual meeting of the Association for the Behavior and Cognitive Therapy, Orlando.

Newman, M. G., & Llera, S. J. (2011). A novel theory of experiential avoidance in generalized anxiety disorder: A review and synthesis of research supporting a contrast avoidance model of worry. *Clinical Psychology Review, 31*(3), 371–382. doi: 10.1016/j.cpr.2011.01.008

Newman, M. G., Llera, S. J., Erickson, T. M., Przeworski, A., & Castonguay, L. G. (2013). Worry and generalized anxiety disorder: A review and theoretical synthesis of evidence on nature, etiology, mechanisms, and treatment. *Annual Review of Clinical Psychology, 9*, 275–297. doi: 10.1146/annurev-clinpsy-050212-185544

Norcross, J. C. (2005). A primer on psychotherapy integration. In J. C. Norcross & M. R. Goldfried (Eds.), *Handbook of psychotherapy integration* (2nd ed., pp. 3–23). New York, NY: Oxford University Press.

Oddli, H. W., & McLeod, J. (2017). Knowing-in-relation: How experienced therapists integrate different sources of knowledge in actual clinical practice. *Journal of Psychotherapy Integration, 27*(1), 107–119. doi: 10.1037/int0000045

Orsillo, S. M., Roemer, L., & Barlow, D. H. (2003). Integrating acceptance and mindfulness into existing cognitive-behavioral treatment for GAD: A case study. *Cognitive and Behavioral Practice, 10*(3), 222–230. doi: 10.1016/S1077-7229(03)80034-2

Öst, L.-G. (1987). Applied relaxation: Description of a coping technique and review of controlled studies. *Behaviour Research and Therapy, 25*(5), 397–409. doi: 10.1016/0005-7967(87)90017-9

Otto, M. W., Smits, J. A. J., & Reese, H. E. (2004). Cognitive-behavioral therapy for the treatment of anxiety disorders. *Journal of Clinical Psychiatry, 65* (Suppl. 5), 34–41.

Paivio, S. C., & Pascual-Leone, A. (2010). *Emotion-focused therapy for complex trauma: An Integrative Approach*. Washington, DC: American Psychological Association.

Paus, T., Keshavan, K., & Giedd, J. N. (2008). Why do many psychiatric disorders emerge during adolescence? *Nature Reviews. Neuroscience, 9*(12), 947–957. doi: 10.1038/nrn2513

Pelligrino, L., Pierce, C., & Walkup, J. T. (2011). Pharmacological management of childhood and adolescent anxiety disorders. In W. K. Silverman & A. P. Field (Eds.), *Anxiety disorders in children and adolescents* (2nd ed., pp. 367–391). New York, NY: Cambridge University Press.

Perls, F. (1969). *Gestalt therapy verbatim*. Moab, UT: Real People Press.

Porensky, E. K., Dew, M. A., Karp, J. F., Skidmore, E., Rollman, B. L., Shear, M. K., & Lenze, E. J. (2009). The burden of late-life generalized anxiety disorder: Effects on disability, health-related quality of life, and healthcare utilization. *The American Journal of Geriatric Psychiatry, 17*(6), 473–482. doi: 10.1097/JGP.0b013e31819b87b2

Rachman, S. (1978). *Fear and courage*. Oxford: Freeman.

Ray, W. J. (2018). *Abnormal psychology*. Thousand Oaks, CA: Sage.

Revicki, D. A., Travers, K., Wyrwich, K. W., Svedsäter, H., Locklear, J., Mattera, M. S., … Montgomery, S. (2012). Humanistic and economic burden of generalized anxiety disorder in North America and Europe. *Journal of Affective Disorders, 140*(2), 103–112. doi: 10.1016/j.jad.2011.11.014

Rodriguez, B. F., Weisberg, R. B., Pagano, M. E., Machan, J. T., Culpepper, L., & Keller, M. B. (2004). Frequency and patterns of psychiatric comorbidity in a sample of primary care patients with anxiety disorders. *Comprehensive Psychiatry, 45*(2), 129–137. doi: 10.1016/j.comppsych.2003.09.005

Roemer, L., & Orsillo, S. M. (2005). An acceptance based behavior therapy for generalized anxiety disorder. In S. M. Orsillo & L. Roemer (Eds.), *Acceptance and mindfulness-based approaches to anxiety Conceptualization and treatment* (pp. 213–240). New York, NY: Springer.

Roemer, L., & Orsillo, S. M. (2007). An open trial of an acceptance-based behavior therapy for generalized anxiety disorder. *Behavior Therapy, 38*(1), 72–85. doi: 10.1016/j.beth.2006.04.004

Roemer, L., Orsillo, S. M., & Barlow, D. H. (2002). Generalized anxiety disorder. In D. H. Barlow, *Anxiety and its disorders: The nature and treatment of anxiety and panic* (2nd ed., pp. 477–515). New York, NY: Guilford Press.

Rogers, C. R. (1951). *Client-centered therapy*. Boston, MA: Houghton Mifflin.

Rollnick, S., Miller, W. R., & Butler, C. C. (2008). *Motivational interviewing in health care: Helping patients change behavior*. New York, NY: Guilford Press.

Schienle, A., Hettema, J. M., Cáceda, R., & Nemeroff, C. B. (2011). Neurobiology and genetics of generalized anxiety disorder. *Psychiatric Annals, 41*(2), 113–123. doi: 10.3928/00485713-20110203-10

Schmidt, N. B., Buckner, J. D., Pusser, A., Woolaway-Bickel, K., Preston, J. L., & Norr, A. (2012). Randomized controlled trial of false safety behavior elimination therapy: A unified cognitive behavioral treatment for anxiety psychopathology. *Behavior Therapy, 43*(3), 518–532. doi: 10.1016/j.beth.2012.02.004

Schottenbauer, M. A., Glass, C. R., & Arnkoff, D. B. (2005). Outcome research on psychotherapy integration. In J. C. Norcross & M. R. Goldfried (Eds.), *Handbook of psychotherapy integration* (2nd ed., pp. 459–493). New York, NY: Oxford University Press.

Segal, Z. V., Williams, J. M. G., & Teasdale, J. D. (2002). *Mindfulness-based cognitive therapy for depression: A new approach for preventing relapse*. New York, NY: Guilford Press.

Sell, C., Möller, H., & Taubner, S. (2018). Effectiveness of integrative imagery- and trance-based psychodynamic therapies: Guided imagery psychotherapy and hypnopsychotherapy. *Journal of Psychotherapy Integration, 28*(1), 90–113. doi: 10.1037/int0000073

Sharf, R. S. (2012). *Theories of psychotherapy and counseling: Concepts and cases* (5th ed.). Pacific Grove, CA: Brooks/Cole.

Shedler, J. (2010). The efficacy of psychodynamic psychotherapy. *American Psychologist, 65*(2), 98–109. doi: 10.1037/a0018378

Stevens, E. S., Jendrusina, A. A., Sarapas, C., & Behar, E. (2014). Generalized anxiety disorder. In P. Emmelkamp & T. Ehring (Eds.), *The Wiley handbook of anxiety disorders, Volume I: Theory and research, Volume II: Clinical assessment and treatment* (pp. 376–423). Hoboken, NJ: Wiley-Blackwell.

Swift, J. K., Greenberg, R. P., Tompkins, K. A., & Parkin, S. R. (2017). Treatment refusal and premature termination in psychotherapy, pharmacotherapy, and their combination: A meta-analysis of head-to-head comparisons. *Psychotherapy, 54*(1), 47–57. doi: 10.1037/pst0000104

Taylor, S., Abramowitz, J. S., & McKay, D. (2012). Non-adherence and non-response in the treatment of anxiety disorders. *Journal of Anxiety Disorders, 26*(5), 583–589. doi: 10.1016/j.janxdis.2012.02.010

Timulak, L., Keogh, D., Chigwedere, C., Wilson, C., Ward, F., Hevey, D., … Irwin, B. (2018). A comparison of emotion-focused therapy and cognitive-behavioural therapy in the treatment of generalised anxiety disorder: Study protocol for a randomised controlled trial. *Trials, 19*(1), 506. doi: 10.1186/s13063-018-2892-0

Timulak, L., & McElvaney, J. (2016). Emotion-focused therapy for generalized anxiety disorder: An overview of the model. *Journal of Contemporary Psychotherapy, 46*(1), 41–52. doi: 10.1007/s10879-015-9310-7

Timulak, L., & McElvaney, J. (2018). *Transforming generalized anxiety: An emotion-focused approach*. New York, NY: Routledge.

Tryon, W. (2014). *Cognitive neuroscience and psychotherapy: Network principles for a unified theory*. Cambridge: Academic Press.

van Rijn, B., & Wild, C. (2013). Humanistic and integrative therapies for anxiety and depression: Practice-based evaluation of transactional analysis, gestalt, and integrative psychotherapies and person-centered counseling. *Transactional Analysis Journal, 43*(2), 150–163. doi: 10.1177/0362153713499545

Wachtel, E. F., & Wachtel, P. L. (1986). *Family dynamics in individual psychotherapy*. New York, NY: Guilford Press.

Wachtel, P. L. (1977). *Psychoanalysis and behavior therapy: Toward an integration*. New York, NY: Basic Books.

Wachtel, P. L. (1997). *Psychoanalysis, behavior therapy, and the relational world*. Washington, DC: American Psychological Association.

Wachtel, P. L. (2014). An integrative relational point of view. *Psychotherapy, 51*(3), 342–349. doi: 10.1037/a0037219

Wachtel, P. L., Kruk, J. C., & McKinney, M. K. (2005). Cyclical psychodynamics and integrative relational psychotherapy. In J. C. Norcross & M. R. Goldfried (Eds.), *Handbook of psychotherapy integration* (2nd ed., pp. 172–195). New York, NY: Oxford University Press.

Watson, D., & Clark, L. A. (1984). Negative affectivity: The disposition to experience aversive emotional states. *Psychological Bulletin, 96*(3), 465–490. doi: 10.1037/0033-2909.96.3.465

Watson, J., Timulak, L., & Greenberg, L. S. (2019). Emotion-focused therapy for generalized anxiety disorder. In L. S. Greenberg & R. N. Goldman (Eds.), *Clinical handbook of emotion-focused therapy* (pp. 315–336). Washington, DC: American Psychological Association.

Watson, J. C., & Greenberg, L. S. (2017). *Emotion-focused psychotherapy for generalized anxiety disorder*. Washington, DC: American Psychological Association.

Wells, A. (1995). Meta-cognition and worry: A cognitive model of generalized anxiety disorder. *Behavioural and Cognitive Psychotherapy, 23*(3), 301–320. doi: 10.1017/S1352465800015897

Wells, A. (1999). A metacognitive model and therapy for generalized anxiety disorder. *Clinical Psychology and Psychotherapy: An International Journal of Theory and Practice, 6*(2), 86–95. doi: 10.1002/(SICI)1099-0879(199905)6:2<86::AID-CPP189>3.0.CO;2-S

Westra, H. A., Constantino, M. J., & Antony, M. M. (2016). Integrating motivational interviewing with cognitive-behavioral therapy for severe generalized anxiety disorder: An allegiance-controlled randomized clinical trial. *Journal of Consulting and Clinical Psychology, 84*(9), 768. doi: 10.1037/ccp0000098

Westra, H. A., & Dozois, D. J. (2006). Preparing clients for cognitive behavioral therapy: A randomized pilot study of motivational interviewing for anxiety. *Cognitive Therapy and Research, 30*(4), 481–498. doi: 10.1007/s10608-006-9016-y

Wittchen, H. U., Jacobi, F., Rehm, J., Gustavsson, A., Svensson, M., Jönsson, B., … Steinhausen, H. C. (2011). The size and burden of mental disorders and other disorders of the brain in Europe 2010. *European Neuropsychopharmacology, 21*(9), 655–679. doi: 10.1016/j.euroneuro.2011.07.018

Wittchen, H. U., Kessler, R. C., Beesdo, K., Krause, P., Höfler, M., & Hoyer, J. (2002). Generalized anxiety and depression in primary care: Prevalence, recognition, and management. *The Journal of Clinical Psychiatry, 63* (Suppl. 8), S24–S34.

Wolfe, B. E. (2003). Integrative psychotherapy of the anxiety disorders. In J. C. Norcross & M. R. Goldfried (Eds.), *Handbook of psychotherapy integration* (2nd ed., pp. 263–280). New York, NY: Oxford University Press.

Wolfe, B. E. (2005). *Understanding and treating anxiety disorders: An integrative approach to healing the wounded self.* Washington, DC: American Psychological Association.

Wolfe, B. E. (2006). An integrative perspective on the anxiety disorders. In G. Stricker & J. Gold (Eds.), *A casebook of psychotherapy integration* (pp. 65–77). Washington, DC: American Psychological Association.

Wolfe, B. E. (2008). Existential issues in anxiety disorders and their treatment. In K. I. Schneider (Ed.), *Existential-integrative psychotherapy* (pp. 204–216). New York, NY: Routledge.

Wolfe, B. E. (2013). Clinical process in an integrative psychotherapy for self- wounds. *Psychotherapy, 50*(3), 326–330. doi: 10.1037/a0032407

Wolitzky-Taylor, K. B., Castriotta, N., Lenze, E. J., Stanley, M. A., & Craske, M. G. (2010). Anxiety disorders in older adults: A comprehensive review. *Depression and Anxiety, 27*(2), 190–211. doi: 10.1002/da.20653

Woodman, C. L., Noyes, R., Black, D. W., Schlosser, S., & Yagia, S. J. (1999). A five-year follow-up study of generalized anxiety disorder and panic disorder. *Journal of Nervous and Mental Disease, 187*(1), 3–9. doi: 10.1097/00005053-199901000-00002

Yalom, I. D. (1980). *Existential psychotherapy.* New York, NY: Basic Books.

Zerbe, K. J. (1990). Through the storm: Psychoanalytic theory in the psychotherapy of the anxiety disorders. *Bulletin of the Menninger Clinic, 54*(2), 171–183.

Zinbarg, R. E., & Barlow, D. H. (1996). Structure of anxiety and the anxiety disorders: A hierarchical model. *Journal of Abnormal Psychology, 105*(2), 181–193. doi: 10.1037/0021-843X.105.2.181

Zinbarg, R. E., Craske, M. G., & Barlow, D. H. (2006). *Mastery of your anxiety and worry: Therapist guide* (2nd ed.). New York, NY: Oxford University Press. doi: 10.1093/med:psych/9780195300024.001.0001

6 Panic Disorder (PD)

Introduction

This chapter focuses on integrated and unified etiology approaches and psychotherapy treatment models for panic disorder. At the end of the chapter, an example of a case study is presented to demonstrate the implementation of an integrated psychotherapy treatment approach for panic disorder (PD). The case shows how an integration of couples and individual as well as cognitive-behavioral and psychodynamic interventions is employed to enhance the therapy process. It presents an integrated psychotherapy treatment approach that includes both individual and couples therapy with CBT methods with a focus on applied relaxation techniques, hypnosis, pharmacotherapy, as well as individual psychodynamic treatment. The case study relies, in part, on Busch, Oquendo, Sullivan, and Sandberg's (2010) psychoanalytic/neurobiological model and draws as well on Scaturo's (1994) integrative therapy work that integrates individual therapy with couples and family therapy.

Symptoms of Panic Disorder (PD)

What are the symptoms of panic disorder? According to DSM-5 (American Psychiatric Association, 2013), the symptoms of panic disorder manifest rapidly and in the absence of a dangerous scenario. Individuals with panic disorder display a great amount of fear, and their attacks may occur repeatedly (Comer, 2015). Physical symptoms can include intense and sudden sweating, shaking, a fast beating heart, shortness of breath, and others (APA, 2013). Individuals with panic disorder tend to report that they feel like they're going crazy, having a stroke, or having a heart attack (Ingersoll & Marquis, 2014).

How do the symptoms of panic disorder compare to the symptoms of other anxiety disorders? There are distinctions between the symptoms of panic disorder and those of other anxiety disorders. According to Craske and Waters (2005), when compared with persons with anxiety disorders other than panic, individuals with panic disorder relate more physical illnesses (e.g., Verburg, Griez, Meijer, & Pols, 1995). Panic disorder and GAD are different in their scope of the object of danger with PD having a more narrow danger object that is relevant to the body (Craske & Waters, 2005). Whereas individuals with panic disorder tend to demonstrate a high degree of anticipatory reactions to threat contexts without reactions of acute stress to particular stimuli that contain threat, individuals with specific phobia tend to exhibit reactions of acute stress to particular stimuli that contain threat without increased anticipatory reactions to threat contexts (Craske & Waters, 2005).

Diagnosis of Panic Disorder

A diagnosis of panic disorder requires that an individual who has a panic attack (with the aforementioned surge of symptoms) will then experience at least a month of either chronic worry that more attacks will occur or serious changes in behavior that can be attributed to the initial panic attack (APA, 2013; Taylor & Asmundson, 2016). Individuals diagnosed with separation anxiety disorder when they are children are more likely to develop panic disorder (Kossowsky et al., 2013).

Prevalence of Panic Disorder (PD)

Prevalence

What is the prevalence of panic disorder? Kessler, Berglund, and Demler (2005) report the lifetime prevalence for panic disorder to be almost 5%, with the 12-month at almost 3%. According to APA (2013), the 12-month rates in the U.S. and Europe range from 2% to 3%. In the U.S., the prevalence of panic is slightly higher in Caucasians than among minorities (Levine et al., 2013; Woodward et al., 2012).

Onset

When does panic disorder occur during an individual's life cycle? Panic disorder can begin at the end of adolescence or at the beginning of adulthood, and it is found, at least, two times more often among women than among men (Comer, 2015; Ray, 2018). Whereas the onset of phobias and separation anxiety disorder can occur in childhood, panic disorder, similar to generalized anxiety disorder, tends to start later, with uncommon onsets prior to early adolescence (Paus, Keshavan, & Giedd, 2008). This finding is consistent with research that reports that panic disorder does not frequently occur in childhood (Sweeney, Levitt, Westerholm, Gaskins, & Lipinski, 2013). According to Craske and Waters (2005), PD's onset frequently can be identified by a first panic attack that is not expected (Barlow, 1988) and usually occurs when an individual is around 25 (Brown, Campbell, Lehman, Grishman, & Mancill, 2001). More recently, Ray (2018) reported that individuals who develop panic disorder usually do so between age 21 and 23. Although, as discussed in Chapter 5, anxiety disorders are prevalent in the elderly, panic disorder is not common (Beekman et al., 1998). In fact, after age 62, panic disorder will develop in fewer than 1% of people (Kessler et al., 2005; Wolitzky-Taylor, Castriotta, Lenze, Stanley, & Craske, 2010).

Comorbidity

Does panic disorder occur with other mental disorders? The onset of panic disorder is frequently accompanied by agoraphobia (Comer, 2015). Other anxiety and depressive disorders tend to accompany panic disorder (Allen et al., 2010).

Heritability

A heritability of 48% has been reported for panic disorder (Hettema, Neale, & Kendler, 2001; Ray, 2018).

An Integrative Etiology of Panic Disorder (PD): Focus, Underpinnings, and Causes of Panic Disorder (PD)

Although DSM-5 classifies panic disorder with its accompanying panic attacks as a disorder in its own right, the different anxiety disorders and other mental disorders can include panic attacks as well (APA, 2013; Ray, 2018). The panic attacks of individuals with panic disorder are triggered by perceptions of intense threats that are connected to negative feelings (Busch et al., 1991; Leichsenring & Salzer, 2014; Shear, Cooper, Klerman, Busch & Shapiro, 1993). This section describes the etiology of panic disorder from an integrated and unified point of view and lays out the implicit and explicit causes implicated in the development and maintenance of panic disorder (PD). This portion discusses the psychological, biological, and environmental causes that are implicated in the etiology of panic disorder (see Figure 6.1).

Psychological Causes of Panic Disorder (PD)

How are psychological causes implicated in the etiology of panic disorder? According to Wolfe's (2003) integrated model for the anxiety disorders (discussed in Chapters 4 and 5), the source of panic disorder is an underlying self-wound. Wolfe (2003) explains that the past experiences of patients with panic disorder (PD) tend to be unconscious, and these individuals can access only small traces of somatic issues that result in cogitation about their physical symptoms, thereby generating further anxiety. Patients with PD, rather than seeking the unconscious meaning of their anxiety, detach, focus on some future tragedy that they perceive will happen, their negative ruminations heighten their perceptions of anxiety, and a vicious cycle begins whereby they start to experience physical manifestations and become sure that they will experience a cardiac arrest or lose control of themselves (Alladin; 2014; Wolfe, 2005). The

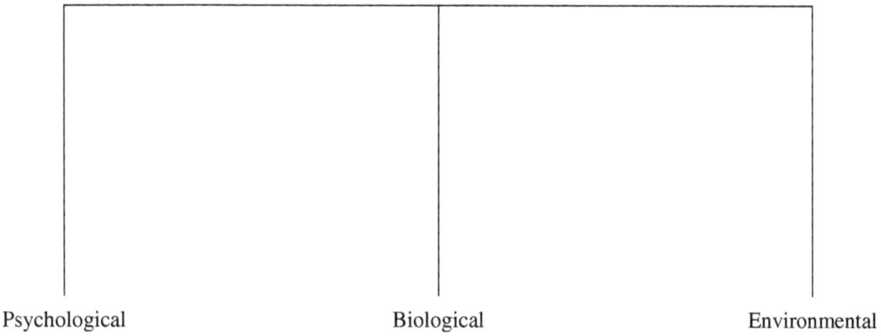

Figure 6.1 The etiology of panic disorder.

vicious cycle culminates in a panic attack, and patients tend to avoid the site of the panic without an understanding of the meaning of the panic (Wolfe, 2003). Anxiety goes hand in hand with the feared future misfortunes that involve pain to the self, which prevents a patient from experiencing the present (Alladin, 2014; Wolfe, 2005). These findings of somatic issues in patients with panic disorder are consistent with research that shows that individuals who panic tend to be sensitive to anxiety and focus a lot on sensations related to their bodies, which they perceive as having a potential to be dangerous (Comer, 2015). Frequently, the panic symptoms, themselves, protect patients with panic disorder from their emotions, which are filled with pain (Wolfe, 2003). Patients with panic disorder employ defenses in an attempt to avoid humiliation and anger (Wolfe, 2003).

According to Wolfe's (2005) integrative model of the etiology of panic disorder, agoraphobic avoidance, an inability to recognize the root of the panic, and a self-wound that has not been repaired can maintain panic disorder with agoraphobia. The theme of insecure attachment plays a prominent role for patients with agoraphobia who tend to seek objects that provide them with security (Bowlby, 1973; Leichsenring and Salzer, 2014). Generally, individuals with panic disorder without agoraphobia have milder symptoms than do individuals with agoraphobia (Wolfe, 2005).

Biological, Physiological, and Genetic Causes of Panic Disorder (PD)

What are the biological, physiological, or genetic causes of panic disorder? There are brain processes that are implicated in anxiety, and others that are implicated in panic (Ray, 2018). Chapter 5 discussed brain circuits related to generalized anxiety disorder (GAD). Different portions of the brain are associated with panic and anxiety, with panic connected to the midbrain as in the limbic and basal ganglia areas of the brain, and anxiety linked to the forebrain, e.g., amygdala (Graeff & Del-Ben, 2008; Ray, 2018). Although the brain circuit that is implicated in panic disorder is different from the one implicated in GAD, there are overlapping brain areas such as the amygdala (Comer, 2015; Henn, 2013). With respect to receptors, the amygdala and cingulate gyrus of individuals with panic have been found to have decreased 5-HT_{1A} density (Greene, Bailey, & Neumeister, 2013; Nash et al., 2008; Neumeister et al., 2004).

Whereas some proponents of biological theories attribute panic disorder to unusual norepinephrine activation in the locus coeruleus, others propose that neurotransmitters are implicated in the development of panic disorder (Comer, 2015; Redmond, 1977, 1981). For example, impairment in serotonin and norepinephrine are related to panic disorder (Busch et al., 2010; Pyke & Greenberg, 1986; Targum & Marshal, 1989).

There are biological and psychological models that can explain the etiology of panic disorder (Busch et al., 2010). For example, included in the biological models of panic disorder is Gorman, Kent, Sullivan, and Coplan's (2000) neuroanatomical model which suggests that panic is related to an impaired fear network in the amygdala. According to Gorman et al.'s (2000) model, environmental experiences can trigger a fear response, or some individuals vulnerable to panic may be more sensitive to trauma because of a hypersensitive system.

Other biological models include separation-distress and suffocation-fear models (Busch et al., 2010; Klein, 1993; Panksepp, 1998). The separation-distress model of the etiology of panic disorder considers that the developmental history of the patient who suffers panic attacks includes many experiences of separation and/or loss or that these experiences predominate prior to the beginning of a panic disorder (Busch et al., 2010; Faravelli & Pallanti, 1989; Kaunonen, Päivi, Paunonen, & Erjanti, 2000). A suffocation model of the etiology of panic disorder posits that the brain can become overly sensitive and can become overly aroused when there isn't a reality of suffocation (Busch et al., 2010; Klein, 1993). In contrast to the integrated model of Alexander and colleagues (2005), which explains the etiology of panic disorder by including an interaction between conditioned fear and amygdala arousal and by focusing on the experience of actual danger while excluding the notion of separation anxiety, the integrated model of panic disorder of Busch and colleagues (2010), a psychoanalytic/neurobiological model that emphasizes psychological, biological and environmental influences, highlights separation anxiety as well as the notion of a hypersensitive suffocation system (Busch et al., 2010; Panksepp, 2005). Individuals who are psychologically vulnerable to intrusion or loss from attachment persons may experience unconscious anger, and an individual's sensitivities that may include trauma can result in panic (Busch et al., 2010). Panic in the brain emerges upon stimulation of separation distress (Busch et al., 2010; Panksepp, 1998, 2005).

There are genetic causes of panic disorder as well. With respect to the genetic etiology of panic disorder, Fyer and colleagues (2006) demonstrated that chromosome regions 15q and 2q are implicated in panic disorder's genetic vulnerability.

Environmental Causes of Panic Disorder (PD)

What role do environmental factors have in the etiology of panic disorder? Although there does not seem to be a single cause for panic disorder, some research has shown that stressful experiences can precede the beginning of an individual's first panic attack (Faravelli, 1985; Ingersoll & Marquis, 2014). For example, with respect to stressors, panic disorder in the elderly is strongly related to the death of a significant other and chronic sickness (Beekman et al., 1998). A source of panic disorder can be death anxiety or fear of loss, and several losses that occur at approximately the same time can cause panic attacks (Wolfe, 2008). Early tragic events were found to be related only to panic disorder in the elderly rather than to other types of anxiety (Beekman et al., 1998).

A Unified Framework for the Etiology of Panic Disorder (PD)

How can a unified model explain the etiology of panic disorder? To describe the etiology of panic disorder, McGinn, Nooner, Cohen, and Leaberry (2015) developed a unified model that relies on the notion of vulnerability. This unified vulnerability model integrates Barlow's (2000, 2002) triple vulnerability model and the theory of expectancy (Reiss & McNally, 1985). In their explanations of how panic develops, both the triple vulnerability model and the theory of expectancy underscore anxiety sensitivity, but Barlow's (2000, 2002) model, in addition, focuses on a perception of low control as characteristic of distal vulnerability (McGin et al., 2015). The unified panic model of McGin and colleagues (2015) includes vulnerability factors arranged in six stages, from proximal to distal. Whereas Stage 2, for example, includes a more distal stage of early learning experiences, Stage 5 focuses on a more proximal factor, a hypervigilance to feelings linked to the body (McGin et al., 2015). The research of McGin and colleagues (2015) suggests that the modeling of the threat of anxiety symptoms by a child's parents may hold more weight than the parents' reinforcement of their offspring's role in being ill, and that the two factors, being sensitive to anxiety and having a perception of low control, may contribute to a more substantial vulnerability for panic in offspring whose parents may have displayed alarm over anxiety symptoms.

Summary

Various psychological theories, frameworks, and models have been proposed to conceptualize panic disorder. What factors comprise the core of panic disorder? A key focus of panic disorder is on what can trigger harm (Ingersoll & Marquis, 2014). This section focused on the integrated and unified models that have contributed to the development and maintenance of panic disorder (see Table 6.1).

Table 6.1 Panic Disorder (PD)

Etiology	*Integrated*	*Unified*
Psychological Causes The source of panic disorder is an underlying self-wound.[a]	An Integrative Four-stage Approach and a Focusing Technique[a,f]	A Unified Model That Underscores Vulnerability[h]
Biological Causes Panic is connected to the midbrain as in the limbic and basal ganglia areas of the brain, and anxiety is linked to the forebrain as in the amygdala.[b,c]	An Integrative Transdiagnostic Model of Emotion-Focused Psychodynamic Psychotherapy (EFPP)[g]	Transdiagnostic Unified Protocol (UP) Unified psychotherapy treatment approaches include the transdiagnostic unified protocol UP where the dropout rate for UP was lower than for the single-disorder protocols. (SDPs)[i,j]
Environmental Stressful experiences can precede the beginning of an person's first panic attack.[d,e]		

[a]Wolfe (2003). [b]Ray (201). [c]Graeff and Del-Ben (2008). [d]Faravelli (1985). [e]Ingersoll and Marquis (2014). [f]Wolfe and Sigl (1998). [g]Beutel, Greenberg, Lane, and Subic-Wrana (2019). [h]McGinn, Nooner, Cohen, and Leaberry (2015). [i]Barlow et al. (2017). [j]Kennedy and Barlow (2018).

Clinical Practice Applications of Integrated and Unified Psychotherapy Treatment Models for Panic Disorder (PD)

This section on clinical practice applications presents treatment models that demonstrate the use of integrated and unified approaches for panic disorder and discusses the relationship between the etiology of panic disorder and its integrated and unified treatment. Although psychodynamic psychotherapy is possibly as effective for treating individuals with panic disorder as is cognitive-behavioral therapy (Leichsenring, Leweke, Klein, & Steinert, 2015), individuals with panic disorder with less emotional awareness did not benefit much from either monotherapy, e.g., psychodynamic therapy or cognitive-behavioral therapy (Beutel et al., 2013). Integrative and unified treatments that address the key issues and emotional components of panic disorder are proposed to treat panic disorder.

Integrated Approaches for Panic Disorder (PD)

An Integrated Self-Wound Approach to Panic Disorder (PD)

What is the focus of integrated models for panic disorder? In his integrative four-stage approach to the anxiety disorders, Wolfe (2003) integrates cognitive-behavioral, psychodynamic, and experiential orientations of psychotherapy. For example, when applying the third stage, uncovering the conflicts or self-wounds of a client with panic disorder, Wolfe (2003) points out that on a conscious level, the client's fears are frequently about physical damage, but the implied threatening image is generally psychological, and, thus, the target of the adjusted imaginal exposure is slightly different from the original. The goal of the felt anxiety is both to learn that the feared catastrophe will not occur and to discover the unconscious self-wound and its felt disaster (Wolfe, 2003). Wolfe (2003) recommends the use of directed imagery, focusing, and insightful interpretations to elicit self-wounds, and he recognizes that although there are clients who prefer to start with insight-based therapy or with cognitive work or behavioral techniques, there are infrequent instances where clients will commence with experiential treatment.

Wolfe (2003) designed an integrative psychotherapy model for the anxiety disorders that includes a type of exposure technique of imagined images. The exposure of imagined material, Wolfe's Focusing Technique, can help a patient with panic disorder focus on key areas of the body that are anxiety provoking in order to learn the meaning of the panic itself (Wolfe, 2003; Wolfe & Sigl, 1998). It is difficult for a patient with panic disorder to access images that are connected to emotions; however, the aforementioned technique has been shown to hold the capability to elicit threatening images that represent patients' self-wounds (Wolfe, 2003).

An Integrative Transdiagnostic Perspective of Panic Disorder (PD)

How can an integrative transdiagnostic model benefit patients with panic disorder? Busch and colleagues (2010) point out that unitary psychological models that can explain the etiology of panic disorder include cognitive-behavioral, psychodynamic, and mentalization. Given that it is difficult for individuals with panic disorder who may not have much emotional insight into their disorder to benefit from either psychodynamic or cognitive-behavioral therapy, two distinct monotherapies which have been used to treat panic disorder, clinicians and researchers have designed integrated interventions for these individuals (Beutel et al., 2013; Leichsenring et al., 2015). For example, to help patients with anxiety disorders who have difficulty accessing and experiencing their emotions, Beutel, Greenberg, Lane, and Subic-Wrana (2019) developed an integrative, transdiagnostic model of emotion-focused psychodynamic psychotherapy (EFPP). The aforementioned integrative model can be helpful for patients with anxiety disorders who tend to avoid affect because of former memories of anxiety (Beutel et al., 2019; Tull & Roemer, 2007). According to Beutel et al.'s (2019) integrative model of emotion-focused psychodynamic psychotherapy, individuals with panic disorder and generalized anxiety disorder are prone to cling to or maintain an ambivalent connection with the therapist as their anxiety symptoms serve as a defense against feelings of painful affect. Therapists who work with an EFPP model can help patients with panic disorder process and re-own their conflict-laden unconscious and conscious emotions both by using interpretations and by chair work which can activate the experiential process (Beutel et al., 2019).

An Integration of Individual and Couples Therapy for Panic Disorder (PD)

How can an integration of individual and couples therapy help patients with panic disorder (PD)? Separation anxiety and abandonment represent key issues for patients with panic disorder (Scaturo, 1994). Pretreatment issues to consider for clients with panic disorder include establishing a therapeutic relationship and a referral to a physician to address the client's physiological symptoms (Scaturo, 1994). The importance of the therapeutic relationship for the treatment of panic disorder (PD) is not to be discounted. Whereas therapist competence has been shown to be a predictor of treatment outcome for clients with PD, the therapeutic relationship was found to be a predictor of treatment outcome and dropout (Haug et al., 2016). For example, when the therapist's competence was high early in the treatment, the outcome from CBT for clients with PD was better, and when the therapist's competence was low, the treatment outcome was poorer (Haug et al., 2016). Furthermore, if the rating of the therapeutic relationship was higher late in the treatment, the outcome was better, and if the rating of the therapeutic relationship was lower late in the treatment, the patient with panic disorder was more likely drop out of therapy (Haug et al., 2016).

Integrative therapy can involve not only the integration of behavioral and psychodynamic perspectives but also the integration of the intrapsychic components of individual therapy with couples and family therapy (Scaturo, 1994). When treating the patient who has panic disorder, it may be important to include a spouse and to recognize that spouses tend to have antithetical defense mechanisms (Goldenberg & Goldenberg, 1980; Scaturo, 1994). For example, the spouse of a patient with panic disorder may have endured past trauma similar to the trauma that represents the key issue for the panic disorder in the client; however, the defense mechanisms in the spouse probably will not manifest as panic and may develop in the opposite way, as a numbing of affect (Scaturo, 1994). According to Scaturo (1994), employing an integrative therapeutic approach that involves the spouse may strengthen the emotional relationship of the pair, may reduce the fears of abandonment of the spouse with panic, and may lead to a decrease in the propensity towards panic as well.

A Combination of Medication and Therapy for Panic Disorder (PD)

How do patients with panic disorder fare with monotherapy, pharmacotherapy, and a combination of monotherapy and pharmacotherapy? In the previous section on the integrated etiology of panic disorder, it was suggested by clinicians and researchers who promote biological theories that panic disorder can be attributed to neurotransmitters or to norepinephrine activation in the locus coeruleus (Comer, 2015; Redmond, 1977, 1981). Which medications adjust this activation, and is psychotherapy preferred to medication? With respect to treatment, it has been shown that antidepressant medications help in the treatment of panic disorder more than do benzodiazepines (Comer, 2015; Klein, 1964; Klein & Fink, 1962), and that these antidepressant medications have been found to restore the correct balance of norepinephrine (NE) in the locus coeruleus and in other sections of the brain circuit implicated in panic disorder (Comer, 2015; Pollack, 2005; Redmond, 1985). Serotonin-specific reuptake inhibitors (SSRIs) and serotonin and norepinephrine reuptake inhibitors (SNRIs) have been shown to be preferred for the treatment of panic disorder (Charney, Kredlow, Bui, Simon, 2013; Hales, Yudofsky, & Gabbard, 2011); however, psychological interventions are preferred to pharmacotherapy given the side effects of drugs and the risk of dependency (Muse, Moore, & Stahl, 2013). Sertraline (Zoloft), for example, has been shown to be effective for panic disorder (Allgulander et al., 2004; Pohl, Wolkow, & Clary, 1998).

Are benzodiazepines effective in the treatment for panic disorder? Although benzodiazepines can have a sedative effect and are not useful for comorbid depression, they have been shown to be effective in the treatment of panic disorder (Charney et al., 2013). Marks et al. (1993) demonstrated that alprazolam was two times less effective than exposure therapy for panic disorder. It has been demonstrated that a combination of benzodiazepines and antidepressants at the beginning of treatment for panic disorder are more effective than only antidepressants (Pollack et al., 2003).

Is a combination of therapy and medication more efficacious than therapy alone in the treatment of panic disorder? There is some support for psychodynamic therapy in the treatment of panic disorder, and in a small sample it was demonstrated that psychodynamic therapy was more efficacious than relaxation training (Milrod et al., 2007). Cognitive-behavioral interventions have been shown to be the most efficacious and cost-effective treatments for panic disorder, and successful outcomes have been maintained for long periods of time (Barlow, 2004; Charney et al., 2013). Although the combined treatment of hypnosis and exposure was not found to be superior to exposure treatment by itself for panic disorder with agoraphobia, cognitive-behavioral hypnotherapy was shown to be beneficial when combined with rational emotive therapy (RE) (Dyck & Spinhoven, 1997; Fredette, El-Baalbaki, Neron, & Palardy, 2013; Singh & Banerjee, 2002). Although it has been shown that cognitive-behavioral interventions are the most efficacious treatments for panic disorder, a combination of antidepressants (e.g., SSRIs) and CBT is more efficacious than either CBT or pharmacotherapy alone (Barlow, 2004; Ray, 2018).

Variables that practitioners need to consider when selecting a treatment plan of therapy by itself, medication alone, or a combination of therapy and pharmacotherapy include the duration of progress as well as patient preference. Some research has shown that the progress of patients with panic disorder who were treated with a combination of cognitive-behavioral therapy and imipramine is not as durable as the progress of those with panic disorder who were treated with therapy by itself (Barlow, Gorman, Shear, & Woods, 2000). With respect to the aforementioned study, Gorman (2016) cautions that other research (e.g., Driessen et al., 2015) shows that the failure to publish negative findings may have resulted in an inflated estimation of the efficacy of the psychological interventions, and that regardless of Barlow et al.'s (2000) findings, other studies (e.g., Marcus, Gorman, & Shear, 2007) found that patients with panic disorder who were treated with combination therapy did not drop out as much and were shown to have less severe negative side effects because of the medication than patients who were treated with only imipramine.

Independent of the issue of durability of treatment is the issue of patient preference. With respect to patient preference, individuals with panic disorder were almost three times more likely to refuse medication over therapy as an intervention (Swift, Greenberg, Tompkins, & Parkin, 2017). Some patients, however, prefer medication to therapy, and patient preference needs to be considered (Muse, Moore, & Stahl, 2013). To manage panic means to encourage patients to confront beliefs about threatening physical symptoms when they face their anxiety (Muse et al., 2013). The use of pharmacotherapy combined with psychosocial intervention needs to further the treatment goal rather than encourage avoidance by reliance on a drug (Muse et al., 2013).

Is there an interaction between treatment and comorbidity for patients with panic disorder? Adults who have panic disorder who receive psychopharmacological interventions have been shown to have poor outcomes if they have symptoms of separation anxiety disorder, and those with panic disorder who are treated with CBT are almost four times less likely to benefit when adult separation anxiety disorder accompanies (Aaronson et al., 2008; Miniati et al., 2012).

Unified Treatment for Panic Disorder (PD)

How have unified models of psychotherapy been used to treat individuals with panic disorder? The unified approach of McGinn and colleagues (2015) was proposed to explain the way in which thoughts about the threat of arousal of anxiety and perceptions of low control can serve as variables of distal vulnerability. (See the section on the etiology of panic disorder that discusses McGinn et al.'s, 2015, unified model.) With respect to the relationship between the etiology of panic disorder and unified treatment, it has been shown that cognitive therapy is associated with better progress than is respiratory therapy for the distal vulnerability variable, perception of low control (Meuret, Rosenfield, Seidel, Bhaskara, & Hofmann, 2010).

How are treatment frameworks that include transdiagnostic unified models linked to dimensional constructs? Other unified psychotherapy treatment approaches include the transdiagnostic unified protocol UP, which when compared with single-disorder protocols (SDPs) for panic disorder with or without agoraphobia (PDA), was found to be as effective a treatment as the

SDPs; however, the dropout rate for UP was lower than for the SDPs (Barlow et al., 2017; Kennedy & Barlow, 2018). Consistent with the UP transdiagnostic approach to psychotherapy treatment, variables such as temperament have been found to contribute to the co-occurrence of panic disorder, generalized anxiety disorder, social phobia, depression, and PTSD (Boettcher & Conklin, 2018; Brown & Barlow, 2009; Ruscio, Borkovec, & Ruscio, 2001). Boettcher and Conklin (2018) offer comorbidity and a tendency towards higher autonomic arousal as a reason for a greater risk of panic attacks in individuals with posttraumatic stress disorder. The aforementioned examples illustrate the UP transdiagnostic approach's emphasis on dimensional constructs (Boettcher & Conklin, 2018).

Summary

The section on clinical practice applications discussed the way in which researchers and therapists have used integrated and unified models of psychotherapy to treat panic disorder (see Table 6.1). The next section, which presents a case study that shows how to implement integrative therapy in clinical practice, concludes the section on panic disorder (PD).

How to Implement Integrative Psychotherapy in Practice for Panic Disorder (PD)

The following case study illustrates how an integration of couples and individual therapy and cognitive-behavioral and psychodynamic interventions are employed to enhance the therapy process. The case material depicts an integrated psychotherapy treatment approach that includes both individual and couples therapy with cognitive-behavioral (CBT) methods and a focus on applied relaxation techniques, pharmacotherapy, hypnosis, assertiveness training, and individual psychodynamic treatment. The case study relies, in part, on Busch et al.'s (2010) psychoanalytic/neurobiological model and draws as well on Scaturo's (1994) integrative therapy work that integrates individual therapy with couples and family therapy.

Henry, age 29, has been experiencing panic attacks for the past several months. He reported that he had been diagnosed with a generalized anxiety disorder (GAD) a year ago and that he left his therapist because he could not tolerate exposure response prevention treatments.

Henry is the eldest of two children, and, as a young boy, he was often left to take care of his brother who is physically disabled. Henry married his wife, Miranda, when he was 24, and he and Miranda have a two-year-old toddler.

Henry co-owns a fine dining restaurant in the city with Ron. He experienced his first panic attack in his new restaurant when Miranda started her medical residency approximately five months ago. Since that time, Miranda has been less available to Henry during evening hours. Henry has difficulty asserting and implementing his ideas and plans when Ron is around. Henry perceives Ron as contrary and, at times, aggressive towards him. His hesitation to assert his needs during planning time for the restaurant irritates Ron, and he fears that Ron will leave him and that he will not be able to cope with managing the restaurant by himself. Related to his distress about communicating with Ron, Henry has had several panic attacks. During one of his panic attacks, he was rushed by ambulance to the hospital because he said that he felt heart palpitations, experienced shallow breathing, and feared that he was having a heart attack. After several tests, the cardiologist at the hospital reassured Henry that his symptoms were not related to his heart.

After the incident at the hospital, Henry's panic attacks escalated, Miranda suggested that Henry see a therapist, and Henry made an appointment with a therapist suggested by a former mentor. The crisis phase offers a therapist an opportunity to begin the integrative approach with an active attempt to help the patient cope with pressing symptoms by reliance on psychoeducation and CBT methods (Scaturo, 1994). At the beginning, the therapist worked on developing trust within the context of the therapeutic relationship and referred Henry to a cardiologist to address Henry's pressing physiological symptoms, e.g., heart palpitations. The cardiologist reassured Henry that he did not have a disorder of the heart and communicated with Henry's therapist. At Henry's request, the therapist referred him to a psychiatrist for medication. Henry mentioned to the psychiatrist that he felt comfortable taking the medication and getting some relief from his symptoms. When Henry felt reassured that his symptoms could be attributed to psychological issues rather than to his heart, he felt ready to continue.

Treatment with cognitive-behavioral therapy has been shown to correct the cortical abnormalities associated with panic disorder and to decrease the activity in the hippocampus, anterior cingulate, and cerebellum of individuals with panic disorder (Busch et al., 2010; Sakai et al., 2006). At the beginning, Henry seemed to have difficulty with some of the CBT techniques. He did not respond well to the aforementioned approach, and, after a few weeks, in no uncertain terms, he decided to refuse CBT interventions. At the same time, Henry expressed to the therapist that he enjoyed participating in the assertiveness training exercises that the therapist taught him.

Rather than insist on continuing CBT methods with Henry, the therapist continued with the assertiveness training, but shifted gears, introduced hypnotherapy, and Henry seemed more receptive. The hypnotherapy portion of the treatment continued for four months. At this point, Henry consented to a trial of CBT methods. The therapist combined hypnotherapy with CBT and was able to teach Henry several CBT methods along with applied relaxation techniques. Henry reported that he was feeling more comfortable, and the therapist treated Henry with CBT methods, e.g., imaginal and in vivo exposure, every week over a seven month period.

Approximately, two months after Henry began therapy, the therapist learned that Henry's wife, Miranda, had been experiencing a lot of stress over difficulties she had been having with her medical residency. While continuing with a combination of hypnotherapy with CBT as well as applied relaxation methods for Henry, the therapist referred Henry to a couples therapist with Miranda.

Henry was pleased to go with Miranda to couples therapy. During the CBT phase of couples therapy, Miranda learned to be supportive to Henry as he attempted to cope with his symptoms of panic and work on his behavioral exercises. Henry, in turn, reciprocated by being more understanding about Miranda's stressors during her residency, and the couple decided to speak to each other on the phone once or twice during the evening when Miranda was at work. Both Henry and Miranda benefited during couples therapy from CBT exercises.

Whereas Henry's panic attacks became less frequent and were not as intense after seven months of individual and couples therapy, Henry was not symptom free. The couple wished to continue with couples therapy, and, at the same time, Henry's individual therapist considered the need to shift gears from CBT work with a focus on symptoms towards a psychodynamic approach that relied on Busch and colleagues' (2010) integrated psychoanalytic/neurobiological psychotherapy model.

During individual psychodynamic therapy, the therapist helped Henry to become aware of the connection between his current perception of Ron as antagonistic to him and his past experience of feeling angry when he was left alone as a child to provide care for his physically disabled and hostile brother while he missed out on childhood activities with his friends. In both situations, Henry perceived that others were aggressive to him, and he felt like he was choking. It was only recently, in therapy, that he became aware of his anger related to feeling stuck and having missed out on childhood opportunities. Without being assertive about communicating his ideas and plans about the restaurant to Ron along with his difficulty in relating his needs to Miranda, Henry was at risk of further irritating Ron and Miranda. When the therapist helped Henry to get in touch with his unconscious needs, he began to feel less like he needed to escape, and he more easily was able to assert himself both at work with Ron and at home with Miranda.

It was revealed during the psychodynamic part of treatment that when Henry was six years old, his father was injured at work, and he could not return to his employment for several years. Henry's father was absent for long periods of time for treatment for fractures at the local hospital. During psychodynamic therapy, Henry became aware of how his present situation, when Miranda returned home at two in the morning for nights at a time when she was on call as a resident, was similar to his past situation when he was left alone for long periods when Henry's father was in the hospital. Being left alone contributed to Henry's feelings of panic, and during individual psychodynamic therapy, he began to recognize how difficult it was for him to be by himself for long periods of time without speaking to Miranda.

Henry reported that his close friend passed away a year ago after a hit-and-run driver left the scene of the accident as his friend was walking across a street near his home. During psychodynamic therapy, Henry explored the recent trauma of losing his close friend, and he began to understand that the effects of this recent tragedy coupled with Miranda's added stressors and involvement at work during the evening as she embarked upon her residency increased his propensity towards panic as he associated current feelings of being left unsupported with past feelings that he experienced as a child when left without his father for long periods of time. During the psychodynamic portion of the therapy, Henry became armed with new insights related to the intersecting themes of attachment, feeling stuck, and panic, and Henry's panic began to subside as he renewed his commitment to work on new behavioral exercises in couples therapy.

After another six months of therapy, Henry felt that he no longer needed to take medication, rarely experienced panic, and he visited the psychiatrist who discontinued pharmacotherapy. Henry and Miranda decided that they had learned how to support each other, and that they no longer needed couples therapy.

Henry, however, decided to continue in individual psychodynamic therapy to work on issues related to impaired attachment and maladaptive interpersonal skills linked to difficulties with assertiveness, which Henry needed to implement both at work and at home. Henry continued in psychodynamic treatment and worked on assertiveness training for another two years before he and the therapist discussed a mutually agreed-upon termination process.

References

Aaronson, C. J., Shear, M. K., Goetz, R. R., Allen, L. B., Barlow, D. H., White, K. S., ... Gorman, J. M. (2008). Predictors and time course of response among panic disorder patients treated with cognitive-behavioral therapy. *Journal of Clinical Psychiatry, 69*(3), 418–424. doi: 10.4088/jcp.v69n0312

Alexander, B., Feigelson, S., & Gorman, J. M. (2005). Integrating the psychoanalytic and neurobiological views of panic disorder. *Neuropsychoanalysis*, 7(2), 129–141. doi: 10.1080/15294145.2005.10773485

Alladin, A. (2014). The wounded self: New approach to understanding and treating anxiety disorders. *American Journal of Clinical Hypnosis, 56*(4), 368–388. doi: 10.1080/00029157.2014.880045

Allen, L. B., White, K. S., Barlow, D. H., Shear, M. K., Gorman, J. M., & Woods, S. W. (2010). Cognitive-behavior therapy (CBT) for panic disorder: Relationship of anxiety and depression comorbidity with treatment outcome. *Journal of Psychopathology and Behavioral Assessment, 32*(2), 185–192. doi: 10.1007/s10862-009-9151-3

Allgulander, C., Dahl, A. A., Austin, C., Morris, P. L., Sogaard, J. A., Fayyad, R., ... Clary, C. M. (2004). Efficacy of sertraline in a 12-week trial for generalized anxiety disorder. *American Journal of Psychiatry, 161*(9), 1642–1649. doi: 10.1176/appi.ajp.161.9.1642

American Psychiatric Association. (2013). *Diagnostic and statistical manual of mental disorders* (5th ed.). Washington, DC: Author.

Barlow, D. H. (1988). *Anxiety and its disorders: The nature and treatment of anxiety and panic.* New York, NY: Guilford Press.

Barlow, D. H. (2000). Unraveling the mysteries of anxiety and its disorders from the perspective of emotion theory. *American Psychologist, 55*(11), 1247–1263. doi: 10.1037/0003-066X.55.11.1247

Barlow, D. H. (2002). *Anxiety and its disorders: The nature and treatment of anxiety and panic* (2nd ed.). New York, NY: Guilford Press.

Barlow, D. H. (2004). *Anxiety and its disorders: The nature and treatment of anxiety and panic* (2nd ed.). New York, NY: Guilford Press.

Barlow, D. H., Farchione, T. J., Bullis, J. R., Gallagher, M. W., Murray-Latin, H., Sauer-Zavala, S., ... Cassiello-Robbins, C. (2017). The unified protocol for transdiagnostic treatment of emotional disorders compared with diagnosis-specific protocols for anxiety disorders: A randomized clinical trial. *JAMA Psychiatry, 74*(9), 875–884. doi: 10.1001/jamapsychiatry.2017.2164

Barlow, D. H., Gorman, J. M., Shear, M. K., & Woods, S. (2000). Cognitive-behavioral therapy, imipramine, or their combination for panic disorder: A randomized controlled trial. *JAMA, 283*(19), 2529–2536. doi: 10.1001/jama.283.19.2529

Beekman, A. T., Bremmer, M. A., Deeg, D. J., van Balkom, A. J., Smit, J. H., de Beurs, E., ... van Tilburg, W. (1998). Anxiety disorders in later life: A report from the Longitudinal Aging Study Amsterdam. *International Journal of Geriatric Psychiatry, 13*(10), 717–726. doi: 10.1002/(sici)1099-1166(1998100)13:10<717::aid-gps857>3.0.co;2-m

Beutel, M. E., Greenberg, L., Lane, R. D., & Subic-Wrana, C. (2019). Treating anxiety disorders by emotion-focused psychodynamic psychotherapy (EFPP)-an integrative, transdiagnostic approach. *Clinical Psychology and Psychotherapy, 26*(1), 1–13. doi: 10.1002/cpp.2325

Beutel, M. E., Scheurich, V., Knebel, A., Michal, M., Wiltink, J., Graf-Morgenstern, M., ... Subic-Wrana, C. (2013). Implementing panic-focused psychodynamic psychotherapy into clinical practice. *The Canadian Journal of Psychiatry, 58*(6), 326–334. doi: 10.1177/070674371305800604

Boettcher, H., & Conklin, L. R. (2018). Transdiagnostic assessment and case formulation: Rationale and application with the unified protocol. In D. H. Barlow & T. J. Farchione (Eds.), *Applications of the unified protocol for transdiagnostic treatment of emotional disorders* (pp. 17–37). New York, NY: Oxford University Press.

Bowlby, J. (1973). *Attachment and loss, Vol. 2. Separation*. New York, NY: Basic Books.

Brown, T. A., & Barlow, D. H. (2009). A proposal for a dimensional classification system based on the shared features of the DSM-IV anxiety and mood disorders: Implications for assessment and treatment. *Psychological Assessment, 21*(3), 256–271.

Brown, T. A., Campbell, L. A., Lehman, C. L., Grishman, J. R., & Mancill, R. B. (2001). Current and life- time comorbidity of the DSM-IV anxiety and mood disorders in a large clinical sample. *Journal of Abnormal Psychology, 110*(4), 585–599.

Busch, F. N., Cooper, A. M., Klerman, G. L., Penzer, R. J., Shapiro, T., & Shear, M., L. (1991). Neurophysiological, cognitive-behavioral and psychoanalytic approaches to panic disorder: Toward an integration. *Psychoanalytic Inquiry, 11*: 316–332.

Busch, F. N., Oquendo, M. A., Sullivan, G. M., & Sandberg, L. S. (2010). An integrated model of panic disorder. *Neuropsychoanalysis, 12*(1), 67–79. doi: 10.1080/15294145.2010.10773631

Charney, M. E., Kredlow, M. A., Bui, E., & Simon, N. M. (2013). Panic disorder. In S. M. Stahl & B. A. Moore (Eds.), *Anxiety disorders: A guide for integrating psychopharmacology and psychotherapy* (pp. 201–220). New York, NY: Routledge.

Comer, R. J. (2015). *Abnormal psychology*. New York, NY: Worth Publisher.

Craske, M. G., & Waters, A. M. (2005). Panic disorder, phobias, and generalized anxiety disorder. *Annual Review of Clinical Psychology, 1*, 197–225. doi: 10.1146/annurev.clinpsy.1.102803.143857

Driessen, E., Hollon, S. D., Bockting, C. L., Cuijpers, P., & Turner, E. H. (2015). Does publication bias inflate the apparent efficacy of psychological treatment for major depressive disorder? A systematic review and meta-analysis of U.S. National Institutes of Health-funded trials. *PLoS ONE, 10*(9), e0137864. doi: 10.1371/journal.pone.0137864

Dyck, R. V., & Spinhoven, P. (1997). Does preference for treatment matter? A study of exposure in vivo with or without hypnosis in the treatment of panic disorder with agoraphobia. *Behavior Modification, 21*(2), 172–186. doi: 10.1177/01454455970212003

Faravelli, C. (1985). Life events preceding the onset of panic disorder. *Journal of Affective Disorders, 9*(1), 103–105. doi: 10.1176/ajp.143.11.1424

Faravelli, C., & Pallanti, S. (1989). Recent life events and panic disorder. *American Journal of Psychiatry, 146*(5), 622–626. doi: 10.1176/ajp.146.5.622

Fredette, C., El-Baalbaki, G., Neron, S., & Palardy, V. (2013). *Using hypnosis in the treatment of anxiety disorders: Pros and cons.* In F. Durbano (Ed.), New insights into anxiety disorders (pp. 343–377). InTech. doi: 10.5772/53768

Fyer, A. J., Hamilton, S. P., Durner, M., Haghighi, F., Heiman, G. A., Costa, R., … Knowles, J. A. (2006). A third-pass genome scan in panic disorder: Evidence for multiple susceptibility loci. *Biological Psychiatry, 60*(4), 388–401. doi: 10.1016/j.biopsych.2006.04.018

Gorman, J. M. (2016). Combining psychodynamic psychotherapy and pharmacotherapy. *Psychodynamic Psychiatry, 44*(2), 183–209. doi: 10.1521/pdps.2016.44.2.183

Gorman, J. M., Kent, J. M., Sullivan, G. M., & Coplan, J. D. (2000). Neuroanatomical hypothesis of panic disorder, revised. *American Journal of Psychiatry, 157*(4), 493–505. doi: 10.1176/appi.ajp.157.4.493

Graeff, F., & Del-Ben, C. (2008). Neurobiology of panic disorder. From animal models to brain neuroimaging. *Neuroscience and Biobehavioral Review, 32*(7), 1326–1335. doi: 10.1016/j.neubiorev.2008.05.017

Greene, A. M., Bailey, C. R., & Neumeister, A. (2013). A biopsychosocial approach to anxiety. In S. M. Stahl & B. A. Moore (Eds.), *Anxiety disorders: A guide for integrating psychopharmacology and psychotherapy* (pp. 25–50). New York, NY: Routledge.

Goldenberg, I., & Goldenberg, H. (1980). *Family therapy. An overview.* Monterey, CA: Brooks/Cole.

Hales, R. E., Yudofsky, S. C., & Gabbard, G. O. (2011). *Essentials of psychiatry* (3rd ed.). Arlington, VA: American Psychiatric Publishing.

Haug, T., Nordgreen, T., Öst, L.-G., Tangen, T., Kvale, G., Hovland, O. J., … Havik, O. E. (2016). Working alliance and competence as predictors of outcome in cognitive behavioral therapy for social anxiety and panic disorder in adults. *Behaviour Research and Therapy*, 77, 40–51. doi: 10.1016/j.brat.2015.12.004

Henn, F. (2013). Using brain imaging to understand the response to cognitive therapy in panic disorder. *American Journal of Psychology, 170*(11), 1235–1236. doi: 10.1176/appi.ajp.2013.13081135

Hettema, J. M., Neale, M. C., & Kendler, K. S. (2001). A review and meta-analysis of the genetic epidemiology of anxiety disorders. *American Journal of Psychiatry, 158*(10), 1568–1578. doi: 10.1176/appi.ajp.158.10.1568

Ingersoll, R. E., & Marquis, A. (2014). *Understanding psychopathology: An integral exploration.* Upper Saddle River, NJ: Pearson Education.

Kaunonen, M., Päivi, A.-K., Paunonen, M., & Erjanti, H. (2000). Death in the Finnish family: Experiences of spousal bereavement. *International Journal of Nursing Practice, 6*(3), 127–134. doi: 10.1046/j.1440-172x.2000.00189.x

Kennedy, K. A., & Barlow, D. (2018). The unified treatment for transdiagnostic treatment of emotional disorders: An introduction. In D. H. Barlow & T. J. Farchione (Eds.), *Applications of the unified protocol for transdiagnostic treatment of emotional disorders* (pp. 1–16). New York, NY: Oxford University Press.

Kessler, R. C., Berglund, P., Demler, O., Jin, R., Merikangas, K. R., & Walters, E. E. (2005). Lifetime prevalence and age-of-onset distributions of DSM-IV disorders in the National Comorbidity Survey Replication. *Archives of General Psychiatry, 62*, 593–602. doi: 10.1001/archpsyc.62.6.593.

Kessler, R. C., Chiu, W. T., Demler, O., Walters, E. E., & Walters, E. E. (2005). Prevalence, severity, and comorbidity of 12-month DSM-IV disorders in the National Comorbidity Survey Replication. *Archives of General Psychiatry, 62*(6), 617–627. doi: 10.1001/archpsyc.62.6.617

Klein, D. F. (1964). Delineation of two drug-responsive anxiety syndromes. *Psychopharmacologia, 5*, 397–408. doi: 10.1007/BF02193476

Klein, D. F. (1993). False suffocation alarms, spontaneous panics, and related conditions: An integrative hypothesis. *Archives of General Psychiatry, 50*(4), 306–317. doi: 10.1001/archpsyc.1993.01820160076009

Klein, D. F., & Fink, M. (1962). Psychiatric reaction patterns to imipramine. *American Journal of Psychiatry, 119*, 432–438. doi: 10.1176/ajp.119.5.432

Kossowsky, J., Pfaltz, M. C., Schneider, S., Taeymans, J., Locher, C., & Gaab, J. (2013). The separation anxiety hypothesis of panic disorder revisited: A meta-analysis. *American Journal of Psychiatry, 170*(7), 768–781. doi: 10.1176/appi.ajp.2012.12070893

Leichsenring, F., Leweke, F., Klein, S., & Steinert, C. (2015). The empirical status of psychodynamic psychotherapy—An update: Bambi's alive and kicking. *Psychotherapy and Psychosomatics, 84*(3), 129–148. doi: 10.1159/000376584

Leichsenring, F., & Salzer, S. (2014). A unified protocol for the transdiagnostic psychodynamic treatment of anxiety disorders: An evidence-based approach. *Psychotherapy, 51*(2), 224–245. doi: 10.1037/a0033815

Levine, D. S., Himle, J. A., Taylor, R. J., Abelson, J. M., Matusko, N., Muroff, J., & Jackson, J. (2013). Panic disorder among African Americans, Caribbean blacks and non-Hispanics whites. *Social Psychiatry and Psychiatric Epidemiology, 48*(5), 711–723.

Marcus, S. M., Gorman, J., Shear, M. K., Lewin, D., Martinez, J., Ray, S., … Woods, S. (2007). A comparison of medication side effect reports by panic disorder patients with and without concomitant cognitive behavior therapy. *American Journal of Psychiatry, 164*(2), 273–275.

Marks, I. M., Swinson, R. P., Başoğlu, M., Kuch, K., Noshirvani, H., O'Sullivan, G., … Wickwire, K. (1993). Alprazolam and exposure alone and combined in panic disorder with agoraphobia: A controlled study in London and Toronto. *The British Journal of Psychiatry, 162*(6), 776–787. doi: 10.1192/bjp.162.6.776

McGinn, L. K., Nooner, K. B., Cohen, J., & Leaberry, K. D. (2015). The role of early experience and cognitive vulnerability: Presenting a unified model of the etiology of panic. *Cognitive Therapy and Research, 39*(4), 508–519. doi: 10.1007/s10608-015-9673-9

Meuret, A. E., Rosenfield, D., Seidel, A., Bhaskara, L., & Hofmann, S. G. (2010). Respiratory and cognitive mediators of treatment change in panic disorder: Evidence for intervention specificity. *Journal of Consulting and Clinical Psychology, 78*(5), 691–704. doi: 10.1037/a0019552.

Milrod, B., Leon, A. C., Busch, F., Rudden, M., Schwalberg, M., Clarkin, J., … Shear, M. K. (2007). A randomized controlled clinical trial of psychoanalytic psychotherapy for panic disorder. *American Journal of Psychiatry, 164*(2), 265–272. doi: 10.1176/ajp.2007.164.2.265

Miniati, M., Calugi, S., Rucci, P., Shear, M. K., Benvenuti, A., Santoro, D., ... Cassano, G. B. (2012). Predictors of response among patients with panic disorder treated with medications in a naturalistic follow-up: The role of adult separation anxiety. *Journal of Affective Disorders, 136*(3), 675–679. doi: 10.1016/j.jad.2011.10.008

Muse, M. D., Moore, B. A., & Stahl, S. M. (2013). Benefits and challenges of integrative treatment. In S. M. Stahl & B. A. Moore (Eds.), *Anxiety disorders: A guide for integrating psychopharmacology and psychotherapy* (pp. 3–24). New York, NY: Routledge.

Nash, J. R., Sargent, P. A., Rabiner, E. A., Hood, S. D., Argyropoulos, S. V., Potokar, J. P., … Nutt, D. J. (2008). Serotonin 5-HT 1A receptor binding in people with panic disorder: Positron emission tomography study. *The British Journal of Psychiatry, 193*(3), 229–234. doi: 10.1192/bjp.bp.107.041186

Neumeister, A., Bain, E., Nugent, A. C., Carson, R. E., Bonne, O., Luckenbaugh, D. A., … Drevets, W. C. (2004). Reduced serotonin type 1A receptor binding in panic disorder. *Journal of Neuroscience, 24*(3), 589–591. doi: 10.1523/JNEUROSCI.4921-03.2004

Panksepp, J. (1998). *Affective neuroscience: The foundations of human and animal emotions*. New York, NY: Oxford University Press.

Panksepp, J. (2005). Commentary on "integrating the psychoanalytic and neurobiological views of panic disorder." *Neuropsychoanalysis*, 7(2), 145–150. doi: 10.1080/15294145.2005.10773490

Paus, T., Keshavan, K., & Giedd, J. N. (2008). Why do many psychiatric disorders emerge during adolescence? *Nature Reviews: Neuroscience, 9*(12), 947–957. doi: 10.1038/nrn2513

Pohl, R. B., Wolkow, R. M., & Clary, C. M. (1998). Sertraline in the treatment of panic disorder: A double-blind multicenter trial. *American Journal of Psychiatry, 155*(9), 1189–1195. doi: 10.1176/ajp.155.9.1189

Pollack, M. H. (2005). The pharmacotherapy of panic disorder. *Journal of Clinical Psychiatry, 66*(4) Suppl. 4, 23–27.

Pollack, M. H., Simon, N. M., Worthington, J. J., Doyle, A. L., Peters, P., Toshkov, F., & Otto, M. W. (2003). Combined paroxetine and clonazepam treatment strategies compared to paroxetine monotherapy for panic disorder. *Journal of Psychopharmacology, 17*(3), 276–282. doi: 10.1177/02698811030173009

Pyke, R. E., & Greenberg, H. S. (1986). Norepinephrine challenges in panic patients. *Journal of Clinical Psychopharmacology, 6*(5), 279–285. doi: 10.1097/00004714-198610000-00004

Ray, W. J. (2018). *Abnormal psychology*. Thousand Oaks, CA: Sage.

Redmond, D. E. (1977). Alterations in the function of the nucleus locus coeruleus: A possible model for studies of anxiety. In I. Hanin & E. Usdin (Eds.), *Animal models in psychiatry and neurology* (pp. 293–306). New York, NY: Pergamon Press.

Redmond, D. E. (1981). Clonidine and the primate locus coeruleus: Evidence suggesting anxiolytic and anti-withdrawal effects. In H. Lal & S. Fielding (Eds.), *Psychopharmacology of clonidine* (pp. 147–168). New York, NY: Alan R. Liss.

Redmond, D. E. (1985). Neurochemical basis for anxiety and anxiety disorders: Evidence from drugs which decrease human fear or anxiety. In A. H. Tuma & J. Maser (Eds.), *Anxiety and the anxiety disorders* (pp. 533–555). Hillsdale, NJ: Lawrence Erlbaum.

Reiss, S., & McNally, R. J. (1985). Expectancy model of fear. In S. Reiss & R. R. Bootzin (Eds.), *Theoretical issues in behavior therapy* (pp. 107–122). New York, NY: Academic Press.

Ruscio, A. M., Borkovec, T. D., & Ruscio, J. (2001). A taxometric investigation of the latent structure of worry. *Journal of Abnormal Psychology, 110*(3), 413–422. doi: 10.1037//0021-843x.110.3.413

Sakai, Y., Kumano, H., Nishikawa, M., Sakano, Y., Kaiya, H., Imabayashi, E., … & Kuboki, T. (2006). Changes in cerebral glucose utilization in patients with panic disorder treated with cognitive–behavioral therapy. *Neuroimage, 33*(1), 218–226. doi: 10.1016/j.neuroimage.2006.06.017

Scaturo, D. J. (1994). Integrative psychotherapy for panic disorder and agoraphobia in clinical practice. *Journal of Psychotherapy Integration*, *4*(3), 253–272. doi: 10.1037/h0101261

Shear, M. K., Cooper, A. M., Klerman, G. L., Busch, F. N., & Shapiro, T. (1993). A psychodynamic model of panic disorder. *American Journal of Psychiatry*, *150*(6), 859–866. doi: 10.1176/ajp.150.6.859

Singh, A. R., & Banerjee, K. R. (2002). Treating panic attack with hypnosis in combination with rational emotive therapy--A case report. *Journal of Projective Psychology and Mental Health*, *9*(2), 105–108.

Sweeney, R. M., Levitt, J., Westerholm, R., Gaskins, C., & Lipinski, C. (2013). Psychosocial treatment of anxiety disorders across the lifespan. In S. M. Stahl & B. A. Moore (Eds.), *Anxiety disorders: A guide for integrating psychopharmacology and psychotherapy* (pp. 71–93). New York, NY: Routledge.

Swift, J. K., Greenberg, R. P., Tompkins, K. A., & Parkin, S. R. (2017). Treatment refusal and premature termination in psychotherapy, pharmacotherapy, and their combination: A meta-analysis of head-to-head comparisons. *Psychotherapy*, *54*(1), 47–57. doi: 10.1037/pst0000104

Targum, S. D., & Marshall, L. E. (1989). Fenfluramine provocation of anxiety in patients with panic disorder. *Psychiatry Research*, *28*(3), 295–306. doi: 10.1016/0165-1781(89)90210-2

Taylor, S., & Asmundson, G. J. G. (2016). Panic disorder and agoraphobia. In A. Carr, A. & M. McNulty (Eds.), *The handbook of adult clinical psychology: An evidence based practice approach* (2nd ed., pp. 467–491). New York, NY: Routledge.

Tull, M. T., & Roemer, L. (2007). Emotion regulation difficulties associated with the experience of uncued panic attacks: Evidence of experiential avoidance, emotional nonacceptance, and decreased emotional clarity. *Behavior Therapy*, *38*(4), 378–391. doi: 10.1016/j.beth.2006.10.006

Verburg, K., Griez, E., Meijer, J., & Pols, H. (1995). Respiratory disorders as a possible predisposing factor for disorder. *Journal of Affective Disorders*, *33*(2), 129–134. doi: 10.1016/0165-0327(94)00083-L

Wolfe, B. E. (2003). Integrative psychotherapy of the anxiety disorders. In J. C. Norcross & M. R. Goldfried (Eds.), *Handbook of psychotherapy integration*. (2nd ed., pp. 263–280). New York, NY: Oxford University Press.

Wolfe, B. E. (2005). *Understanding and treating anxiety disorders: An integrative approach to healing the wounded self.* Washington, DC: American Psychological Association.

Wolfe, B. E. (2008). Existential issues in anxiety disorders and their treatment. In K. I. Schneider (Ed.), *Existential-integrative psychotherapy* (pp. 204–216). New York, NY: Routledge.

Wolfe, B. E., & Sigl, P. (1998). Experiential psychotherapy of the anxiety disorders. In L. S. Greenberg J. C. Watson & G. Lietaer (Eds.), *Handbook of experiential psychotherapy* (pp. 272–294). New York, NY: Guilford Press.

Wolitzky-Taylor, K. B., Castriotta, N., Lenze, E. J., Stanley, M. A., & Craske, M. G. (2010). Anxiety disorders in older adults: A comprehensive review. *Depression and Anxiety*, *27*(2), 190–211. doi: 10.1002/da.20653

Woodward, A. T., Taylor, R. J., Bullard, K. M., Aranda, M. P., Lincoln, K. D., & Chatters, L. M. (2012). Prevalence of life-time DSM-IV affective disorders among older African Americans, Black Carribeans, Latinos, Asians and non-Hispanic White people. *International Journal of Geriatric Psychiatry*, *27*(8), 816–827. doi: 10.1002/gps.2790

7 Phobias

Social Anxiety Disorder (SAD) (Social Phobia) and Specific Phobia (SP)

Introduction

Chapter 7 discusses the integrated and unified etiology approaches and psychotherapy treatment models for social anxiety disorder (SAD) (social phobia) and specific phobia (SP) (see Table 7.1). The first case study demonstrates the use of Magnavita and Anchin's (2014) unifying psychotherapy model for social anxiety, and the second case study employs an integrated psychotherapy approach that relies on Wolfe's (2006) integrative self-wound approach and incorporates Gold's (1993) model for specific phobias that derives from attachment theory (Bowlby, 1980; Guidano, 1987).

Are some anxiety disorders more common than others? Social anxiety disorder (SAD) or social phobia is the most common of the anxiety disorders and presents a substantial emotional health concern (Bener, Ghuloum, & Dafeeah, 2011; Ingersoll & Marquis, 2014; Kessler et al., 1994). SAD is a large concern because it can lead to impairment in social and employment situations (Wong, Sarver, & Beidel, 2012).

Symptoms of Social Anxiety Disorder (SAD) (Social Phobia)

What are the symptoms of social anxiety disorder (SAD) or social phobia? Note that this disorder is now referred to as social anxiety disorder (SAD) since it has replaced the term, social phobia (Ray, 2018). According to the *Diagnostic and Statistical Manual of Mental Disorders, 5th edition* (DSM-5), individuals with social anxiety disorder may have enduring anxiety about participating in social activities, intense trepidations about their performance, and they are fearful that other individuals are evaluating them (American Psychiatric Association, 2013). The following are two kinds of social phobia: (1) Generalized (where patients are afraid of most social contexts, and (2) specific (where patients are frightened about a specific situation, e.g., speaking in front of others) (Fredette et al., 2013). The aforementioned conceptualization is consistent with Fraser (2018) who views social anxiety disorder as distress that is confined to a restricted range of scenarios, e.g., speaking in public, but frequently, the fear extends

Table 7.1 Social Anxiety Disorder (SAD) (Social Phobia) and Specific Phobia (SP)

Etiology	*Integrated/Unified Therapy*	*Etiology*	*Integrated/Unified Therapy*
Social Anxiety	Social Anxiety	Specific Phobia	Specific Phobia
Shame and Separation Anxiety[a,b]	An Integrated Cognitive-Behavioral (CBT) and Interpersonal Model[i,j,k]	The Interaction Between Learning Theory and Biology[p,q]	An Integrative Attachment Framework[s,t,u]
An Integrative Self-Wounds Framework[c]	An Assimilative Integrative Approach[l]	Integrative Theory and Self-Wounds[c,r]	A Transtheoretical Integration Model[v]
A View from a Neuroscientific Window	An Integrated Treatment: Cognitive-Behavioral Hypnotherapy (CBH)[m]		A Self-Wound Framework and a Focusing Technique[w,r,x]
Amygdala[d], Insula[e,f,g]			
An Integrated Aetiological and Maintenance Model[h]	A Transdiagnostic Unified Protocol[n,o]		

[a]Gabbard (1992). [b]Leichsenring and Salzer (2014). [c]Wolfe (2005). [d]Birbaumer et al. (1998). [e]Miskovic and Schmidt (2012). [f]Ray (2018). [g]Tillfors et al. (2001). [h]Wong and Rapee (2016). [i]Lipsitz (2012). [j]Macarthur (2013). [k]Newman, Castonguay, Borkovec, Fisher, and Nordberg, (2008). [l]Macarthur (2013). [m] Schoenberger, Kirsch, Gearan, Montgomery, and Pastyrnak (1997). [n]Barlow et al. (2017). [o]Kennedy and Barlow (2018). [p]Antony and Barlow (2002). [q] Shearer, Harmon, Younger, and Brown (2013). [r]Wolfe (2006). [s]Bowlby (1980). [t]Gold (1993). [u]Guidano (1987). [v]Prochaska and DiClemente (2005). [w]Wolfe (2003). [x]Wolfe and Sigl (1998).

to broader social contexts such as parties. Individuals with social phobia may fear being exposed as imposters, may be afraid that they will appear as lower in front of others, their own feelings of humiliation related to their perceived inadequacy overwhelm them, and it seems easier to have a panic attack than to confront their own painful affect related to humiliation (Wolfe, 2003, 2008). The social fear symptoms of these individuals can have a negative impact on their school, job, and social activities, and largely decrease their quality of life (Aderka et al., 2012; Forstner et al., 2017).

Diagnosis of Social Anxiety Disorder (SAD) or Social Phobia

Individuals with social anxiety disorder (SAD) (social phobia) often have an unbalanced concern about social situations as they tend to perceive evaluation from others when, in reality, it may not occur (APA, 2013). To receive a diagnosis of SAD, an individual's symptoms need to ensue for a period of six months or longer (APA, 2013). Individuals with this disorder are frequently hypervigilant in their perception of negative reviews from others, and their hypervigilance may result in difficulties in performance (Fraser, 2018). Often individuals with SAD feel shame in social situations, and they experience anxiety about and tend to avoid social events (APA, 2013; Shahar, Bar-Kalifa, & Alon, 2017).

Prevalence of Social Anxiety Disorder (SAD) or Social Phobia

Prevalence

What is the prevalence rate of social anxiety disorder (SAD)? The lifetime prevalence rate of social anxiety disorder has been reported to be approximately 12% (Kessler et al., 2005). More recently, the prevalence of social anxiety disorder was reported as a range from approximately 3% to 13% (Fredette et al., 2013). According to the DSM-5, the 12-month prevalence for the U.S. is estimated at around 7% (APA, 2013).

Onset

When does social anxiety disorder begin? Social anxiety disorder can begin when individuals are older children or adolescents, and this disorder may persist when they are adults (Comer, 2015; Ray, 2018;). Although the rates of occurrence for social anxiety disorder are the most elevated when individuals are children and adolescents (Beesdo et al., 2007; Wittchen, Stein, Kessler, 1999), after age 52, social anxiety disorder will develop in fewer than 1% of people (Kessler et al., 2005; Wolitzky-Taylor, Castriotta, Lenze, Stanley, & Craske, 2010).

Social anxiety disorder tends to occur more frequently in different populations. For example, more women have been found to have social anxiety disorder than men (APA, 2013; Ray, 2018), and researchers have found that Hispanics have a lower lifetime prevalence rate for this disorder than do African Americans and Whites (Cohen et al., 2017; Morreale, Tancer, & Uhde, 2010). There are some disorders found in other parts of the world that appear to be similar to social anxiety disorder. For example, the disorder, "*taijin kyofusho*," frequently found in Japan and Korea, refers to a fear about triggering discomfort in other individuals; however, today, clinicians are of the opinion that those with this disorder are overly concerned about hearing negative comments about themselves from others (Comer, 2015).

Heritability and Comorbidity

To what degree is social anxiety heritable, is there a relationship between a specific gene and social anxiety disorder, and which emotional disorders can accompany social anxiety disorder? Social anxiety disorder is somewhat heritable; however, with respect to genetic factors affecting the development of the disorder, genetic investigations are not common, and only a few genes are implicated (Forstner et al., 2017). In their investigation of the contribution of genes to the development of anxiety, Forstner and colleagues (2017) reported a relationship between the rs140701 allele in SLC6A4, the serotonin transporter gene, and social anxiety disorder. The heritability of SAD ranges from approximately 20% to 50% (Kendler, Myers, Prescott, Neale, 2001; Skre et al., 2000). There is a partial overlap between the genetic risk for SAD and the risk for generalized anxiety disorder and between the genetic risk for SAD and the risk for panic disorder, and it has been suggested that there is an overlap that is genetic between the anxiety disorders themselves (Forstner, 2017; Hettema, Prescott, Myers, Neale, & Kendler, 2005; Jensen et al., 2014).

SAD frequently is accompanied by other anxiety disorders (Fehm, Pelissolo, Furmark, & Wittchen, 2005). For example, social anxiety disorder has been shown to have a high comorbidity rate with bipolar disorder (Merikangas et al., 2007; Queen, Donaldson, & Luiselli, 2015), with major depression (APA, 2013), and with substance abuse (APA, 2013).

An Integrative Etiology of Social Anxiety Disorder (SAD) (Social Phobia): Focus, Underpinnings, and Causes of SAD

This section discusses the etiology of social anxiety disorder (SAD) and explains how it is developed and maintained. It takes an integrative view of the etiology of social anxiety disorder, and presents examples of models that explain the etiology of the disorder from an integrative perspective.

Various factors affect the etiology of social anxiety disorder (SAD). SAD is a complex psychiatric disorder where environmental and genetic variables affect an individual's vulnerability to develop the disorder (Bandelow et al.,

2004). A core feature of social anxiety disorder is that it takes place in situations where an individual is noticed by others (Kariuki & Stein, 2013). Individuals with social anxiety disorder fear that they appear anxious, stupid, or that they may have insulted others (Kariuki & Stein, 2013). The underlying issue for individuals with SAD is fear of evaluation, and this evaluation can occur in social interactions, in situations where an individual can be observed, or when an individual is performing (Ray, 2018). Past experiences, e.g., negative social incidents experienced as a child, seem to play a more prominent role in individuals with social anxiety disorder than they do in individuals with other anxiety disorders, e.g., panic disorder and obsessive-compulsive disorder (McCabe & Antony, 2005; Ray, 2018). More recently, it has been found that the use of computers, e.g., social networking on Facebook, can trigger social anxiety (Comer, 2015; Smith, 2014). In short, individuals with social anxiety tend to avoid social interactions at all costs.

Shame, Separation Anxiety, and Social Anxiety Disorder (SAD)

How do the concepts of shame and separation anxiety contribute to the etiology of social anxiety disorder? Researchers found that shame and separation anxiety underlie the development of social anxiety disorder (Gabbard, 1992; Leichsenring & Salzer, 2014). In order to prevent or to protect against separation anxiety, the fear of losing another's acceptance and love, individuals with social anxiety disorder tend to avoid people in the world at large (Leichsenring & Salzer, 2014).

Self-Wounds and Social Anxiety Disorder (SAD)

Chapter 5 describes Wolfe's (2003) integrative etiological model for the anxiety disorders. When applied to social phobia, this integrative model can explain the beginning of a cycle for a child who experiences a high degree of critical behavior, chronic negative criticism that is not constructive, from a parent, particularly when the child reveals a weakness. According to Wolfe (2003), a child who is the target of chronically negative criticism adopts a severely poor view of the self by internalizing the harsh criticism, and experiences a feeling of a self-wound, accompanied by feelings of inadequacy or inferiority. Wolfe's (2003) integrative model predicts how settings that include public speaking or social situations may begin to generate a perception of self-endangerment, and the individual may begin to avoid the felt humiliation by experiencing a sense of anxiety or panic instead. The person's self-preoccupation with social constraints accompanied by perceived rejection from others ensues, and the vicious cycle ends with the individual's inability to navigate social situations (Wolfe, 2003). According to Wolfe's (2005) integrative framework, the origin of social phobia involves self-wounds associated with an individual's perception of the self as deficient. Wolfe (2006) explains that social phobia disorder is maintained by excessive cogitation, avoidance of social situations, and the management of impressions.

A View From a Neuroscientific Window: The Amygdala and Social Anxiety Disorder (SAD)

According to Barlow (2004), the etiology of social anxiety disorder can be attributed to an interaction between genetic, biological, psychological, and environmental variables. Chapters 5 and 6 delineated the brain circuits involved in generalized anxiety disorder and panic disorder. A physiological variable that is implicated in the etiology of social anxiety disorder is the amygdala (Birbaumer et al., 1998). For example, researchers found that in response to pictures of angry faces, the amygdala of persons with social anxiety disorder is activated, and the amount of activity in the amygdala has been found to be positively associated with the degree of social anxiety rather than with general anxiety (Phan, Fitzgerald, Nathan, & Tancer, 2006; Ray, 2018).

In addition to the excessive activation in the amygdala, another area of the brain that is implicated in social anxiety disorder is the insula (Miskovic & Schmidt, 2012; Ray, 2018; Tillfors et al., 2001). It is possible that the insula, a portion of the cerebral cortex, is overactive in individuals with social anxiety disorder (Ray, 2018).

An Integrated Aetiological and Maintenance Model (IAM) and Social Anxiety Disorder (SAD)

Are there integrated models that are evidence-based that can explain the etiology of social anxiety disorder (SAD)? Wong and Rapee (2016) developed an evidence-based integrated model that explains the etiology and maintenance of social anxiety disorder. This evidence-based integrated model, the integrated aetiological and maintenance (IAM) model, proposes that there is a "social-evaluative threat" principle, the SET principle, that explains the degree to which stimuli that are social-evaluative threaten a patient's daily living (Wong & Rapee, 2016, p. 87). According to their integrated model of social anxiety disorder, manifestations of this principle occur both on a neurobiological level and a cognitive level. For example, according to this model of social anxiety disorder, there exists a relationship between the SET principle and the amygdala. Results of fMRI investigations show that the SET principle manifests in a neurobiological way in that patients with social anxiety disorder, when compared to controls without SAD, display a higher degree of activity in the amygdala when confronted with social-evaluative material that is perceived as dangerous (Phan et al., 2006; Wong et al., 2016). The SET principle manifests in a cognitive way as well in that the cognitions or thoughts of individuals with SAD underscore that stimuli perceived as social-evaluative threaten the self (Wong & Rapee, 2016). Wong and Rapee (2016) explain that aetiological variables can affect the threat value itself. They offer examples of variables such as temperament, behaviors of parents, peer and life experiences, and culture, and suggest that duration, intensity, and timing of the variable can have an impact on the threat value. For example, they explain that if one of the variables or factors takes place during a sensitive time, it will have a higher impact on the threat value. In summary, the SET principle and its parts tend to create a self-continuing cycle that culminates in feelings of anxiety associated with settings that are social-evaluative, and the higher the threat value, the greater the tendency for an individual to be diagnosed with SAD (Wong & Rapee, 2016).

An Integrative Experiential Approach: Emotion-Schemes and Social Anxiety Disorder (SAD)

Chapter 5 discussed how emotion-schemes relate to generalized anxiety disorder. This section explains how emotion-schemes relate to social anxiety disorder. According to emotion-focused therapy (EFT) (Elliott, Watson, Goldman, & Greenberg, 2004), an integrative humanistic treatment framework, the etiology underlying social anxiety disorder includes the notion of emotion schemes (Elliot & Shahar, 2017). Dysfunctional emotion schemes, which emerge as a consequence of shaming or bullying during a time when the patient was a child or adolescent, can result in the patient's experience of interpersonal contacts as situations that involve threat where the patient may be exposed as socially impaired (Elliot & Shahar, 2017). For example, the patient's emotion scheme of a lack of trust signals the patient to engage in behaviors aimed at safety, e.g., rather than speaking spontaneously, an individual who prepares verbatim what to say in order to avoid rejection (Elliot & Shahar, 2017).

Summary

Symptoms of social anxiety disorder can include a broad range of fears, e.g., from speaking in front of others to eating and performing poorly in front of other individuals (Comer, 2015). This section concludes the portion on the etiology of integrated frameworks for social anxiety disorder (SAD). The next section discusses the connection between the development and maintenance of social anxiety disorder and integrated and unified treatment for social anxiety disorder (see Table 7.1).

Clinical Practice Applications of Integrated and Unified Psychotherapy Treatment Models for Social Anxiety Disorder (SAD) (Social Phobia)

How helpful are standard, unitary treatments for social anxiety disorder (SAD)? Individuals with SAD are not prone to seek treatment (Weiller et al., 1996). Whereas cognitive therapy has been shown to decrease patients' fears about social settings, social skills training rather than cognitive interventions have been found to assist patients to perform adequately in social settings (Comer, 2015; Kim, Parr, & Alfano, 2011; Sarver, Beidel, & Spitalnick, 2014). Exposure therapy, included in CBT, is a key treatment element for social anxiety (Heimberg, 2002). Although cognitive-behavioral therapy (CBT) has been shown to be highly effective for the treatment of social anxiety disorder, it is often limited in use by clinicians (McHugh, & Barlow, 2010; Shafran et al., 2009). It was found that therapists with lower levels of therapist competence deleteriously affect CBT treatment for social anxiety disorder (Haug et al., 2016). Other researchers have suggested that CBT does not help many individuals with social anxiety disorder (Hofmann & Bögels, 2006; Leichsenring et al., 2013; Moscovitch, 2009). Moscovitch (2009) recommends that rather than addressing the social situations that patients fear, exposure needs to address patients' self attributes. e.g., patients' perceptions of impairment in personality.

Can an integrative psychotherapy approach help patients with social anxiety disorder? The first therapist to propose integrative psychotherapy may have been Freud (1912) who asserted that a patient with social phobia (social anxiety) may be using psychoanalytic exploration of past interpersonal problems as an intellectualized defense, as a means to avoid enacting newly learned social behaviors, and there may be a point when an analyst needs to confront the patient with social phobia (social anxiety) to face the feared object, social situations (Stricker & Gold, 2005). At this point, a time for an assimilative shift, it is important for the therapist to recommend active treatment, e.g., social skills training accompanied by in vivo homework, so that the patient can learn to try fresh skills (Stricker & Gold, 2005). Stricker and Gold (2005) explain that a patient's resistance to an assimilative shift, e.g., to a cognitive, experiential, or behavioral treatment, might be avoided by an exploration of the psychodynamic meaning of the patient's social anxiety symptoms for which the aforementioned assimilative integrative treatment techniques are planned. Research has demonstrated that cognitive-behavioral therapists integrated more than did psychodynamic therapists and that cognitive-behaviors therapists used a greater degree of treatment of a psychodynamic type than psychodynamic therapists used treatment of a cognitive-behavioral nature (Leichsenring et al., 2013).

An Integrated Cognitive-Behavioral (CBT) and Interpersonal Model for Social Anxiety Disorder (SAD)

Chapter 2 explored the concept of assimilative integration. What is the rationale for using an assimilative integrative approach for social anxiety disorder (SAD), and how can this type of integration assist patients with SAD? An assimilative integrative approach that introduces other treatment components, e.g., interpersonal, while at the same time drawing on the effective aspects of cognitive behavioral therapy may appeal to therapists who treat individuals with social anxiety (Macarthur, 2013). Chapter 5 described the difficulty that individuals with generalized anxiety have with avoidance and relationships. Individuals with social anxiety disorder, similar to those with generalized anxiety disorder, have similar difficulties (Newman, Castonguay, Borkovec, Fisher, & Nordberg, 2008). Whereas cognitive-behavioral therapy does not place a lot of weight on the aforementioned elements that hold difficulty for patients with social anxiety, an integrative treatment can utilize the beneficial parts of cognitive-behavioral treatment for social anxiety while integrating interpersonal therapy that focuses on interpersonal relationships for patients with social anxiety disorder (Lipsitz, 2012; Macarthur, 2013). It has been established that a CBT-directed integrative psychotherapy treatment is helpful for patients with generalized anxiety disorder, and given certain similarities (e.g., emotional avoidance and interpersonal relationships) between generalized anxiety disorder and social anxiety disorder, a similar CBT-directed integrative treatment approach may be helpful for those with social anxiety disorder (Macarthur, 2013; Newman et al., 2008). Social anxiety disorder has been shown to have a high comorbidity rate with bipolar disorder, and it has been suggested that an integrated psychotherapy approach of CBT and interpersonal therapy (IPT) be used in treating social anxiety disorder for patients with bipolar disorder (Merikangas et al., 2007; Queen et al., 2015).

Macarthur's (2013) Assimilative Integrative Approach and Social Anxiety Disorder (SAD)

Using an assimilative integrative framework for social anxiety, how can therapists integrate core beliefs into their own integration approaches as they treat patients with social anxiety disorder (SAD)? Theoretical integration models need to include ongoing integration along with exploration and flexibility (Macarthur, 2013; Stricker, 2010). Similar to Marquis (2018), Macarthur (2013) views integration as a process that proceeds from one moment to another. Rather than accepting a predetermined rigid approach, integrative psychotherapists need to be flexible as they consider the unique needs of each patient (Macarthur, 2013). At the same time that integration is continuous, and proceeds from one moment to another, models of integration have a directed core principle that shape psychotherapy (Macarthur, 2013; Stricker, 2010). For Macarthur's (2013) assimilative integrative approach to psychotherapy, the directed core principle or theme that guides is Clark and Wells' (1995) belief system of social anxiety, which includes high-standard, conditional, and unconditional beliefs. For example, if individuals with high-standard beliefs do not meet their own standards, they may become anxious (Macarthur, 2013; Van Yperen & Hagedoorn, 2008).

Macarthur (2013) considers his integrated approach to be similar to interpersonal therapy (IPT) and to Wolfe's (1992) integrative model of social anxiety in that each of the models (for the sake of theoretical stability) focuses on a few major core aspects of integration. Macarthur (2013) explains that the core of Wolfe's (1992) integrative approach, which derives principles from different theoretical orientations, e.g., psychodynamic, experiential, CBT, is the experience of the self, which facilitates a patient's minute-to-minute experience. Macarthur (2013) explains that whereas IPT and Wolfe's (1992) model focus on a product, Macarthur's (2013) integrative social anxiety model, which incorporates a core belief system (Clark & Wells, 1995), focuses on an ongoing process. Utilizing a psychotherapy integration model for social anxiety,

Macarthur (2013) offers examples of how the core beliefs of Clark & Wells (1995) can be integrated into other theoretical models, e.g., narrative therapy, solution focused brief therapy, and he encourages therapists to integrate the core beliefs into their own integration approaches as they treat patients with social anxiety disorder.

An Integrated Cognitive-Behavioral Hypnotherapy (CBH) Framework and Social Anxiety Disorder (SAD), and a Transdiagnostic Unified Protocol (UP) and SAD

How do integrated psychotherapy approaches for social anxiety disorder (SAD) compare to single-disorder protocols (SDPs)? The integrated treatment, cognitive-behavioral hypnotherapy (CBH), was shown to be more effective than CBT, by itself, for patients with social anxiety disorder (Schoenberger, Kirsch, Gearan, Montgomery, & Pastyrnak, 1997). When the transdiagnostic unified protocol (UP) was compared with single-disorder protocols (SDPs) for social phobia, it was found that the UP was as effective a treatment as the SDPs; however, the dropout rate for UP was lower than for the SDPs (Barlow et al., 2017; Kennedy & Barlow, 2018).

Emotion-Focused Therapy (EFT): An Integrative Humanistic Treatment Model and Social Anxiety Disorder (SAD)

Are there alternative integrated treatments to monotherapies, e.g., cognitive-behavioral therapy, client-centered therapy, for social anxiety? Are there integrative, humanistic treatment orientations for individuals with social anxiety who do not respond to cognitive-behavioral therapy (CBT)? Emotion-focused therapy (EFT) (Elliott et al., 2004; Greenberg, 2015), an integrative experiential treatment framework, has been proposed as a treatment that may be offered to individuals who do not respond to the monotherapy, CBT (Shahar, 2014; Shahar et al., 2017). A key feature of EFT (Elliot et al., 2004) is the notion of emotion schemes, the behavior style that individuals adopt in the face of experiencing specific emotions (Watson, 2006). Chapter 5 discussed the use of emotion schemes and emotion-focused therapy (EFT) for generalized anxiety disorder (GAD). Emotion-focused therapy (EFT) (Elliott et al., 2004), which derives from several theories (e.g., Rogers, 1951; Bowlby's attachment theory, 1969) and focuses on the exploration of emotional processing, may be appropriate for patients with social anxiety disorder (Shahar, 2014; Watson, 2006). For example, EFT may be incorporated into cognitive therapy for social anxiety, e.g., rescripting of images related to trauma (Wild & Clark, 2011). Shahar et al.'s (2017) study, which showed empirically that EFT is effective for individuals with social anxiety disorder, was the first research study to investigate the use of EFT for social anxiety disorder. EFT helps patients with social anxiety disorder to discover their emotions, decrease their avoidance of their experience of their emotions, and lessen shame by decreasing self-criticism and increasing compassion for the self (Shahar, 2014). The integrative EFT has been found to be more effective than the unitary therapy, client-centered therapy, in the treatment of social anxiety disorder (Elliott, 2013). A robust interpersonal alliance, the two-chair and empty chair methods, and the facilitation of self-soothing are important for patients with SAD (Elliott, 2013; Goldman, 2019; Goldman & Fox-Zurawic, 2012).

Medication for Social Anxiety Disorder (SAD)

What medications or combinations of therapy and medication have benefited patients with social anxiety disorder (SAD)? Psychopharmacological interventions such as antidepressant medications and/or cognitive-behavioral interventions such as exposure therapy have been found to be effective in treating individuals with social anxiety disorder (Comer, 2015; Heimberg & Magee, 2014). SSRIs or SSNRIs are the preferred treatment for social anxiety disorder (Guastella, Howard, Dadds, Mitchell, & Carson, 2009; Kariuki & Stein, 2013). The selective serotonin reuptake inhibitors (SSRIs), paroxetine and sertraline, and the serotonin and norepinephrine reuptake inhibitor (SNRI), venlafaxine, have been shown to be beneficial for individuals with social anxiety disorder (Ray, 2018).

Other medications for social anxiety disorder include antiepileptic medications (Feltner, Liu-Dumaw, Schweizer, & Bielski, 2011; Julien, 2013). In contrast to the SSRIs and SSNRIs, Kariuki and Stein (2013) concluded that the benzodiazepines, although relievers of the physical issues related to social anxiety disorder, are not preferred for SAD because of the potential for dependence (Connor et al., 1998; Stein et al., 2010). CBT treatments that include exposure and social skills training as well as group CBT have been shown to be effective for individuals with SAD, and CBT has been demonstrated to be as effective as pharmacotherapy (Heimberg, 2002; Ray, 2018). In contrast to the aforementioned positive findings for the SSRIs and SSNRIs (Guastella et al., 2009) and for CBT (Heimberg, 2002), Cohen et al. (2017) reported that 42% of individuals who have received CBT terminated therapy prematurely or did not show improvement (Heimberg et al., 1998) and that selective serotonin reuptake inhibitors (SSRIs) did not fare much better (Liebowitz, Gelenberg, & Munjack, 2005; Van Ameringen et al., 2001). Limitations of psychotropics include the late onset of some medications, side effects, and relapse after patients with social anxiety stop taking the medication (Kariuki & Stein, 2013). Individuals with social anxiety disorder were almost two times more likely to refuse medication over therapy as an intervention (Swift, Greenberg, Tompkins, & Parkin, 2017).

The Therapeutic Relationship and Integration for Social Anxiety Disorder

The value of the therapeutic relationship cannot be underestimated across treatments and theoretical orientations. Is the quality of the relationship between patients and therapists different depending upon the specific anxiety disorder? Patients with social anxiety disorder have been found to have a poorer therapeutic relationship than individuals with panic disorder (Haug et al., 2016). It was found that low therapist competence was related to premature termination from CBT therapy among patients with SAD (Haug et al., 2016). A stronger therapeutic relationship may increase the likelihood that patients with SAD would adhere to medication by enhancing their willingness to be exposed to situations that are fearful (Cohen et al., 2017). Furthermore, a stronger therapeutic relationship may help an individual with SAD feel safe, a feeling that individuals with SAD do not often feel with others (Cohen et al., 2017; Taylor & Alden, 2005; Weiss, Dodge, Bates, & Pettit, 1992). Whereas therapist competence has been shown to be a predictor of premature termination for clients with SAD, the therapeutic relationship was found to be a predictor of treatment outcome and dropout (Haug et al., 2016). For example, when the therapist's competence was low, premature termination from CBT for clients with SAD was more likely (Haug et al., 2016). Furthermore, if the rating of the therapeutic relationship was higher late in the treatment, the outcome was better, and if the rating of the therapeutic relationship was lower late in the treatment, the patient with social anxiety was more likely drop out of therapy (Haug et al., 2016).

How is the therapeutic relationship related to an integral approach? Relational techniques such as attunement can help individuals with past failures in the relational realm, especially when these early failures impede the process of relating in an intersubjective dimension (Rodriguez, 2018; Stern, 1985). The integral psychotherapy quadratic model includes the Lower Left (LL), the culture or the intersubjective component of a group (Ingersoll & Marquis, 2014; Marquis & Elliot, 2015; Wilber, 2000). Recently, Rodriguez (2018) shows how relational levels of relationships, e.g., non-verbal relating, within an intersubjective sphere can have an impact on psychotherapy integration. Rather than simply observing and diagnosing patients, psychotherapists need to recognize that psychotherapy occurs inside a therapeutic alliance where therapists participate within an intersubjective context (Rodriguez, 2018). In order to promote integration, a therapist needs to attend to the relation levels in the relationship that are conscious, to those that are nonverbal, and to those that are preverbal or non-linguistic (Erskine, 2010; Rodriguez, 2018). To access integration of patients' earlier experiences, it is suggested that the therapist utilize empathy to facilitate a therapeutic alliance that stays open to the aforementioned relation levels (Clark, 1991; Rodriguez, 2018). Within the development of the therapist–patient dyadic relationship, patients have opportunities to find expression for their past thwarted needs as therapists employ the relational technique of courteous inquiry along with attunement and involvement (Erskine, 1991; Rodriguez, 2018). Integrative psychotherapy's intersubjective focus is critical for helping patients access their deepest experiences during therapeutic encounters when preverbal memories of past relational failures emerge (Rodriguez, 2018). Furthermore, the aforementioned focus can assist individuals with social interaction difficulties who have experienced past relational failures that impede their ability to effectively engage in intersubjective communication (Rodriguez, 2018).

How to Implement Unified Psychotherapy in Practice for Social Anxiety Disorder

The following is a case study that applies Magnavita and Anchin's (2014) unifying psychotherapy model to treat a patient with social anxiety disorder (SAD). Chapter 1 describes Magnavita and Anchin's (2014) unifying psychotherapy model, which suggests a biopsychosocial model where a patient's symptoms of social anxiety comprise an interaction of intrapsychic-biological, interpersonal-dyadic, triadic relational, and sociocultural variables.

Corey, a 26-year-old male began psychotherapy after he experienced several incidents of social anxiety when he attempted to present a project in front of a group of people at a university's architecture program. Corey enrolled in an architecture program a year ago and is living in a residence hall of a university. Two of his fellow graduate students often feud with each other, and each tries to get Corey to side with him during department meetings. Two weeks ago, Corey reported that he tried to present his work at one of the department meetings, but felt ill in the middle, and needed to excuse himself. He said that next week the graduate students of his department will be attending a party for one of his professors, but he thinks that he will not go because there is a lot of fighting between the professors in his department. Corey reported to the therapist that he often fears that people are angry at him.

Corey's parents who live about two hours from the university recently told him that they were having difficulty with his older sister whom they had recently accompanied to an emergency room because she felt anxious and had difficulty breathing. Corey reported that his siblings picked on him when he was a child, but his parents were preoccupied and unavailable to help him. He related that when he was in elementary school, he was shamed and bullied by another boy. He recalled that the bullying took place when he would present his work in class and on the playground in front of his classmates. Corey reported that his father tends to become intense about his chronic worries, has recently become more agitated because he lost his job, and has been diagnosed with generalized anxiety disorder. Corey mentioned that as a child, his mother repeatedly criticized him, and he felt inferior to his siblings and friends. Corey's younger brother was recently diagnosed with panic disorder with agoraphobia.

The patient wants to keep his scholarship at the architecture program, but is having difficulty presenting his work during department meetings. He says that he fears negative reviews from others, and becomes very anxious before meetings. At the same time, he mentioned that he is not willing to try pharmacotherapy. He is trying to keep a small work study position which requires that he attend eight hours a week, but finds his supervisor to be overly demanding, and he often deprecates Corey's work in front of others. Corey tends to stay in his room at the residence hall, to avoid participating in many of the activities offered at the university, and he tries to avoid social situations where he feels awkward.

Relying on Magnavita and Anchin's (2014) unifying psychotherapy model, the therapist views Corey's social anxiety disorder within the context of a biopsychosocial framework where Corey's symptoms of social anxiety manifest as an unhealthy interaction of intrapsychic-biological, interpersonal-dyadic, triadic relational, and sociocultural variables. At the level of the intrapsychic-biological, Corey may have inherited a tendency towards anxiety, has memories of being bullied, feels wounded, inferior, inadequate, humiliated, particularly in social situations, and is hypervigilant that others are criticizing him. At the level of the interpersonal-dyadic, Corey works for a supervisor that denigrates him and his work. At the level of the triadic-relational, Corey is concerned about his feuding peers, each of whom, tries to get Corey to side with him. At the sociocultural level, Corey is part of an architecture program, a milieu for sounding out his work and for developing future endeavors, a setting where the professors and students in the architecture community are competitive with each other.

It has been suggested that a dialogic perspective that focuses on mutuality be employed with patients who are prone to shame because this approach offers them an opportunity to become involved in a relationship at their own pace (Evans, 1994; Gilbert & Orlans, 2011). To help Corey with his symptoms of social avoidance and difficulty with relationship building, Corey's therapist used an assimilative integrative approach that introduces interpersonal treatment while at the same time drawing on the effective aspects of cognitive behavioral therapy to help Corey decrease his symptoms of social anxiety. The therapist used cognitive methods to help Corey decrease his fears of social situations and to help him decrease his feelings of awkwardness and distress in public. To increase his ability to perform adequately in social settings, Corey's therapist suggested that Corey join a group where the therapist uses evidence-based CBT with a focus on social skills training. Along with the CBT methods, the therapist used relaxation training and hypnosis to alleviate some of the physical anxiety effects of Corey's symptoms.

Once some of the symptoms decreased and Corey attained some relief from his distress, the therapist began to explore the psychodynamic meaning of Corey's social anxiety symptoms for which assimilative integrative treatment techniques were planned. A focus was on addressing Corey's perception of impaired self-attributes.

In the context of Magnavita and Anchin's (2014) unified approach, the therapist facilitated awareness of the external stressors, e.g., a hypercritical boss, Corey's feuding peers, that contributed to Corey's social difficulties, and the therapist taught him assertiveness training. After a few sessions of assertiveness training, Corey was able to plan a strategy to cope by increasing his assertiveness at the level of interpersonal-dyadic (e.g., deprecating boss) and at the level of the triadic-relational (e.g., feuding peers).

After a year of individual treatment, it was suggested that Corey participate in an integrated group treatment in order to maintain the treatment effects and to prevent relapse. In addition to attending to the reduction of symptoms and to the presence of external stressors, the therapist considered Corey's overall personality dysfunction where he is prone to feelings of inferiority, inadequacy, and vulnerability, which contribute to his social anxiety. In this sense, the therapist facilitated Corey's awareness of his tendency to escape and to employ avoidance of social situations as a defense mechanism against being flooded by feelings of inferiority. When Corey was more assertive at the level of the interpersonal-dyadic (e.g., deprecating boss) and the triadic relational (e.g., feuding peers), the therapist proceeded to deepen Corey's experiential feelings of his new confidence at the sociocultural level so that Corey began to feel that he fit in as he continued to pursue his program in architecture. After two years of therapy, Corey reported that he was on his way to accepting a fellowship to teach students in the architecture program and that he was well able to present several innovative work products both at the university and at a company associated with the university.

Summary

To manage social anxiety means to encourage patients to confront ideas of threat to their being, their social life, and/or their career, e.g., nervousness about public speaking (Muse, Moore, & Stahl, 2013). This section demonstrated clinical practice applications of integrated and unified psychotherapy treatment models for social anxiety disorder (see Table 7.1). It concluded with a case study that employed Magnavita and Anchin's (2014) unifying psychotherapy model for a patient with social anxiety disorder.

Symptoms of Specific Phobia (SP)

A specific phobia refers to an unrelenting and irrational fear or avoidance of a particular situation or object, and the individual with social phobia is aware that the fear is disproportionate to the situation (APA, 2013; Comer, 2015; Shearer, Harmon, Younger, & Brown, 2013). For example, when individuals intensely fear a specific type of insect, they will strongly avoid that insect (APA, 2013; Comer, 2015). If they are exposed to the insect, they may develop a panic attack.

Diagnosis of Specific Phobia (SP)

According to DSM-5, an individual diagnosed with specific phobia has excessive anxiety related to a particular situation or object, and the anxiety continues for six months or more while causing a great deal of distress (APA, 2013). Whereas the categories of specific phobia, animal, natural environment, blood–injection–injury, begin when an individual is a child, the category of specific phobia, situational, has a later onset (usually in one's 20's) (Craske & Waters, 2005; Öst & Treffers, 2001). In contrast to the other anxiety disorders, the breadth of specific phobia disorder's threat response is very narrow, and the persistent fear of individuals with this disorder is related to distinct situations or objects (Craske & Waters, 2005, Kessler et al., 1994).

Prevalence of Specific Phobia (SP)

Prevalence

What is the prevalence of specific phobia? For the U.S., the 12-month prevalence rate for specific phobia is given as 7% to 9% (APA, 2013). The prevalence, dysfunction, and period length of specific phobia were shown to be more elevated in countries with a high income than in those with a low income, and females were twice as likely to develop specific phobia than males (APA, 2013; Wardenaar et al., 2017). The elderly are the least likely to develop specific phobia (Sigström, Skoog, Karlsson, Nilsson, & Östling, 2016; Stinson et al., 2007). The lifetime prevalence for animal phobia was found to be the highest among the specific phobias, and the lowest prevalence was found for flying phobia (Wardenaar et al., 2017).

Onset

When in the life cycle do individuals become afflicted with specific phobia? Whereas the onset of generalized anxiety disorder is later, phobias begin in childhood (Paus, Keshavan, Giedd, 2008; Ray, 2018). In fact, specific phobia's median onset is age eight (Wardenaar et al., 2017). After age 64, specific phobia will develop in fewer than 1% of people (Kessler et al., 2005; Wolitzky-Taylor, 2010).

Heritability

Does the type of specific phobia influence heritability? For specific phobia, a heritability of 47% has been reported for animal phobia, a heritability of 59% has been reported for blood phobia, and a heritability of 46% has been found for situational phobia (Ray, 2018).

Comorbidity

Do patients with specific phobia have other anxiety disorders? Frequently, specific phobia (SP) paves the way for other emotional disorders, thus rendering it a potential marker for vulnerability (Wardenaar et al., 2017). More than half of the cases of lifetime specific phobia were found to have another lifetime emotional disorder, with almost 50% having an anxiety disorder (Wardenaar et al., 2017). In the elderly, specific phobia is connected to depression (APA, 2013).

An Integrative Etiology of Specific Phobia (SP): Focus, Underpinnings, and Causes of Specific Phobia (SP)

The Interaction Between Learning Theory and Biology

What are the sources of the etiology of the development and maintenance of specific phobia (SP) (see Table 7.1)? The etiology of the development and maintenance of specific phobia does not emerge from one source. Rather, Shearer and colleagues (2013) proposed that the etiology of specific phobia derives from different sources such as learning theory, e.g., Rachman's (1977) conditioning, Poulton, Pine, & Harrington's (2009) biological explanations, and Craske and Waters's (2005) informational sources about a threatening stimulus, such as other individuals warning the patient.

What is the relationship between learning theory and the etiology of specific phobia? Explanations for the etiology of specific phobia derive from learning theory's classical conditioning and modeling where stimuli are conditioned to anxiety responses, and avoidance behaviors then maintain the phobia (Comer, 2015; Ingersoll & Marquis, 2014). Observational learning that may result in the formation of a phobia takes place when an individual observes another person's fear of an object (Ray, 2018).

When compared to generalized anxiety disorder and panic disorder, distinct variables contribute to more variance in specific phobia disorder (Craske & Waters, 2005). Specifically, the distinct learning experiences of traumatic conditioning, the observation of a traumatized model, and the relating potentially of dangerous information contribute substantially in specific phobia disorder (Craske & Waters, 2005).

How does biology and genetics affect the etiology of specific phobia? Poulton and colleagues (2009) propose a biological perspective where specific phobia develops internally. Hyperactivity is seen in the amygdala, the cingulate cortex, and in the insula of individuals with specific phobia when they viewed snakes or spiders (Etkin & Wager, 2007). Some individuals may have a diathesis or a biological or genetic vulnerability to acquire specific phobia (Gabbay, 1992; Gray, 1987).

Is there an interaction between a learning framework and biology that contributes to the etiology of specific phobia? According to Ingersoll and Marquis (2014), the causes of specific phobia are consistent with Barlow's (2004) triple vulnerability model given that there is an interaction between a general tendency towards anxiety and a nonspecific psychological tendency towards anxiety along with particular learned events. Learning may interact with biological and/or genetic variables to generate a specific phobia (Antony & Barlow, 2002, Shearer et al., 2013).

Psychodynamic theorists view phobias as deriving from an unconscious source related to early trauma and as rooted in the neglect of caregivers (Marquis, 2018). Wolfe (2005) explains that when individuals transfer their worries to a concrete phenomenon, they are in a better position to cope with the anxiety.

Wolfe's (2005, 2006) Integrative Theory and Self-Wounds

This chapter described how Wolfe's (2003) integrative etiological model can be applied to social phobia. Wolfe's (2005, 2006) idea of a wounded self can extend on the existing explanations for specific phobia as well. According to Wolfe's (2005) integrative theory of the etiology of anxiety, a specific phobia can develop when a child experiences a traumatic event related to a specific object that represents a danger to the child's well-being. Avoidance reinforces the specific phobia, and the phobia can endure until the self-wound is repaired (Wolfe, 2005).

Specific Phobia and the Elderly

What factors contribute to the development and maintenance of specific phobia in the elderly? Lindesay (1991) studied phobic disorders in older individuals and found that whereas a decline in physical health and the early death of parents were related to anxiety disorders in the elderly, socioeconomic status and intimacy within the social network were not associated with phobic disorders. It has been found, however, that there is both a relationship between phobic disorders in the elderly and a network that has a small size and a connection between phobic disorders in the elderly and less emotional support (Beekman et al., 1998).

Clinical Practice Applications of Single-School and Integrated Psychotherapy Treatment Models for Specific Phobia (SP)

Do individuals with specific phobia tend to seek treatment, is the treatment effective, and how effective is it when compared to other anxiety disorders? The length of time that it takes for patients with specific phobia to seek treatment is more extensive than the length of time it takes for patients with other anxiety disorders to seek therapy (Iza et al., 2013; ten Have, de Graaf, van Dorsselaer, & Beekman, 2013). Research has shown that although specific phobia is the most treatable of the emotional disorders (Barlow, 2004), most individuals seek to avoid the feared objects or situations (Comer, 2015). The treatment rates of specific phobia were shown to be more elevated in countries with a high income than in those with a low income (Wardenaar et al., 2017). In general, post-treatment, phobias have higher success rates than does generalized anxiety disorder (Ray, 2018).

Single-School Cognitive-Behavioral Therapy (CBT) and Integrated CBT with Hypnotherapy

Although phobias can be treated by exposure to the object or situation that evokes dread (Antony & Barlow, 2002), Wolfe (2005) found that exposure treatments led to a quick decrease in symptoms of phobia only about 30% of the time, that patients were unable to complete the treatment because of intense fear, that the treatment effects were not enduring, and that although there was a decrease in avoidance, patients became anxious when faced with the object or situation that induced fear. Some researchers found that although exposure is highly beneficial for specific phobia, the rate of attrition is high (Shearer et al., 2013). An integrated psychotherapy approach, cognitive-behavioral hypnotherapy, an alternative to CBT by itself, has been shown to be effective in the treatment of specific phobia (Fredette et al., 2013).

Alternative Integrated Approaches for Specific Phobia (SP)

An Integrative Attachment Framework for Phobias

Gold (1993) developed an integrative psychotherapy approach to phobias and anxiety disorders that incorporates ideas and methods from cognitive, psychodynamic, humanistic, and behavioral perspectives. Gold's (1993) theoretical and technical model derives from attachment theory (Bowlby, 1980; Guidano, 1987). An adult with a clinical diagnosis of a phobia (and other anxiety disorders) is recognized to have had difficulty with attachment figures, e.g., conflictual, rejecting caregivers (Gold, 1993). The child views the relationship with a rejecting or a conflictual early attachment figure as impaired, and separation from the attachment figure is perceived to be dangerous. In the case of a specific (or formerly, simple) phobia, the symptoms are linked to a pattern of attachment that was, for the most part, satisfying, but which included only particular ideas and situations of danger (Gold, 1993).

A Transtheoretical Integration Model for Phobias

Prochaska and DiClemente's (2005) transtheoretical model, an approach that emphasizes theoretical integration, underscores the notion of the stages of change. They proposed that a transtheoretical model focuses on an individual approach for each patient, and that therapists need to consider that prior to recommending counterconditioning as the best therapy intervention for phobias, it is better to first analyze the stages of change.

A Self-Wound Framework and Wolfe's Focusing Technique for Phobias (Wolfe, 2003; Wolfe & Sigl, 1998)

Wolfe's (2006) integrative psychotherapy that includes a self-wound framework of the etiology of phobic disorders can help patients with phobias address their self-wounds on the following three levels: (1) Behavioral, (2) cognitive, and (3) emotional. The behavior and cognitions of patients with phobias may improve as they move towards and alter their thoughts about the feared object(s); however, the changes may not endure permanently without a corrective emotional relationship that helps to alter self-perceptions (Wolfe, 2006). Whereas the behavioral symptoms may remit in a short period of time, the unconscious components may require a psychodynamic and/or experiential/humanistic approach that takes place over a longer period of time (Wolfe, 2006).

Wolfe's Focusing Technique is a diagnostic method for discovering the meaning of the symptoms of a specific phobia (Wolfe, 2003; Wolfe & Sigl, 1998). For patients with specific phobia, Wolfe's Focusing Technique involves a deep attention to the object that is feared (Wolfe, 2003). According to Wolfe (2003), therapy involves less structure in the exploratory phase when there is a focus on the source of the phobia; however, when the exploration phase reveals a self-wound, it is suggested that the therapist use a more structured, cognitive method. It is the adept therapist that can shift between greater and lesser periods of structure during the therapy session suggested by Wolfe's (2003) integrative model.

Medication and Combined Treatment for Specific Phobia

Is a combination of medication and therapy more effective than single-school therapy for specific phobia? Antidepressant medication has been shown to have an anxiolytic effect for patients with phobias (Comaty and Advokat, 2013); however, medication for specific phobia has produced only modest results, at best (Shearer et al., 2013). Antidepressants and other medications combined with exposure do not yield a greater long-term positive outcome than does CBT, by itself, for cases of specific phobia that are not complex (Norberg, Korstel, & Tolin, 2008; Shearer et al., 2013).

How to Implement Integrative Psychotherapy in Practice for Specific Phobia

The following integrative psychotherapy is a case study of cognitive behavioral and psychodynamic therapy with a patient with a needle phobia where shifts take place during the therapy with the facilitation of more structure within the context of a cognitive-behavioral intervention to less structure within the context of a psychodynamic psychotherapy approach. The integrated psychotherapy approach that the therapist employed in the following case underscores a shift from CBT to a psychodynamic approach and relies on Wolfe's (2006) integrative psychotherapy that includes a self-wound framework for the etiology of phobic disorders. This approach incorporates Gold's (1993) model that derives from attachment theory which suggests that the patient with a specific phobia may have had difficulty with attachment figures (Bowlby, 1980; Guidano, 1987).

The patient, Liz, a 21-year old waitress, presented with a needle phobia. In the past, she had canceled several appointments with her physician because of her phobia. Research has shown that exposure treatments have been effective for decreasing needle phobias (McMurtry et al., 2015). The therapist used a cognitive behavioral therapy approach, exposure and applied muscle tension, to help Liz alleviate her panic related to needles. After the fourth session of exposure, Liz reported that she was able to walk to her physician's office while she experienced only minor symptoms of anxiety as she received a routine examination and a flu vaccine. She reported that during the vaccine she had mild fears of fainting, but did not faint. Recently, however, during an eighth CBT therapy session, Liz related that she had been on her way, walking with her friend, Mia, to her internist's office last week when she had a panic attack when Mia informed her that she intended to pick something up at a bakery shop while Liz proceeded to walk to her internist's office to receive a blood test. Although Liz found cognitive-behavioral therapy and walking with her friend, Mia, to be somewhat helpful in that she was able to gain some relief by setting out to walk towards her internist's office, she ended up canceling her appointment when Mia decided to stop off at the bakery for a short time. Whereas the behavioral symptoms may remit somewhat in a short period of time, the unconscious components may require a psychodynamic and/or experiential/humanistic approach that takes place over a longer period of time (Wolfe, 2006).

Upon learning that Liz's needle phobia was not entirely resolved with CBT, the therapist shifted her approach during the therapy session from a highly structured cognitive-behavioral approach to a psychodynamic focus with a decrease in structure, and facilitated exploration of the unconscious self-wounds and emotions (related to Liz's underlying attachment issues) that had been avoided. During psychodynamic therapy, it was discovered that Liz's panic attack was related to panic that she had experienced at age 11. When she was 11, Liz had been sitting in the waiting room of her pediatrician's office while her older sister, Adrian, age 17, was gaming on her computer. Adrian accidentally poked a child in the head with her pencil, and the child was injured. Shocked by what she had done, Adrian, ran out of the office and left Liz to fend for herself at the pediatrician's office. Commotion ensued with nurses attending to the child whom Adrian accidentally wounded. One of the nurses administered a tetanus shot to the distressed child. The children in the pediatrician's office seemed startled, and Liz observed how their parents comforted them. Liz's sister, Adrian, was nowhere to be found. Liz was left by herself sitting next to the injured child. During the psychodynamic portion of the therapy, Liz was able to get in touch with her emerging self-wounds (related to attachment figures), and after a year of psychodynamic therapy, she was able to go to her physician without anyone accompanying her.

Summary

Unlike generalized anxiety disorder, the precipitants of social anxiety disorder (SAD) and specific phobia (SP) can be identified (Watson & Greenberg, 2017). This chapter offered explanations for the development and maintenance of social anxiety disorder (SAD) and specific phobia (SP) and described the integrated and unified etiology approaches and psychotherapy treatment models for SAD and SP (see Table 7.1).

References

Aderka, I. M., Hofmann, S. G., Nickerson, A., Hermesh, H., Gilboa-Schectman, E., & Marom, S. (2012). Functional impairment in social anxiety disorder. *Journal of Anxiety Disorders, 26*(3), 393–400. doi: 10.1016/j.janxdis.2012.01.003

American Psychiatric Association. (2013). *Diagnostic and statistical manual of mental disorders* (5th ed.). Washington, DC: Author.

Antony, M. M., & Barlow, D. H. (2002). Specific phobias. In D. H. Barlow (Ed.), *Anxiety and its disorders: The nature and treatment of anxiety and panic* (2nd ed., pp. 380–417). New York, NY: Guilford Press.

Bandelow, B., Charimo Torrente, A., Wedekind, D., Broocks, A., Hajak, G., & Rüther, E. (2004). Early traumatic life events, parental rearing styles, family history of mental disorders, and birth risk factors in patients with social anxiety disorder. *European Archives of Psychiatry and Clinical Neuroscience, 254*(6), 397–405. doi: 10.1007/s00406-004-0521-2

Barlow, D. H. (2004). *Anxiety and its disorders: The nature and treatment of anxiety and panic* (2nd ed.). New York: Guilford Press.

Barlow, D. H., Farchione, T. J., Bullis, J. R., Gallagher, M. W., Murray-Latin, H., Sauer-Zavala, S., … Cassiello-Robbins, C. (2017). The unified protocol for transdiagnostic treatment of emotional disorders compared with diagnosis-specific protocols for anxiety disorders: A randomized clinical trial. *JAMA Psychiatry, 74*(9), 875–884. doi: 10.1001/jamapsychiatry.2017.2164

Beekman, A. T., Bremmer, M. A., Deeg, D. J., Van Balkom, A. J., Smit, J. H., De Beurs, E., … van Tilburg, W. (1998). Anxiety disorders in later life: A report from the Longitudinal Aging Study Amsterdam. *International journal of geriatric psychiatry, 13*(10), 717–726. doi:10.1002/(sici)1099-1166(1998100)13:10<717::aid-gps857>3.0.co;2-m

Beesdo, K., Bittner, A., Pine, D. S., Stein, M. B., Höfler, M., Lieb, R., & Wittchen, H.-U. (2007). Incidence of social anxiety disorder and the consistent risk for secondary depression in the first three decades of life. *Archives of General Psychiatry, 64*(8), 903–912. doi: 10.1001/archpsyc.64.8.903

Bener, A., Ghuloum, S., & Dafeeah, E. E. (2011). Prevalence of common phobias and their socio-demographic correlates in children and adolescents in a traditional developing society. *African Journal of Psychiatry, 14*(2), 140–145. doi: 10.4314/ajpsy.v14i2.6

Birbaumer, N., Grodd, W., Diedrich, O., Klose, U., Erb, M., Lotze, M., … Flor, H. (1998). fMRI reveals amygdala activation to human faces in social phobics. *NeuroReport, 9*(6), 1223–1226. doi: 10.1097/00001756-199804200-00048

Bowlby, J. (1969). *Attachment and loss, Vol. 1. Attachment*. New York, NY: Basic Books.

Bowlby, J. (1980). *Attachment and loss, Vol. 3. Loss*. New York, NY: Basic Books.

Clark, B. D. (1991). Empathic transactions in the deconfusion of child ego states. *Transactional Analysis Journal, 21*(2), 92–98. doi: 10.1177/036215379102100204

Clark, D. M., & Wells, A. (1995). A cognitive model of social phobia. In R. Heimberg, M. Liebowitz, D. A. Hope & Schneier, F. R. (Eds.), *Social phobia: Diagnosis, assessment and treatment* (pp. 69–93). New York, NY: Guilford Press.

Cohen, J. N., Drabick, D. A., Blanco, C., Schneier, F. R., Liebowitz, M. R., & Heimberg, R. G. (2017). Pharmacotherapy for social anxiety disorder: Interpersonal predictors of outcome and the mediating role of the working alliance. *Journal of Anxiety Disorders, 52,* 79–87. doi: 10.1016/j.janxdis.2017.10.004

Comaty, J. E., & Advokat, C. (2013). Generalized anxiety disorder. In S. M. Stahl & B. A. Moore (Eds.), *Anxiety disorders: A guide for integrating psychopharmacology and psychotherapy* (pp. 97–132). New York, NY: Routledge.

Comer, R. J. (2015). *Abnormal psychology.* New York, NY: Worth Publisher.

Connor, K. M., Davidson, J. R., Potts, N. L., Tupler, L. A., Miner, C. M., Malik, M. L., … Ferrell, F. (1998). Discontinuation of clonazepam in the treatment of social phobia. *Journal of Clinical Psychopharmacology, 18*(5), 373–378. doi: 10.1097/00004714-199810000-00004

Craske, M. G., & Waters, A. M. (2005). Panic disorder, phobias, and generalized anxiety disorder. *Annual Review of Clinical Psychology, 1,* 197–225. doi: 10.1146/annurev.clinpsy.1.102803.143857

Elliott, R. (2013). Person-centered/experiential psychotherapy for anxiety difficulties: Theory, research and practice. *Person-Centered and Experiential Psychotherapies, 12*(1), 16–32. doi: 10.1080/14779757.2013.767750

Elliott, R., & Shahar, B. (2017). Social anxiety. *Person-Centered and Experiential Psychotherapies, 16*(2), 140–158. doi: 10.1080/14779757.2017.1330701

Elliott, R., Watson, J. C., Goldman, R. N., & Greenberg, L. S. (2004). *Learning emotion-focused therapy: The process-experiential approach to change.* Washington, DC: American Psychological Association.

Erskine, R. G. (1991). Transference and transactions: Critique from an intrapsychic and integrative perspective. *Transactional Analysis Journal, 21*(2), 63–76. doi: 10.1177/036215379102100202

Erskine, R. G. (2010). Life scripts, unconscious relational patterns and psychotherapeutic involvement. In R. G. Erskine (Ed.), *Life scripts. A transactional analysis of unconscious relational patterns* (pp. 1–28). London: Karnac Books Ltd.

Etkin, A., & Wager, T. D. (2007). Functional neuroimaging of anxiety: A meta-analysis of emotional processing in PTSD, social anxiety disorder, and specific phobia. *The American Journal of Psychiatry, 164,* 1476–1488. doi: 10.1176/appi.ajp.2007.07030504

Evans, K. R. (1994). Healing shame: A gestalt perspective. *Transactional Analysis Journal, 24*(2), 103–120. doi: 10.1177/036215379402400205

Fehm, L., Pelissolo, A., Furmark, T., & Wittchen, H. U. (2005). Size and burden of social phobia in Europe. *European Neuropsychopharmacology, 15*(4), 453–462. doi: 10.1016/j.euroneuro.2005.04.002

Feltner, D. E., Liu-Dumaw, M., Schweizer, E., & Bielski, R. (2011). Efficacy of pregabalin in generalized social anxiety disorder: Results of a double-blind, placebo-controlled, fixed-dose study. *International Clinical Psychopharmacology, 26*(4), 213–220. doi: 10.1097/YIC.0b013e32834519bd

Forstner, A. J., Rambau, S., Friedrich, N., Ludwig, K. U., Böhmer, A. C., Mangold, E., … Conrad, R. (2017). Further evidence for genetic variation at the serotonin transporter gene SLC6A4 contributing toward anxiety. *Psychiatric Genetics, 27*(3), 96–102. doi: 10.1097/YPG.0000000000000171

Fraser, J. (2018). *Unifying effective psychotherapies: Tracing the process of change.* Washington, DC: American Psychological Association.

Fredette, C., El-Baalbaki, G., Neron, S., & Palardy, V. (2013). Using hypnosis in the treatment of anxiety disorders: Pros and cons. In F. Durbano (Ed.), *New insights into anxiety disorders* (pp. 343–377). InTech. doi: 10.5772/53768

Freud, S. (1912). Recommendations to physicians practicing psychoanalysis. In J. Strachey (Ed. and trans.), *The standard edition of the complete works of Sigmund Freud,* (Vol. 12, pp. 111–120). London: Hogarth Press.

Gabbard, G. O. (1992). Psychodynamics of panic disorder and social phobia. *Bulletin of the Menninger Clinic, 56*(2)(Suppl. A), A3–A13.

Gilbert, M., & Orlans, V. (2011). *Integrative therapy: 100 key points and techniques*. London, England: Routledge.

Gold, J. R. (1993). An integrated approach to the treatment of anxiety disorders and phobias. In G. Stricker & J. R. Gold (Eds.), *Comprehensive handbook of psychotherapy integration* (pp. 293–301). New York, NY: Plenum Press.

Goldman, R. N. (2019). History and overview of emotion-focused therapy. In L. S. Greenberg & R. N. Goldman (Eds.), *Clinical handbook of emotion-focused therapy* (pp. 3–35). Washington, DC: American Psychological Association.

Goldman, R. N., & Fox-Zurawic, A. (2012, July). *Working with self-soothing for anxiety in EFT*. Paper presented at the conference of the World Association for Person-Centered and Experiential Psychotherapy and Counseling, Antwerp, Belgium.

Gray, J. A. (1987). *The psychology of fear and stress* (2nd ed.). Cambridge, UK: Cambridge University Press.

Greenberg, L. S. (2015). *Emotion-focused therapy* (2nd ed.). Washington, DC: American Psychological Association.

Guastella, A. J., Howard, A. L., Dadds, M. R., Mitchell, P., & Carson, D. S. (2009). A randomized controlled trial of intranasal oxytocin as an adjunct to exposure therapy for social anxiety disorder. *Psychoneuroendocrinology, 34*(6), 917–923. doi: 10.1016/j.psyneuen.2009.01.005

Guidano, V. (1987). *The development of the self.* New York, NY: Guilford Press.

Haug, T., Nordgreen, T., Öst, L., Tangen, T., Kvale, G., Hovland, O. J., ... Havik, O. E. (2016). Working alliance and competence as predictors of outcome in cognitive behavioral therapy for social anxiety and panic disorder in adults. *Behaviour Research and Therapy*, 77, 40–51. doi: 10.1016/j.brat.2015.12.004

Heimberg, R. G. (2002). Cognitive-behavioral therapy for social anxiety disorder: Current status and future directions. *Biological Psychiatry, 51*(1), 101–108. doi: 10.1016/S0006-3223(01)01183-0

Heimberg, R. G., Liebowitz, M. R., Hope, D. A., Schneier, F. R., Holt, C. S., Welkowitz, L. A., ... Klein, D. F. (1998). Cognitive behavioral group therapy vs phenelzine therapy for social phobia: 12-week outcome. *Archives of General Psychiatry, 55*(12), 1133–1141. doi: 10.1001/archpsyc.55.12.1133

Heimberg, R. G., & Magee, L. (2014). Social anxiety disorder. In D. H. Barlow (Ed.), *Clinical handbook of psychological disorders: A step-by-step treatment manual* (5th ed., pp. 114–154). New York, NY: Guilford Press.

Hettema, J. M., Prescott, C. A., Myers, J. M., Neale, M. C., & Kendler, K. S. (2005). The structure of genetic and environmental risk factors for anxiety disorders in men and women. *Archives of General Psychiatry, 62*(2), 182–189. doi: 10.1001/archpsyc.62.2.182

Hofmann, S. G., & Bögels, S. M. (2006). Recent advances in the treatment of social phobia: Introduction to the special issue. *Journal of Cognitive Psychotherapy, 20*(1), 3–5. doi: 10.1891/jcop.20.1.3

Ingersoll, R. E., & Marquis, A. (2014). *Understanding psychopathology: An integral exploration.* Upper Saddle River, NJ: Pearson Education.

Iza, M., Olfson, M., Vermes, D., Hoffer, M., Wang, S., & Blanco, C. (2013). Probability and predictors of first treatment contact for anxiety disorders in the United States: Analysis of data from the National Epidemiologic Survey on Alcohol and Related Conditions (NESARC). *Journal of Clinical Psychiatry, 74*(11), 1093–1100. doi: 10.4088/JCP.13m08361

Jensen, K. P., Stein, M. B., Kranzler, H. R., Yang, B. Z., Farrer, L. A., & Gelernter, J. (2014). The α-endomannosidase gene (MANEA) is associated with panic disorder and social anxiety disorder. *Translational Psychiatry, 4*, e353. doi: 10.1038/tp.2013.122

Julien, R. M. (2013). Pharmacological treatment of anxiety disorders across the lifespan. In S. M. Stahl & B. A. Moore (Eds.), *Anxiety disorders: A guide for integrating psychopharmacology and psychotherapy* (pp. 51–70). New York, NY: Routledge.

Kariuki, C. M., & Stein, D. J. (2013). Social anxiety disorder. In S. M. Stahl & B. A. Moore (Eds.), *Anxiety disorders: A guide for integrating psychopharmacology and psychotherapy* (pp. 221–239). New York, NY: Routledge.

Kendler, K. S., Myers, J., Prescott, C. A., & Neale, M. C. (2001). The genetic epidemiology of irrational fears and phobias in men. *Archives of General Psychiatry, 58*(3), 257–265. doi: 10.1001/archpsyc.58.3.257

Kennedy, K. A., & Barlow, D. (2018). The unified treatment for transdiagnostic treatment of emotional disorders: An introduction. In D. H. Barlow & T. J. Farchione (Eds.), *Applications of the unified protocol for transdiagnostic treatment of emotional disorders* (pp. 1–16). New York, NY: Oxford University Press.

Kessler, R. C., Berglund, P., Demler, O., Jin, R., Merikangas, K. R., & Walters, E. E. (2005). Lifetime prevalence and age-of-onset distributions of DSM-IV disorders in the National Comorbidity Survey Replication. *Archives of General Psychiatry, 62*(6), 593–602. doi: 10.1001/archpsyc.62.6.593

Kessler, R. C., McGonagle, K. A., Zhao, S., Nelson, C. B., Hughes, M., Eshleman, S., … Kendler, K. S. (1994). Lifetime and 12- month prevalence of DSM-III-R psychiatric disorders in the United States: Results from the National Comorbidity Survey. *Archives of General Psychiatry, 51*(1), 8–19. doi: 10.1001/archpsyc.1994.03950010008002

Kim, K. L., Parr, A. F., & Alfano, C. A. (2011). Behavioral and cognitive behavioral treatments for social anxiety disorder in adolescents and young adults. In C. A. Alfano & D. C. Beidel (Eds.), *Social anxiety in adolescents and young adults: Translating developmental science into practice* (pp. 245–264). Washington, DC: American Psychiatric Publishing.

Leichsenring, F., & Salzer, S. (2014). A unified protocol for the transdiagnostic psychodynamic treatment of anxiety disorders: An evidence-based approach. *Psychotherapy, 51*(2), 224–245. doi: 10.1037/a0033815

Leichsenring, F., Salzer, S., Beutel, M. E., Herpertz, S., Hiller, W., Hoyer, J., … Leibing, E. (2013). Psychodynamic therapy and cognitive-behavioral therapy in social anxiety disorder: A multicenter randomized controlled trial. *American Journal of Psychiatry, 170*(7), 759–767. doi: 10.1176/appi.ajp.2013.12081125

Liebowitz, M. R., Gelenberg, A. J., & Munjack, D. (2005). Venlafaxine extended release vs placebo and paroxetine in social anxiety disorder. *Archives of General Psychiatry, 62*(2), 190–198. doi: 10.1001/archpsyc.62.2.190

Lindesay, J. (1991). Phobic disorders in the elderly. *British Journal of Psychiatry, 159*, 531–541. doi: 10.1192/bjp.159.4.531

Lipsitz, J. D. (2012). Interpersonal psychotherapy for social anxiety disorder. In J. C. Markowitz & M. M. Weissman (Eds.), *Casebook of interpersonal psychotherapy* (pp. 169–184). New York, NY: Oxford University Press.

Macarthur, J. (2013). An integrative approach to addressing core beliefs in social anxiety. *Journal of Psychotherapy Integration, 23*(4), 386–396. doi: 10.1037/a0035043

Magnavita, J. J., & Anchin, J. C. (2014). *Unifying psychotherapy: Principles, methods, and evidence from clinical science*. New York, NY: Springer.

Marquis, A. (2018). *Integral psychotherapy: A unifying approach*. New York, NY: Routledge.

Marquis, A., & Elliot, A. (2015). Integral psychotherapy in practice, Part 2: Revisions to the metatheory of integral psychotherapy based on therapeutic practice. *Journal of Unified Psychotherapy and Clinical Science, 3*(1), 1–40.

McCabe, R. E., & Antony, M. M. (2005). Panic disorder and agoraphobia. In M. M. Antony, D. R. Ledley & R. G. Heiberg (Eds.), *Improving outcomes and preventing relapse in cognitive-behavioral therapy* (pp. 1–37). New York, NY: Guilford Press.

McHugh, R. K., & Barlow, D. H. (2010). The dissemination and implementation of evidence- based psychological treatments. *American Psychologist, 65*(2), 73–84. doi: 10.1037/a0018121

McMurtry, C. M., Noel, M., Taddio, A., Antony, M. M., Asmundson, G. J., Riddell, R. P., … HelpinKids&Adults Team. (2015). Interventions for individuals with high levels of needle fear: Systematic review of randomized controlled trials and quasi-randomized controlled trials. *The Clinical Journal of Pain, 31*(10)(Suppl. 10), S109–S123. doi: 10.1097/AJP.0000000000000273

Merikangas, K. R., Akiskal, H. S., Angst, J., Greenberg, P. E., Hirschfeld, R. A., Petukhova, M., & Kessler, R. C. (2007). Lifetime and 12-month prevalence of bipolar spectrum disorder in the National Comorbidity Survey Replication. *Archives of General Psychiatry, 64*(5), 543–552. doi: 10.1001/archpsyc.64.5.543

Miskovic, V., & Schmidt, L. (2012). Social fearfulness in the human brain. *Neuroscience and Biobehavioral Reviews, 36*(1), 459–478. doi: 10.1016/j.neubiorev.2011.08.002

Morreale, M., Tancer, M. E., & Uhde, T. W. (2010). Pathogenesis of social anxiety disorder. In D. J. Stein, E. Hollander & B. O. Rothbaum (Eds.), *Textbook of anxiety disorders* (2nd ed., pp. 453–469). Washington, DC: American Psychiatric Publishing, Inc.

Moscovitch, D. A. (2009). What is the core fear in social phobia? A new model to facilitate individualized case conceptualization and treatment. *Cognitive and Behavioral Practice, 16*(2), 123–134. doi: 10.1016/j.cbpra.2008.04.002

Muse, M. D., Moore, B. A., & Stahl, S. M. (2013). Benefits and challenges of integrative treatment. In S. M. Stahl & B. A. Moore (Eds.), *Anxiety disorders: A guide for integrating psychopharmacology and psychotherapy* (pp. 3–24). New York, NY: Routledge.

Newman, M. G., Castonguay, L. G., Borkovec, T. D., Fisher, A. J., & Nordberg, S. S. (2008). An open trial of integrative therapy for generalized anxiety disorder. *Psychotherapy: Theory, Research, Practice, Training, 45*(2), 135–147. doi: 10.1037/0033-3204.45.2.135

Norberg, M. M., Krystal, J. H., & Tolin, D. F. (2008). A meta-analysis of D-cycloserine and the facilitation of fear extinction and exposure therapy. *Biological Psychiatry, 63*(12), 1118–1126. doi: 10.1016/j.biopsych.2008.01.012

Öst, L.-G., & Treffers, P. D. A. (2001). Onset, course, and outcome for anxiety disorders in children. In W. K. Silverman & P. D. A. Treffers (Eds.), *Cambridge child and adolescent psychiatry. Anxiety disorders in children and adolescents: Research, assessment and intervention* (pp. 293–312). New York, NY: Cambridge University Press.

Paus, T., Keshavan, K., & Giedd, J. N. (2008). Why do many psychiatric disorders emerge during adolescence? *Nature Reviews: Neuroscience, 9*(12), 947–957. doi: 10.1038/nrn2513

Phan, K. L., Fitzgerald, D. A., Nathan, P. J., & Tancer, M. E. (2006). Association between amygdala hyperactivity to harsh faces and severity of social anxiety in generalized social phobia. *Biological Psychiatry, 59*(5), 424–429. doi: 10.1016/j.biopsych.2005.08.012

Poulton, R., Pine, D. S., & Harrington, H. (2009). Continuity and etiology of anxiety disorders: Are they stable across the life course? In G. Andrews, D. S. Charney, P. J. Sirovatka & D. A. Regier (Eds.), *Stress-induced and fear circuitry disorders: Advancing the research agenda for DSM-5* (pp. 105–123). Arlington, VA: American Psychiatric Publishing Inc.

Prochaska, J. O., & DiClemente, C. C. (2005). The transtheoretical approach. In J. C. Norcross & M. R. Goldfried (Eds.), *Handbook of psychotherapy integration* (2nd ed., pp. 147–171). New York, NY: Oxford University Press.

Queen, A. H., Donaldson, D. L., & Luiselli, J. K. (2015). Interpersonal psychotherapy and cognitive-behavioral therapy as an integrated treatment approach for co-occurring bipolar and social anxiety disorder. *Clinical Case Studies, 14*(6), 434–448. doi: 10.1177/1534650115571663

Rachman, S. (1977). The conditioning theory of fear-acquisition: A critical examination. *Behaviour Research and Therapy, 15*(5), 375–387. doi: 10.1016/0005-7967(77)90041-9

Ray, W. J. (2018). *Abnormal psychology*. Thousand Oaks, CA: Sage.

Rodriguez, J. M. M. (2018). Three relational and intersubjective levels in integrative psychotherapy. *International Journal of Integrative Psychotherapy, 8*, 16–25.

Rogers, C. R. (1951). *Client-centered therapy*. Boston, MA: Houghton-Mifflin.

Sarver, N. W., Beidel, D. C., & Spitalnick, J. S. (2014). The feasibility and acceptability of virtual environments in the treatment of childhood social anxiety disorder. *Journal of Clinical Child and Adolescent Psychology, 43*(1), 63–73. doi: 10.1080/15374416.2013.843461

Schoenberger, N. E., Kirsch, I., Gearan, P., Montgomery, G., & Pastyrnak, S. L. (1997). Hypnotic enhancement of a cognitive behavioral treatment for public speaking anxiety. *Behavior Therapy, 28*(1), 127–140. doi: 10.1016/S0005-7894(97)80038-X

Shafran, R., Clark, D. M., Fairburn, C. G., Arntz, A., Barlow, D. H., Ehlers, A., . . . Wilson, G. T. (2009). Mind the gap: Improving the dissemination of CBT. *Behaviour Research and Therapy, 47*(11), 902–909. doi: 10.1016/j.brat.2009.07.003

Shahar, B. (2014). Emotion-focused therapy for the treatment of social anxiety: An overview of the model and a case description. *Clinical Psychology and Psychotherapy, 21*(6), 536–547. doi: 10.1002/cpp.1853

Shahar, B., Bar-Kalifa, E., & Alon, E. (2017). Emotion-focused therapy for social anxiety disorder: Results from a multiple-baseline study. *Journal of Consulting and Clinical Psychology, 85*(3), 238–249. doi: 10.1037/ccp0000166

Shearer, D. S., Harmon, C., Younger, R. D., & Brown, C. S. (2013). Specific phobia. In S. M. Stahl & B. A. Moore (Eds.), *Anxiety disorders: A guide for integrating psychopharmacology and psychotherapy* (pp. 240–259). New York, NY: Routledge.

Sigström, R., Skoog, I., Karlsson, B., Nilsson, J., & Östling, S. (2016). Nine-year follow-up of specific phobia in a population sample of older people. *Depression and Anxiety, 33*(4), 339–346. doi: 10.1002/da.22459

Skre, I., Onstad, S., Torgersen, S., Philos, D. R., Lygren, S., & Kringlen, E. (2000). The heritability of common phobic fear: A twin study of a clinical sample. *Journal of Anxiety Disorders, 14*(6), 549–562. doi: 10.1016/S0887-6185(00)00049-9

Smith, A. (2014). *6 new facts about Facebook*. Washington, DC: Pew Research Center.

Stein, M. B., Ravindran, L. N., Simon, N. M., Liebowitz, M. R., Khan, A., Brawman-Mintzer, O., … Pollak, M. H. (2010). Levetiracetam in generalized social anxiety disorder: A double-blind, randomized controlled trial. *Journal of Clinical Psychiatry, 71*(5), 627–631. doi: 10.4088/JCP.08m04949gre

Stern, D. N. (1985). *The interpersonal world of the infant. A view from psychoanalysis and developmental psychology*. New York, NY: Basic Books.

Stinson, F. S., Dawson, D. A., Chou, S. P., Smith, S., Goldstein, R. B., Ruan, W. J., & Grant, B. F. (2007). The epidemiology of DSM-IV specific phobia in the USA: Results from the National Epidemiologic Survey on Alcohol and Related Conditions. *Psychological Medicine, 7*(7), 1047–1059. doi: 10.1017/S0033291707000086

Stricker, G. (2010). A second look at psychotherapy integration. *Journal of Psychotherapy Integration, 20*(4), 397–405. doi: 10.1037/a0022037

Stricker, G., & Gold, J. (2005). Assimilative psychodynamic psychotherapy. In J. C. Norcross & M. R. Goldfried (Eds.), *Handbook of psychotherapy integration* (2nd ed., pp. 221–240). New York, NY: Oxford University Press.

Swift, J. K., Greenberg, R. P., Tompkins, K. A., & Parkin, S. R. (2017). Treatment refusal and premature termination in psychotherapy, pharmacotherapy, and their combination: A meta-analysis of head-to-head comparisons. *Psychotherapy*, *54*(1), 47–57. doi: 10.1037/pst0000104

Taylor, C. T., & Alden, L. E. (2005). Social interpretation bias and generalized social phobia: The influence of developmental experiences. *Behaviour Research and Therapy*, *43*(6), 759–777. doi: 10.1016/j.brat.2004.06.006

ten Have, M., de Graaf, R., van Dorsselaer, S., & Beekman, A. (2013). Lifetime treatment contact and delay in treatment seeking after first onset of a mental disorder. *Psychiatric Services*, *64*(10), 981–989. doi: 10.1176/appi.ps.201200454

Tillfors, M., Furmark, T., Marteinsdottir, I., Fischer, H., Pissiota, A., Långström, B., & Fredrikson, M. (2001). Cerebral blood flow in subjects with social phobia during stressful speaking tasks: A PET study. *American Journal of Psychiatry*, *158*(8), 1220–1226. doi: 10.1176/appi.ajp.158.8.1220

Van Ameringen, M. A., Lane, R. M., Walker, J. R., Bowen, R. C., Chokka, P. R., Goldner, E. M., … & Swinson, R. P. (2001). Sertraline treatment of generalized social phobia: A 20-week, double-blind, placebo-controlled study. *American Journal of Psychiatry*, *158*(2), 275–281. doi: 10.1176/appi.ajp.158.2.275

Van Yperen, N. W., & Hagedoorn, M. (2008). Living up to high standards and psychological distress. *European Journal of Personality*, *22*(4), 337–346. doi: 10.1002/per.681

Wardenaar, K. J., Lim, C. C., Al-Hamzawi, A. O., Alonso, J., Andrade, L. H., Benjet, C., … de Jonge, P. (2017). The cross-national epidemiology of specific phobia in the World Mental Health Surveys. *Psychological Medicine*, *47*(10), 1744–1760. doi: 10.1017/S0033291717000174

Watson, J. C. (2006). Resolving trauma in process-experiential therapy. In G. Stricker & J. Gold (Eds.), *A casebook of psychotherapy integration* (pp. 89–106). Washington, DC: American Psychological Association.

Watson, J. C., & Greenberg, L. S. (2017). *Emotion focused psychotherapy for generalized anxiety disorder*. Washington, DC: American Psychological Association.

Weiller, E., Bisserbe, J. C., Boyer, P., Lepine, J. P., & Lecrubier, Y. (1996). Social phobia in general health care: An unrecognised undertreated disabling disorder. *The British Journal of Psychiatry*, *168*(2), 169–174. doi: 10.1192/bjp.168.2.169

Weiss, B., Dodge, K. A., Bates, J. E., & Pettit, G. S. (1992). Some consequences of early harsh discipline: Child aggression and a maladaptive social information processing style. *Child Development*, *63*(6), 1321–1335. doi: 10.2307/1131558

Wilber, K. (2000). *Integral psychology: Consciousness, spirit, psychology, therapy*. Boston, MA: Shambala.

Wild, J., & Clark, D. M. (2011). Imagery rescripting of early traumatic memories in social phobia. *Cognitive and Behavioral Practice*, *18*(4), 433–443. doi: 10.1016/j.cbpra.2011.03.002

Wittchen, H. U., Stein, M. B., & Kessler, R. C. (1999). Social fears and social phobia in a community sample of adolescents and young adults: Prevalence, risk factors and co-morbidity. *Psychological Medicine*, *29*(2), 309–323. doi: 10.1017/s0033291798008174

Wolfe, B. E. (1992). Self-experiencing and the integrative treatment of the anxiety disorders. *Journal of Psychotherapy Integration*, *2*(1), 29–43. doi: 10.1037/h0101237

Wolfe, B. E. (2003). Integrative psychotherapy of the anxiety disorders. In J. C. Norcross & M. R. Goldfried (Eds.), *Handbook of psychotherapy integration* (2nd ed., pp. 263–280). New York, NY: Oxford University Press.

Wolfe, B. E. (2005). *Understanding and treating anxiety disorders: An integrative approach to healing the wounded self.* Washington, DC: American Psychological Association.

Wolfe, B. E. (2006). An integrative perspective on the anxiety disorders. In G. Stricker & J. Gold (Eds.), *A casebook of psychotherapy integration* (pp. 65–77). Washington, DC: American Psychological Association.

Wolfe, B. E. (2008). Existential issues in anxiety disorders and their treatment. In K. I. Schneider (Ed.), *Existential-integrative psychotherapy* (pp. 204–216). New York, NY: Routledge.

Wolfe, B. E., & Sigl, P. (1998). Experiential psychotherapy of the anxiety disorders. In L. S. Greenberg J. C. Watson & G. Lietaer (Eds.), *Handbook of experiential psychotherapy* (pp. 272–294). New York, NY: Guilford Press.

Wolitzky-Taylor, K. B., Castriotta, N., Lenze, E. J., Stanley, M. A., & Craske, M. G. (2010). Anxiety disorders in older adults: A comprehensive review. *Depression and Anxiety, 27*(2), 190–211. doi: 10.1002/da.20653

Wong, N., Sarver, D. E., & Beidel, D. C. (2012). Quality of life impairments among adults with social phobia: The impact of subtype. *Journal of Anxiety Disorders, 26*(1), 50–57. doi: 10.1016/j.janxdis.2011.08.012

Wong, Q. J., & Rapee, R. M. (2016). The aetiology and maintenance of social anxiety disorder: A synthesis of complementary theoretical models and formulation of a new integrated model. *Journal of Affective Disorders, 203*, 84–100. doi: 10.1016/j.jad.2016.05.069

8 Separation Anxiety Disorder (SAD) and Adult Separation Anxiety Disorder (ASAD)

Introduction

Separation anxiety disorder, a disorder that has been recently grouped under the Anxiety Disorders section of the DSM-5 (American Psychiatric Association, 2013), develops prior to any other anxiety disorder (American Psychiatric Association, 2013; Carmassi, Gesi, Massimetti, Shear, & Dell'Osso, 2015; Ray, 2018). The DSM-5 (APA, 2013) has removed the criterion for age of onset for separation anxiety disorder given that this disorder can begin in childhood, adolescence, or adulthood, and it is not usual for separation anxiety disorder to occur for the first time in adulthood (APA, 2013; Carmassi et al., 2015). Chapter 8 focuses on integrated and unified etiology approaches and psychotherapy treatment models for separation anxiety disorder (see Table 8.1). At the end of the chapter, a case study is presented to demonstrate how a therapist integrated attachment theory and individual cognitive-behavioral therapy (CBT) along with emotion-focused cognitive-behavioral group therapy in the treatment of a patient with separation anxiety disorder.

Symptoms of Separation Anxiety Disorder (SAD) and Adult Separation Anxiety Disorder (ASAD)

Symptoms of separation anxiety disorder include chronic distress when an individual separates from home or from primary attachment persons (APA, 2013). Individuals with separation anxiety disorder may be afraid to be by themselves or without their primary attachment persons either when they are at home or when they are in other settings (Carmassi et al., 2015). Children with symptoms of separation anxiety disorder frequently display behaviors that are disruptive or avoidant that disturb their own academic and social development as well as the daily life of the family unit (Pincus, Santucci, Ehrenreich, & Eyberg, 2008). Children with separation anxiety disorder frequently refuse to attend school, and, generally, do not participate in age appropriate activities such as birthday parties and sleepovers (Doobay, 2008; Kapalka & Peters,

Table 8.1 Separation Anxiety Disorder (SAD) and Adult Separation Anxiety Disorder (ASAD)

Etiology (SAD)	*Etiology (ASAD)*	*Integrated Psychotherapy*
Biological and Genetic From a biological perspective, children with SAD may inherit a predisposition towards anxiety, and in the context of certain environmental stressors, symptoms may manifest as issues related to separation.[a,b] An individual with SAD may have a genetic predisposition towards the development of anxiety along with biological and temperamental propensities.[c]	Adult Separation Anxiety Disorder (ASAD): The Continuity Model[f] The continuity model seeks to revise the separation anxiety–panic disorder/agoraphobia hypothesis (SA-PD/Ag). The continuity framework holds that children with SAD may experience symptoms of separation anxiety when they become adults; however, symptoms will be adjusted according to each person's level of maturity.[f]	Integrated Cognitive Behavioral Therapy (CBT) Integrated Cognitive-Behavioral Therapy (CBT) with a Family and an Attachment Framework Cognitive-behavioral therapy that is integrated with a family approach based in attachment can be beneficial in alleviating the symptoms of separation anxiety disorder.[g,h]
Environmental Separation anxiety is affected by environmental variables more so than any other anxiety disorder of childhood.[d,e]		Integrated Cognitive Behavioral Therapy (CBT) with Eye Movement Desensitization and Reprocessing (EMDR)[i,j] An Integration of Parent-Child Interaction Therapy (PCIT) and Bravery Directed Interaction (BDI)[k,l,b]

[a]Barlow (2002). [b]Pincus, Santucci, Ehrenreich, and Eyberg (2008). [c]Goldsmith and Gottesman (1981). [d]Ehrenreich, Santucci, and Weiner (2008). [e]Eley (2001). [f]Silove and Rees (2014). [g]Bowlby (1988). [h]Cunningham and Renk (2017). [i]Morrissey (2013). [j]Tofani (2007). [k]Brinkmeyer & Eyberg, (2003). [l]Pincus, Eyberg, and Choate (2005).

2013). They tend to report somatic symptoms such as nausea and stomach pains more frequently than do children with phobias (Last, 1991). Reports of somatic symptoms suggest avoidance or physiological distress, and these children may find it hard to sleep in the absence of a parent as well (Albano, Chorpita, & Barlow, 1996; Black, 1995; Tonge, 1994;). Whereas, generally, the attachment figures of children with separation anxiety disorder are their parents, and symptoms include school refusal, tantrums, and crying, the attachment figures of adults are a child or a spouse, and symptoms include repeated attempts to stay in close contact even when not practical (Pini et al., 2010; Rochester & Baldwin, 2015).

Diagnosis of Separation Anxiety Disorder (SAD) and Adult Separation Anxiety Disorder (ASAD)

According to the DSM-5 (APA, 2013), the symptoms need to endure in children and adolescents for at least four weeks in order for them to receive a diagnosis of separation anxiety disorder (SAD). It was found that children who received a diagnosis of juvenile separation anxiety disorder were 11 times more likely to have a parent who was diagnosed with adult separation anxiety disorder (Manicavasagar et al., 2009). Key symptoms of separation anxiety disorder include anxiety that doesn't go away or avoidance when an individual separates from attachment figures (Mowlaie, Hajloo, Sadeghi Hashjin, Mikaeili, & Heidari, 2018). If the aforementioned symptoms do not remit for a period of six months in adults, the patient would receive a diagnosis of adult separation anxiety disorder (ASAD) (Rochester & Baldwin, 2015).

According to DSM-5 (APA, 2013), adult separation anxiety disorder (ASAD) is a diagnosis that is distinct from the diagnosis of separation anxiety disorder of childhood. A diagnosis of adult separation anxiety disorder (ASAD) can be assigned both to individuals whose symptoms began when they were adults and to those whose symptoms began when they were children and continue when they are adults (Rochester & Baldwin, 2015). Formerly, an individual with adult separation anxiety disorder was frequently given a diagnosis of panic disorder; however, today, it seems that the diagnosis of adult separation anxiety disorder is acceptable, and the panic attacks are to be considered as symptoms of adult separation anxiety disorder (Rochester & Baldwin, 2015).

Prevalence of Separation Anxiety Disorder (SAD) and Adult Separation Anxiety Disorder (ASAD)

Prevalence

What is the prevalence of separation anxiety disorder? It has been shown that for children, the 12-month prevalence is reported at approximately 4%; for adolescents, at approximately 1.6%; and for adults, the range is between 0.9% and 1.9% (APA, 2013; Ray, 2018). Separation anxiety disorder is a key and damaging anxiety disorder of childhood, and its presence makes up 50% of psychological referrals (Bell-Dolan, 1995; Cartwright-Hatton, McNicol, & Doubleday, 2006; Santucci et al., 2009). According to the World Health Organization (WHO), the lifetime prevalence rates are 4.8% across countries, and almost 50% of lifetime onsets of separation anxiety disorder take place after an individual reaches the age of 18 (Carmassi et al., 2015; Silove et al., 2015). In the U.S., ASAD's lifetime prevalence is 6.6% (Shear, Jin, Ruscio, Walters, & Kessler, 2006; Silove & Rees, 2014).

Onset

The most frequent anxiety disorder in childhood, for those under age 12, is separation anxiety disorder (Ray, 2018; Sweeney, Levitt, Westerhom, Gaskins,

& Lapinski, 2013). When does separation anxiety disorder begin? Separation anxiety disorder can begin in children who are in preschool (Kapalka & Peters, 2013). Separation anxiety disorder is a disorder of childhood, but can continue into adolescence and, at times, adulthood (Carmassi et al., 2015; Alladin, 2016). Separation anxiety disorder is classified among the anxiety disorders, and for many years has been thought of as a disorder that occurs in childhood; however, practitioners are not completely cognizant of its prevalence for adults (Carmassi et al., 2015). Separation anxiety disorder can persist throughout an individual's lifespan and can constrict an individual's social and emotional functioning (Kapalka & Peters, 2013; Masi, Mucci, & Millipiedi, 2001).

Bögels, Knappe, and Clarke (2013) distinguish between the following types of adult separation anxiety disorder (ASAD): Adult-onset and childhood-onset. Whereas adult-onset involves individuals who have not fulfilled the criteria of childhood separation anxiety disorder, childhood-onset includes those with a history of separation anxiety disorder in childhood (Bögels et al., 2013). Approximately 40% of individuals with separation anxiety report that their symptoms began when they were adults (Milrod, 2015; Silove et al., 2015). Separation anxiety disorder (SAD) in childhood can lead to adult separation anxiety disorder (ASAD) (Bögels et al., 2013; Silove, Marnane, Wagner, Manicavasagar, & Rees, 2010).

It has been shown that there is a strong relationship between separation anxiety disorder and being female, having a childhood characterized by a dysfunctional family, and an assortment of traumatic incidents throughout the lifespan (Carmassi et al., 2015). It has been found that separation anxiety disorder (SAD) is comorbid with generalized anxiety disorder (GAD) and specific phobia (SP) (APA, 2013). ASAD is comorbid with several anxiety disorders including post-traumatic stress disorder (PTSD) (APA, 2013; Silove, Manicavasagar, & Drobny, 2002), grief (Pini et al., 2012), and bipolar disorder (APA, 2013).

An Integrative Etiology of Separation Anxiety Disorder (SAD) and Adult Separation Anxiety Disorder (ASAD): Focus, Underpinnings, and Causes of SAD and ASAD

What contributes to the development of separation anxiety disorder (SAD)? Genetic variables as well as distinctive and shared environmental characteristics contribute to the etiology of separation anxiety disorder (SAD) (Scaini, Ogliari, Eley, Zavos, & Battaglia, 2012). This section discusses the integrative etiology of separation anxiety disorder (SAD) and adult separation anxiety disorder (ASAD).

Separation Anxiety Disorder (SAD)

How do biological and environmental variables contribute to the development of SAD? From a biological perspective, children with SAD may inherit a predisposition towards anxiety, and in the context of certain environmental stressors, symptoms may manifest as issues related to separation (Barlow, 2002; Pincus et al., 2008). An individual with SAD may have a genetic predisposition towards the development of anxiety along with biological and temperamental propensities (Goldsmith & Gottesman, 1981).

Separation anxiety is affected by environmental variables more so than any other anxiety disorder of childhood (Ehrenreich, Santucci, & Weiner, 2008; Eley, 2001). From an environmental perspective, research on parents' interactions with their children has shown that children with anxiety tend to have parents who are critical, controlling, colder, and/or overprotective (Eisen, Engler, & Geyer, 1998). Particularly at risk are children with parents who are intrusive (Wood, 2006). At times, because of a lack of harmony between parents, reliable limits are not set for children with SAD (Ziegler, 1996).

Locus of control is implicated in the etiology of anxiety symptoms in that if children perceive that there is an external locus or that they do not have a lot of control over their environment, they will be more prone to develop anxiety (Chorpita & Barlow; 1998; Ehrenreich et al., 2008). External locus of control and perceived inadequacy are characteristics of children with separation anxiety disorder (Ceyhan & Ceyhan, 2009).

Žvelc (2010) developed an integrated framework of attachment theory and object relations to describe interpersonal relationships. According to this integrated model, separation anxiety is a basic human fear that is part of adult and child relationships. Whereas separation anxiety is healthy when it facilitates forming an attachment to another person, it is not adaptive when it is intense and manifests at the slightest hint of separation (Žvelc, 2010). Consistent with Kohut's (1971) theory that underscores the relationship between adequate parenting and the integration of self-object processes, Žvelc's (2010) integrated framework of attachment theory and object relations proposes that individuals who suffer from separation anxiety tend to be overly dependent, cling to the object, fear being alone, do not integrate regulatory behaviors of caregivers, and do not have a sense of their own internal balance. Consistent with Žvelc's (2010) integrated framework is Rochester and Baldwin's (2015) proposal that the ability of individuals to establish and maintain relationships rests at the core of separation anxiety disorder.

Adult Separation Anxiety Disorder (ASAD)

There is a paucity of findings on the antecedents of adult separation anxiety disorder; however, it has been shown that there exists a stronger relationship between symptoms of separation anxiety and neuroticism and its associative features (e.g., attachment that is insecure) than the relationship between the symptoms of other anxiety disorders and neuroticism (Bögels et al., 2013; Manicavisigar et al., 2009; Silove, Marnane et al., 2010). It has been suggested that individuals' exposure to trauma may be related to their developing adult separation disorder (Silove, Momartin, Marnane, Steel, & Manicavasagar, 2010).

Various models have been proposed to explain the etiology of separation anxiety disorder. Silove and Rees (2014) proposed a continuity model that seeks to revise the separation anxiety–panic disorder/agoraphobia hypothesis (SA-PD/Ag). Their continuity framework holds that children with SAD may experience symptoms of separation anxiety when they become adults; however, symptoms will be adjusted according to each person's level of maturity. Chronic symptoms of separation anxiety trigger a propensity towards the occurrence of other mental disorders that tend to manifest when children become adults, e.g., panic disorder with agoraphobia (Milrod et al., 2014; Silove & Rees, 2014). The persistent symptoms of separation anxiety of individuals who are adults tend to mediate the link between childhood separation anxiety and later panic disorder with agoraphobia (Silove & Rees, 2014). Both separation anxiety disorder and panic disorder have a common pattern of an oversensitivity to carbon dioxide when inhaled, which suggests that both diagnoses share a common factor, a pathophysiological core (Atli, Bayin, & Alkin, 2012).

Clinical Practice Applications of Single-School and Integrated Psychotherapy for Separation Anxiety Disorder (SAD) and Adult Separation Anxiety Disorder (ASAD)

The Therapeutic Alliance

Researchers have emphasized the importance of the therapeutic relationship. For example, the therapeutic relationship, as early as the third session, is specifically associated with outcome (Creed and Kendall, 2005; Horvath, 1994; O'Malley, Suh, & Strupp, 1983), and the findings for these alliances have been consistent across types of therapy (e.g. psychodynamic, CBT) and patient diagnoses (Shirk & Karver, 2003). Differences in the therapeutic alliance depend on whether the patient is an adult, an adolescent, or a child (Creed & Kendall, 2005). Whereas in the case of adult patients, improvement in the relationship between therapist and patient occurred when disruptions, e.g., conversations about patients feeling negative towards therapist, were addressed, in the case of adolescent patients, disruptions were negatively related to the strength of the therapeutic relationship. (Creed & Kendall, 2005; DiGiuseppe, Linscott, & Jilton, 1996; Safran, Muran, & Wallner Samstag, 1994). A greater number of therapeutic alliance type behaviors or specific levels of client-centered alliance factors (e.g., warmth, on target empathy; Rogers, 1951) were correlated with increased benefits for the internalizing emotional disorders of children (Creed & Kendall, 2005; Truax, Altmann, Wright, & Mitchell, 1973). Coercing patients who are children to address their anxiety before they are ready is related negatively to a therapeutic alliance (Creed & Kendall, 2005).

Single-School Cognitive-Behavioral Therapy (CBT) and Integrated Cognitive-Behavioral Therapy (CBT) with Parent-Training for Separation Anxiety Disorder (SAD)

Younger children do not benefit as much as older children from the monotherapy, cognitive-behavioral therapy (CBT), because CBT requires the use of cognitions that may not be targeted to the developmental stage of young children (Bennett & Gibbons, 2000; Grave & Blisset, 2004; Pincus et al., 2008). Recommendations for treatments to include the parents of children with anxiety disorders may result in a decrease of symptoms of anxiety in children, and suggestions to teach parents how to interact with children who are anxious are critical given that over 60% of children with social anxiety disorder have a parent with anxiety (Cartwright-Hatton, McNally &White, 2005; Manicavasagar, Silove, Rapee, Waters, & Momartin, 2001; Pincus et al., 2008).

It has been suggested that family members become involved in the interventions for separation anxiety disorder given the parent's contribution to the continuation of the separation distress of children (Ehrenreich et al., 2008). For example, Eisen, Raleigh, and Neuhoff (2008) found that an integrated CBT parent-training treatment for parents of children with separation anxiety disorder was effective for eliminating the symptoms of separation anxiety disorder in children and was beneficial in decreasing the distress and increasing the self-efficacy of parents.

Integrated Cognitive-Behavioral Therapy (CBT) with a Family and an Attachment Framework for Separation Anxiety Disorder (SAD)

Recently, Cunningham and Renk (2017) found cognitive-behavioral therapy that is integrated with a family approach based in attachment theory (Bowlby, 1988) to be beneficial in alleviating the symptoms of separation anxiety disorder. It is recognized that interventions that target young children require the development of a stable therapeutic relationship with the child's parents since children look to their parents or caregivers for the fulfillment of their mental and physiological needs (Cunningham & Renk, 2017). An integrative therapeutic model of treatment for separation anxiety disorder that includes the context of the family can help clinicians to determine the messages that children receive from their parents (Cunningham & Renk, 2017).

Integrated Cognitive Behavioral Therapy (CBT) with Eye Movement Desensitization and Reprocessing (EMDR) for Separation Anxiety Disorder (SAD)

Can eye movement desensitization and reprocessing (EMDR) benefit individuals with separation anxiety disorder (SAD)? During therapeutic work with children, the integration of eye movement desensitization and reprocessing (EMDR) with cognitive-behavioral therapy along with family therapy has been suggested by several researchers (Morrissey, 2013; Tofani, 2007). Morrissey (2013) used eye movement desensitization and reprocessing (EMDR) as an integrative treatment for separation anxiety disorder. She demonstrated the use of EMDR in combination with family therapy to alleviate symptoms of separation anxiety disorder and to facilitate developmentally suitable activities.

An Integration of Parent-Child Interaction Therapy (PCIT) and Bravery Directed Interaction (BDI) for Separation Anxiety Disorder (SAD)

Children who were treated with traditional Parent-Child Interaction Therapy (PCIT) (Brinkmeyer & Eyberg, 2003), an intervention with empirical support that consists of a Child-Directed Interaction (CDI) and a Parent-Directed Interaction (PDI), showed a mild decrease in symptoms of separation anxiety disorder (SAD); however, the SAD symptoms did not decrease to a nonclinical position after the PCIT intervention (Pincus et al., 2008). Given that children who received PCIT treatment demonstrated some positive benefits, but did not reach a nonclinical level for their symptoms of anxiety, the Bravery Directed Interaction (BDI) (Pincus, Eyberg, & Choate, 2005), an intervention phase aimed at addressing particular anxiety issues noted by parents, was integrated into PCIT and was successful in increasing the relevance of PCIT for young children with SAD by helping these children confront situations that had been avoided in the past (Pincus et al., 2008).

Pharmacotherapy and a Combination of Medication with Psychological Interventions for Separation Anxiety Disorder (SAD)

Results of studies with pharmacological interventions for childhood anxiety are mixed (Ehrenreich et al., 2008). Selective serotonin reuptake inhibitors (SSRIs) may benefit youth with anxiety disorders (Reinblatt & Riddle, 2007). Fluvoxamine (Luvox) was shown to be more effective than placebo in reducing anxiety in youth with SAD (Research Unit on Pediatric Psychopharmacology Anxiety Study Group , 2001), and fluoxetine (Prozac) was demonstrated to be more effective than placebo in improving the symptoms of SAD (Birmaher et al., 2003). Utilizing a randomized trial, Schneider et al. (2011) showed that a CBT intervention benefits young children with SAD. Some research shows that pharmacological treatment for separation anxiety disorder is not a first choice; however, it can be beneficial for those who do not respond to CBT (Masi et al., 2001). Treatment that combines psychosocial interventions along with pharmacotherapy has been found to be beneficial (Kapalka & Peters, 2013).

An Integrated Framework of Attachment Theory and Object Relations and Separation Anxiety Disorder

The section on the etiology of separation anxiety disorder presented Žvelc's (2010) integrated framework of attachment theory and object relations and explained that individuals who suffer from separation anxiety tend to be overly dependent. Žvelc's (2010) integrated approach can be used to develop an in-depth psychotherapy treatment planning approach. For example, whereas object relations involve the right pole, dependence, of interpersonal relationships, subject relations describe the opposing pole, independence (Žvelc, 2010). It is suggested that therapists use the interpersonal dimension of Independence-Dependence to assess a patient's level of relationships (Žvelc, 2010).

Adult Separation Anxiety Disorder (ASAD)

Separation anxiety disorder is complex. There is a paucity of evidence related to the interventions for adult separation anxiety disorder, and the disorder does not tend to respond neatly to conventional CBT and medication utilized for panic disorder, a disorder that may occur with separation anxiety disorder (Manicavasagar et al., 2010; Miniati et al., 2012; Silove & Rees, 2014). In fact, it has been shown that adult patients with separation anxiety disorder have a lot of impairment and do not tend to improve much with conventional psychological interventions or with medication (Silove & Rees, 2014).

Up until 2017, there has been no research that has offered an assessment of the effectiveness of pharmacotherapy or therapy treatment for patients with a main diagnosis of adult separation anxiety disorder (ASAD). In 2017, Schneier et al. presented preliminary findings that the SSRI, vilazodone, which has been shown to be beneficial for generalized anxiety disorder (Khan et al., 2016) may be effective for ASAD, but they caution that further study is required.

In short, individuals with ASAD do not respond as well as individuals with other anxiety disorders to either psychotherapy or medication (Copeland, Angold, & Shanahan, 2014; Miniati et al., 2012; Mowlaie et al., 2018). Both brief empathic psychotherapy (BEP) and affect phobia therapy (APT) have been shown to decrease anxiety in individuals with ASAD (Mowlaie et al., 2018).

How to Implement Integrative Psychotherapy in Practice for Separation Anxiety Disorder (SAD)

Interventions for anxiety in children and adolescents that are evidenced-based include CBT; however, it has been shown that despite the robust evidence for CBT, up to half of children and adolescents have symptoms of an anxiety disorder after a complete course of a CBT intervention (Compton et al., 2004; Rapee, Schniering, & Hudson, 2009; Silverman, Pina, & Viswesvaran, 2008). In the following case study, the therapist integrated attachment theory and individual cognitive-behavioral therapy (CBT) along with emotion-focused cognitive-behavioral group therapy in the treatment of an eight-year-old girl with separation anxiety disorder (SAD). The aforementioned integrated treatment relies upon Weems and Carrion's (2003) intervention, which includes the incorporation of an attachment focus into a CBT model. Research continues to support treatment for anxiety disorders that includes exposure within a setting of an affectively solid therapeutic alliance that can repair ruptures in the therapeutic relationship (Cunningham & Renk, 2017; Kendall et al., 2009).

Shannon is an eight-year-old girl who lives with her grandmother, her grandfather, and two older sisters in a small apartment. Shannon's parents died in a car accident approximately three years ago. She has been experiencing moderate fears about separation from her grandparents for the last three years. Prior to her parents' death, there were marital difficulties, and Shannon experienced mild anxiety about going to play group and preschool. After the death of her parents, Shannon's fears escalated, and she refused to go to school, displayed much anxiety about sleeping over her best friend's house, and cried when asked to stay in the room with the therapist without her grandmother. Her disruptive home situation where her parents experienced a difficult marital relationship and the subsequent death of her parents contributed to a serious attachment disruption for Shannon.

According to attachment theory, children develop a lasting bond with their caregivers, and when caregivers are attuned to children's needs, the emotional attachment facilitates a feeling of security both at times when the caregivers are present and when they are not present (Bowlby, 1977; Weems & Carrion, 2003). It has been demonstrated that the therapist–child alliance is associated with greater motivation for psychotherapy, increased participation in tasks, and more beneficial outcomes (Chu et al., 2004). A better therapist–parent collaboration results in more substantial benefit for both the child's outcome and for parenting (Kazdin, Whitley, & Marciano, 2006; Kendall et al., 2009).

The therapist began by fostering a therapeutic relationship with Shannon, empathized at every session with Shannon over the loss of her parents, and explained to both grandparents and to Shannon the importance of bonding with attachment figures. The therapist treated Shannon for separation anxiety with CBT methods, e.g., psychoeducation and exposure, beginning with a first step when the therapist explained to grandparents and child that Shannon's grandparents would leave the room, but would hold Shannon's hands while they stood out the door, followed by Shannon's grandparents leaving Shannon alone with the therapist for three minutes with the door open. Minimal exposures within the setting of increased bonding with the therapist continued until Shannon felt able to tolerate the door closed for longer periods of time.

The therapist set up a behavioral contract with Shannon's grandparents to reinforce separations between the two at appropriate times, e.g., for short times of separation during the therapy sessions, when Shannon went to school, and when Shannon slept over her best friend's house. Initially, the therapist suggested to the school psychologist that Shannon be allowed to make five FaceTime calls to her grandmother during the day. These calls helped Shannon stay in school during each day, and were eventually decreased to one a day.

According to attachment theory, caretakers' sensitivity, attunement, and availability help to facilitate bonding and to decrease distress (Kobak, 1999; Weems & Carrion, 2003). The therapist recommended that the behavioral contract between Shannon and her grandparents include grandparent–child interaction reinforcers for separations. The therapist suggested that reinforcers for going to school and sleeping over a friend's house need to include extra and responsive activity time with Shannon's grandmother and grandfather (at times other than therapy, school, and sleepovers with a friend), e.g., miniature golfing with grandparents, joint activities such as bike riding, going on picnics with grandparents, extra trips with grandparents to Shannon's favorite ice cream shop. The behavioral contract between Shannon and her grandparents used caregiver-child attachment activity reinforcers that helped Shannon feel more secure, that taught Shannon that her grandparents are available for her and responsive to her concerns, and that Shannon needs to comply with contracted separations for school time and therapy.

Emotion-focused cognitive behavioral therapy (ECBT) targets emotion dysregulation in youth with separation anxiety by employing strategies aimed at emotion regulation (Afshari, Neshat-Doost, Maracy, Ahmady, & Amiri, 2014; Suveg, Kendall, Comer, & Robin, 2006). ECBT differs from CBT in that emotion ideas and skills that emphasize regulation are integrated into ECBT (Suveg et al., 2006). Children with separation anxiety disorder often utilize oppositional behaviors, e.g., temper tantrums, to avoid being separated from their parents (Afshari et al., 2014). When Shannon's grandparents requested that she get dressed for school, Shannon would start to scream and cry while retching and throwing up. After three months of the integration of attachment theory and individual CBT, Shannon's therapist suggested that Shannon attend an emotion-focused cognitive behavioral therapy group (ECBT) designed to target Shannon's emotionally dysregulated behaviors, e.g., screaming upon requests for separation. The therapist relied on the suggested integrated ECBT group interventions of Suveg and colleagues (2006) and Afshari and colleagues (2014) to regulate Shannon's angry outbursts that were disruptive to her family. During the first part of the ECBT group, the therapist introduced the group to various emotions, e.g., feeling sad, feeling nervous, and Shannon learned along with other children to identify these emotions in herself and in other children. During the second portion of the ECBT group, Shannon more easily learned to tolerate exposures to situations that are anxiety producing, which Shannon finds hard to regulate. During this time, the group therapist trained the children to manage their experiences of escalating emotions. After four months of group ECBT, Shannon's anxiety, in general, and her separation anxiety symptoms, e.g., screaming upon requests for separation, decreased.

Individual therapy continued as Shannon attended the ECBT group. The integration of attachment theory into an individual behavioral protocol taught Shannon's grandparents the importance of fostering security and availability for Shannon. The attachment approach whereby Shannon spent extra time with her grandmother and grandfather at appropriately selected times reinforced a decrease in Shannon's fears about separations during other necessary periods, e.g., during therapy, school, and when sleeping over her friend's house. Shannon was symptom free after two years of weekly therapy. Shannon's grandparents benefited from the integration of the attachment approach into the CBT protocol in that it helped them to understand the concept of separation anxiety disorder, the importance of attachment figures and bonding, and the need to increase quality time with Shannon along with a behavioral contract for reinforced separations. The integrated protocol of CBT along with the attachment approach facilitated Shannon's compliance with exposure therapy during therapy and school hours as well.

References

Afshari, A., Neshat-Doost, H. T., Maracy, M. R., Ahmady, M. K., & Amiri, S. (2014). The effective comparison between emotion-focused cognitive behavioral group therapy and cognitive behavioral group therapy in children with separation anxiety disorder. *Journal of Research in Medical Sciences, 19*(3), 221–227.

Albano, A. M., Chorpita, B. R., & Barlow, D. H. (1996). Childhood anxiety disorders. In E. J. Mash & R. A. Barkley (Eds.), *Child psychopathology* (pp. 196–241). New York, NY: Guilford Press.

Alladin, A. (2016). *Integrative CBT for anxiety disorders: An evidence-based approach to enhancing cognitive behavioral therapy with mindfulness and hypnotherapy*. Chichester, UK: Wiley Blackwell.

American Psychiatric Association. (2013). *Diagnostic and statistical manual of mental disorders* (5th ed.). Washington, DC: American Psychiatric Association.

Atli, O., Bayin, M., & Alkin, T. (2012). Hypersensitivity to 35% carbon dioxide in patients with adult separation anxiety disorder. *Journal of Affective Disorders, 141*(2–3), 315–323. doi: 10.1016/j.jad.2012.03.032

Barlow, D. H. (2002). *Anxiety and its disorders: The nature and treatment of anxiety and panic* (2nd ed.). New York, NY: Guilford Press.

Bell-Dolan, D. (1995). Separation anxiety disorder. In R. T. Ammerman & M. Hersen (Eds.), *Handbook of child behavior therapy in the psychiatric setting* (pp. 217–298). New York: John Wiley and Sons.

Bennett, D. S., & Gibbons, T. A. (2000). Efficacy of child cognitive–behavioral interventions for antisocial behavior: A meta-analysis. *Child and Family Behavior Therapy, 22*(1), 1–15. doi: 10.1300/J019v22n01_01

Birmaher, B., Axelson, D. A., Monk, K., Kalas, C., Clark, D. B., Ehmann, M., ... Brent, D. A. (2003). Fluoxetine for the treatment of childhood anxiety disorders. *Journal of the American Academy of Child and Adolescent Psychiatry, 42*(4), 415–423. doi: 10.1097/01.CHI.0000037049.04952.9F

Black, B. (1995). Separation anxiety disorder and panic disorder. In J. S. March (Ed.), *Anxiety disorders in children and adolescents* (pp. 212–234). New York, NY: Guilford Press.

Bögels, S. M., Knappe, S., & Clark, L. A. (2013). Adult separation anxiety disorder in DSM-5. *Clinical Psychology Review, 33*(5), 663–674. doi: 10.1016/j.cpr.2013.03.006

Bowlby, J. (1977). The making and breaking of affectional bonds: Aetiology and psychopathology in the light of attachment theory. *British Journal of Psychiatry, 130*(3), 201–210. doi: 10.1192/bjp.130.3.201

Bowlby, J. (1988). *A secure base: Clinical applications of attachment theory*. London, England: Routledge.

Brinkmeyer, M. Y., & Eyberg, S. M. (2003). Parent-child interaction therapy for oppositional children. In A. E. Kazdin (Ed.), *Evidence-based psychotherapies for children and adolescents* (pp. 204–223). New York, NY: The Guilford Press.

Carmassi, C., Gesi, C., Massimetti, E., Shear, M. K., & Dell'Osso, L. (2015). Separation anxiety disorder in the DSM-5 era. *Journal of Psychopathology, 21*, 365–371.

Cartwright-Hatton, S., McNally, D., & White, C. (2005). A new cognitive behavioural parenting intervention for families of young anxious children: A pilot study. *Behavioural and Cognitive Psychotherapy, 33*(2), 243–248. doi: 10.1017/S1352465804002036

Cartwright-Hatton, S., McNicol, K., & Doubleday, E. (2006). Anxiety in a neglected population: Prevalence of anxiety disorders in pre-adolescent children. *Clinical Psychology Review, 26*, 817–833. doi: 10.1016/j.cpr.2005.12.002

Ceyhan, A., & Ceyhan, E. (2009). Relationship between early separation anxiety and depressive symptoms: The mediating role of locus of control and problem solving skills. *Pakistan Journal of Social and Clinical Psychology*, 7(1), 3–17.

Chorpita, B. E., & Barlow, D. H. (1998). The development of anxiety: The role of control in the early environment. *Psychological Bulletin, 124*(1), 3–21. doi: 10.1037/0033-2909.124.1.3

Chu, B. C., Choudhury, M. S., Shortt, A. L., Pincus, D. B., Creed, T. A., & Kendall, P. C. (2004). Alliance, technology, and outcome in the treatment of anxious youth. *Cognitive and Behavioral Practice, 11*(1), 44–55. doi: 10.1016/S1077-7229(04)80006-3

Compton, S. N., March, J. S., Brent, D., Albano, A. M., Weersing, V. R., & Curry, J. (2004). Cognitive-behavioral psychotherapy for anxiety and depressive disorders in children and adolescents: An evidence-based medicine review. *Journal of the American Academy of Child and Adolescent Psychiatry, 43*(8), 930–959. doi: 10.1097/01.chi.0000127589.57468.bf

Copeland, W. E., Angold, A., & Shanahan, L. (2014). Longitudinal patterns of anxiety from childhood to adulthood: The Great Smoky Mountains Study. *Journal of American Academic Child Adolescence Psychiatry, 53*(1), 21–33. doi: 10.1016/j.jaac.2013.09.017

Creed, T. A., & Kendall, P. C. (2005). Therapist alliance-building behavior within a cognitive- behavioral treatment for anxiety in youth. *Journal of Consulting and Clinical Psychology, 73*(3), 498–505. doi: 10.1037/0022-006X.73.3.498

Cunningham, A., & Renk, K. (2017). I'm uncomfortable, you're uncomfortable, we're uncomfortable: An integrative family approach to the treatment of Tourette's disorder and separation anxiety disorder in a young child. *Clinical Case Studies, 16*(6), 446–463. doi: 10.1177/1534650117732143p

DiGiuseppe, R., Linscott, J., & Jilton, R. (1996). Developing the therapeutic alliance in child–adolescent psychotherapy. *Applied and Preventive Psychology, 5*(2), 85–100. doi: 10.1016/S0962-1849(96)80002-3

Doobay, A. F. (2008). School refusal behavior associated with separation anxiety disorder: A cognitive-behavioral approach to treatment. *Psychology in the Schools, 45*(4), 261–272. doi: 10.1002/pits.20299

Ehrenreich, J. T., Santucci, L. C., & Weiner, C. L. (2008). Separation anxiety disorder in youth: Phenomenology, assessment, and treatment. *Psicologia Conductual, 16*(3), 389–412. doi: 10.1901/jaba.2008.16-389

Eisen, A. R., Engler, L. B., & Geyer, B. (1998). Parent training for separation anxiety disorder. In J. M. Briesmeister & C. E. Schaefer (Eds.), *Handbook of parent training: Parents as co-therapists for children's behavior problems* (2nd ed., pp. 205–224). New York, NY: John Wiley and Sons.

Eisen, A. R., Raleigh, H., & Neuhoff, C. C. (2008). The unique impact of parent training for separation anxiety disorder in children. *Behavior Therapy, 39*(2), 195–206. doi: 10.1016/j.beth.2007.07.004

Eley, T. C. (2001). Contributions of behavioral genetics research: Quantifying genetic, shared environment and nonshared environmental influences. In M. W. Vasey & M. R. Dadds (Eds.), *The developmental psychopathology of anxiety* (pp. 45–59). New York, NY: Oxford University Press.

Goldsmith, H., & Gottesman, I. (1981). Origins of variation in behavioral style: A longitudinal study of temperament in young twins. *Child Development, 52*(1), 91–103. doi: 10.2307/1129218

Grave, J., & Blissett, J. (2004). Is cognitive behavior therapy developmentally appropriate for young children? A critical review of the evidence. *Clinical Psychology Review, 24*(4), 399–420. doi: 10.1016/j.cpr.2004.03.002

Horvath, A. O. (1994). Empirical validation of Bordin's pantheoretical model of the alliance: The working alliance inventory perspective. In A. O. Horvath & L. S. Greenberg (Eds.), *The working alliance: Theory, research, and practice* (pp. 109–128). New York, NY: Wiley.

Kapalka, G. M., & Peters, C. (2013). Separation anxiety disorder. In S. M. Stahl & B. A. Moore (Eds.), *Anxiety disorders: A guide for integrating psychopharmacology and psychotherapy* (pp. 260–284). New York, NY: Routledge.

Kazdin, A. E., Whitley, M., & Marciano, P. L. (2006). Child–therapist and parent–therapist alliance and therapeutic change in the treatment of children referred for oppositional, aggressive, and antisocial behavior. *Journal of Child Psychology and Psychiatry, 47*(5), 436–445. doi: 10.1111/j.1469-7610.2005.01475.x

Kendall, P. C., Comer, J. S., Marker, C. D., Creed, T. A., Puliafico, A. C., Hughes, A. A., … Hudson, J. (2009). In-session exposure tasks and therapeutic alliance across the treatment of childhood anxiety disorders. *Journal of Consulting and Clinical Psychology, 77*(3), 517–525. doi: 10.1037/a0013686

Khan, A., Durgam, S., Tang, X., Ruth, A., Mathews, M., & Gommoll, C. P. (2016). Post hoc analyses of anxiety measures in adult patients with generalized anxiety disorder treated with vilazodone. *Primary Care Companion for CNS Disorders, 18*(2). Retrieved from https://doi.org/10.4088/PCC.15m01904 doi: 10.4088/PCC.15m01904

Kobak, R. (1999). The emotional dynamics of disruptions in attachment relationships. In J. Cassidy & P. R. Shaver (Eds.), *Handbook of attachment: Theory, research and clinical applications* (pp. 21–43). New York, NY: Guilford Press.

Kohut, H. (1971). *The analysis of the self.* New York, NY: International Universities Press.

Last, C. G. (1991). Somatic complaints in anxiety disordered children. *Journal of Anxiety Disorders, 5*(2), 125–138. doi: 10.1016/0887-6185(91)90024-N

Manicavasagar, V., Marnane, M., Pini, S., Abelli, M., Rees, S., Eapen, V., & Silove, D. (2010). Adult separation anxiety disorder: A disorder comes of age. *Current Psychiatry Reports, 12*(4), 290–297. doi: 10.1007/s11920-010-0131-9

Manicavisigar, V., Silove, D., Marnane, C., & Wagner, R. (2009). Adult attachment styles in panic disorder with and without adult separation anxiety disorder. *Australian and New Zealand Journal of Psychiatry, 43*, 167–172. doi: 10.1080/00048670802607139

Manicavasagar, V., Silove, D., Rapee, R., Waters, F., & Momartin, S. (2001). Parent–child concordance for separation anxiety: A clinical study. *Journal of Affective Disorders, 65*(1), 81–84. doi: 10.1016/S0165-0327(00)00241-X

Masi, G., Mucci, M., & Millepiedi, S. (2001). Separation anxiety disorder in children and adolescents. *CNS Drugs, 15*(2), 93–104. doi: 10.2165/00023210-200115020-00002

Milrod, B. (2015). An epidemiological contribution to clinical understanding of anxiety. *American Journal of Psychiatry, 72*(7), 601–6022. doi: 10.1176/appi.ajp.2015.15030312

Milrod, B., Markowitz, J. C., Gerber, A. J., Cyranowski, J., Altemus, M., Shapiro, T., … Glatt, C. (2014). Childhood separation anxiety and the pathogenesis and treatment of adult anxiety. *American Journal of Psychiatry, 171*(1), 34–43. doi: 10.1176/appi.ajp.2013.13060781

Miniati, M., Calugi, S., Rucci, P., Shear, M. K., Benvenuti, A., Santoro, D., … Cassano, G. B. (2012). Predictors of response among patients with panic disorder treated with medications in a naturalistic follow-up: The role of adult separation anxiety. *Journal of Affective Disorders, 136*(3), 675–679. doi: 10.1016/j.jad.2011.10.008

Morrissey, M. (2013). EMDR as an integrative therapeutic approach for the treatment of separation anxiety disorder. *Journal of EMDR Practice and Research*, 7(4), 200–207. doi: 10.1891/1933-3196.7.4.200

Mowlaie, M., Hajloo, N., Sadeghi Hashjin, G., Mikaeili, N., & Heidari, S. (2018). The effectiveness of empathic dynamic psychotherapy and anxiety-regulating psychodynamic therapy in treating adult separation anxiety disorder. *Practice in Clinical Psychology, 6*(3), 143–152.

O'Malley, S. S., Suh, C. S., & Strupp, H. H. (1983). The Vanderbilt Psychotherapy Process Scale: A report on scale development and a process-outcome study. *Journal of Consulting and Clinical Psychology, 51*(4), 581–586. doi: 10.1037/0022-006X.51.4.581

Pincus, D. B., Eyberg, S., & Choate, M. L. (2005). Adapting parent-child interaction therapy for children with separation anxiety disorder. *Education and Treatment of Children, 28*, 163–181. doi: 10.1016/j.chc.2012.05.005

Pincus, D. B., Santucci, L. C., Ehrenreich, J. T., & Eyberg, S. M. (2008). The implementation of modified parent-child interaction therapy for youth with separation anxiety disorder. *Cognitive and Behavioral Practice, 15*(2), 118–125. doi: 10.1016/j.cbpra.2007.08.002

Pini, S., Abelli, M., Shear, K. M., Cardini, A., Lari, L., Gesi, C., ... Cassano, G. B. (2010). Frequency and clinical correlates of adult separation anxiety in a sample of 508 outpatients with mood and anxiety disorders. *Acta Psychiatrica Scandinavica, 122*(1), 40–46. doi: 10.1111/j.1600-0447.2009.01480.x

Pini, S., Gesi, C., Abelli, M., Muti, Lari, L., Cardini, A., ... Shear, K. M. (2012). The relationship between adult separation anxiety disorder and complicated grief in a cohort of 454 outpatients with mood and anxiety disorders. *Journal of Affective Disorders, 143*(1–3), 64–68.

Rapee, R. M., Schniering, C. A., & Hudson, J. L. (2009). Anxiety disorders during childhood and adolescence: Origins and treatment. *Annual Review of Clinical Psychology, 5*, 311–341. doi: 10.1146/annurev.clinpsy.032408.153628

Ray, W. J. (2018). *Abnormal psychology*. Thousand Oaks, CA: Sage.

Reinblatt, S. P., & Riddle, M. A. (2007). The pharmacological management of childhood anxiety disorders: A review. *Psychopharmacology, 191*(1), 67–86. doi: 10.1007/s00213-006-0644

Research Unit on Pediatric Psychopharmacology Anxiety Study Group (2001). Fluvoxamine for the treatment of anxiety disorders in children and adolescents. *New England Journal of Medicine, 344*(17), 1279–1285. doi: 10.1056/NEJM200104263441703

Rochester, J., & Baldwin, D. S. (2015). Adult separation anxiety disorder: Accepted but little understood. *Human Psychopharmacology: Clinical and Experimental, 30*(1), 1–3. doi: 10.1002/hup.2452

Rogers, C. R. (1951). *Client-centered therapy: Its current practice, implications, and theory*. Boston, MA: Houghton Mifflin.

Safran, J. D., Muran, J. C., & Wallner Samstag, L. (1994). Resolving therapeutic alliance ruptures: A task analytic investigation. In A. O. Horvath & L. S. Greenberg (Eds.), *The working alliance: Theory, research, and practice* (pp. 225–255). New York, NY: Wiley.

Santucci, L. C., Ehrenreich, J. T., Trosper, S. E., Bennett, S. M., & Pincus, D. B. (2009). Development and preliminary evaluation of a one-week summer treatment program for separation anxiety disorder. *Cognitive and Behavioral Practice, 16*(3), 317–331. doi: 10.1016/j.cbpra.2008.12.005

Scaini, S., Ogliari, A., Eley, T. C., Zavos, H. M. S., & Battaglia, M. (2012). Genetic and environment contributions to separation anxiety: A meta-analytic approach to twin data. *Depression and Anxiety, 29*(9), 754–761. doi: 10.1002/da.21941

Schneider, S., Blatter-Meunier, J., Herren, C., Adornetto, C., In-Albon, T., & Lavallee, K. (2011). Disorder-specific cognitive-behavioral therapy for separation anxiety disorder in young children: A randomized waiting-list-controlled trial. *Psychotherapy and Psychosomatics, 80*(4), 206–215. doi: 10.1159/000323444

Schneier, F. R., Moskow, D. M., Choo, T. H., Galfalvy, H., Campeas, R., & Sanchez-Lacay, A. (2017). A randomized controlled pilot trial of vilazodone for adult separation anxiety disorder. *Depression and Anxiety, 34*(12), 1085–1095. doi: 10.1002/da.22693

Shear, K., Jin, R., Ruscio, A. M., Walters, E. E., & Kessler, R. C. (2006). Prevalence and correlates of estimated DSM-IV child and adult separation anxiety disorder in the National Comorbidity Survey Replication. *The American Journal of Psychiatry, 163*(6), 1074–1083. doi: 10.1176/ajp.2006.163.6.1074

Shirk, S. R., & Karver, M. (2003). Prediction of treatment outcome from relationship variables in child and adolescent therapy: A meta-analytic review. *Journal of Consulting and Clinical Psychology, 71*(3), 452–464. doi: 10.1037/0022-006X.71.3.452

Silove, D., Alonso, J., Bromet, E., Gruber, M., Sampson, N., Scott, K., … Kessler, R. C. (2015). Pediatric-onset and adult-onset separation anxiety disorder across countries in the World Mental Health Survey. *American Journal of Psychiatry, 172*(7), 647–656. doi: 10.1176/appi.ajp.2015.14091185.

Silove, D., Manicavasagar, V., & Drobny, J. (2002). Associations between juvenile and adult forms of separation anxiety disorder: A study of volunteers with histories of school refusal. *Journal of Nervous and Mental Diseases, 190*(6), 413–415. doi: 10.1097/00005053-200206000-00013

Silove, D., Marnane, C., Wagner, R., Manicavasagar, V., & Rees, S. (2010). The prevalence and correlates of adult separation anxiety disorder in an anxiety clinic. *BMC Psychiatry, 10*, 21–27. doi: 10.1186/1471-244X-10-21

Silove, D., Momartin, S., Marnane, C., Steel, Z., & Manicavasagar, V. (2010). Adult separation anxiety disorder among war-affected Bosnian refugees: Comorbidity with PTSD and associations with dimensions of trauma. *Journal of Traumatic Stress, 23*(1), 169–172. doi: 10.1002/jts.20490

Silove, D., & Rees, S. (2014). Separation anxiety disorder across the lifespan: DSM-5 lifts age restriction on diagnosis. *Asian Journal of Psychiatry, 11*, 98–101. doi: 10.1016/j.ajp.2014.06.021

Silverman, W. K., Pina, A. A., & Viswesvaran, C. (2008). Evidence-based psychosocial treatments for phobic and anxiety disorders in children and adolescents. *Journal of Clinical Child and Adolescent Psychology, 37*(1), 105–130. doi: 10.1080/15374410701817907.

Suveg, C., Kendall, P. C., Comer, J. S., & Robin, J. (2006). Emotion-focused cognitive-behavioral therapy for anxious youth: A multiple-baseline evaluation. *Journal of Contemporary Psychotherapy: On the Cutting Edge of Modern Developments in Psychotherapy, 36*(2), 77–85. doi: 10.1007/s10879-006-9010-4

Sweeney, M., Levitt, J., Westerhom, R., Gaskins, C., & Lapinski, C. (2013). Pharmacological treatment of anxiety disorders across the lifespan. In S. M. Stahl & B. A. Moore (Eds.), *Anxiety disorders: A guide for integrating psychopharmacology and psychotherapy* (pp. 71–93). New York, NY: Routledge.

Tofani, L. R. (2007). Complex separation, individuation processes, and anxiety disorders in young adulthood. In F. Shapiro, F. W. Kaslow & L. Maxfield (Eds.), *Handbook of EMDR and family therapy processes* (pp. 265–283). Hoboken, NJ: John Wiley and Sons.

Tonge, B. (1994). Separation anxiety disorder. In T. H. Ollendick, N. J. King & W. Yule (Eds.), *International handbook of phobic and anxiety disorders in children and adolescents* (pp. 145–167). New York, NY: Plenum Press.

Truax, C. B., Altmann, H., Wright, L., & Mitchell, K. M. (1973). Effects of therapeutic conditions in child therapy. *Journal of Community Psychology, 1*, 313–318. doi: 10.1002/1520-6629(197307)1:3<313::AID- JCOP2290010319>3.0.CO;2-T

Weems, C. F., & Carrion, V. G. (2003). The treatment of separation anxiety disorder employing attachment theory and cognitive behavior therapy techniques. *Clinical Case Studies, 2*(3), 188–198. doi: 10.1177/1534650103253818

Wood, J. J. (2006). Parental intrusiveness and children's separation anxiety in a clinical sample. *Child Psychiatry and Human Development, 37*(1), 73–87. doi: 10.1007/ s10578-006-0021-x

Ziegler, (1996). Anxiety disorders in children: Applying a cognitive-behavioral technique that can be integrated with pharmacotherapy or other psychosocial interventions. In J. M. Ellison (Ed.), *Integrative treatment of anxiety disorders* (pp.153–197). Washington, DC: American Psychiatric Press.

Žvelc, G. (2010). Object and subject relations in adulthood–towards an integrative model of interpersonal relationships. *Psychiatria Danubina, 22*(4), 498–508.

Part III

Integrated and Unified Psychotherapy Approaches for Obsessive-Compulsive Disorder (OCD) and Posttraumatic Stress Disorder (PTSD)

Part III discusses the integrated and unified etiological and psychotherapy treatment models as they apply to obsessive-compulsive disorder (OCD) and posttraumatic stress disorder (PTSD). The third part consists of Chapter 9, "Obsessive-Compulsive Disorder (OCD)," and Chapter 10, "Posttraumatic Stress Disorder (PTSD)."

9 Obsessive-Compulsive Disorder (OCD)

Introduction

Prior to DSM-5 (American Psychiatric Association, 2013), obsessive-compulsive disorder (OCD) was listed with the anxiety disorders. DSM-5 no longer lists OCD with the anxiety disorders; however, it has been found that individuals with OCD and those with anxiety disorders share similar distorted perceptions that maintain their fears (Ingersoll & Marquis, 2014). A distinction between obsessive-compulsive disorder and other anxiety disorders is one of a conscious versus an unconscious source (Comer, 2015). Whereas in the other anxiety disorders, patients struggle between id impulses that produce anxiety and their defenses exist in the unconscious, the struggles of patients with obsessive-compulsive disorder manifest in explicit ideation and actions (Comer, 2015).

This chapter focuses on integrated and unified etiology approaches and psychotherapy treatment models for obsessive-compulsive disorder (see Table 9.1). At the end of the chapter, a case study is presented to demonstrate the implementation of an integrated emotional schema therapy model along with cognitive therapy in the treatment of an adult with OCD. Basile, Luppino, Mancini, and Tenore (2018) proposed an integrated model whereby cognitive therapy (CT) is combined with schema therapy (ST) and aimed towards the treatment of OCD. The integrated psychotherapy treatment approach of an individual with OCD presented in the case study relies on Basile et al.'s (2018) integrative framework of schema therapy to help a patient understand the emotional schemas comprising her OCD. The treatment relies as well on the integrative model of schema treatment of Sookman and Steketee (2007), which can combine with exposure response prevention (ERP) to reinforce learning that is meaningful.

Symptoms of Obsessive-Compulsive Disorder (OCD)

What features characterize obsessive-compulsive disorder (OCD)? At times, most people have obsessions or intrusive thoughts and/or compulsions or repetitive behaviors that are neutralizing (Barlow, 2004; Ingersoll & Marquis,

Table 9.1 Obsessive-Compulsive Disorder (OCD)

Etiology: Neuroscience	*Etiology*	*Integrated and Unified Psychotherapy*
A Genetic Perspective[a,b,c]	A Psychological Perspective[i]	An Integration of a Cognitive Approach with Self Theories[n,o,p]
A Biological Perspective[d,a,e]	Psychoanalytic or Psychodynamic Approaches[j,k]	An Integration of Cognitive-Behavioral Therapy (CBT) with Motivational Interviewing (MI)[q]
The Interaction of Biological and Environmental[f,g,h]	Self-Wounds Individuals with OCD have internalized the shame and idea that they, in reality, are bad people.[l,m]	An Integration of Cognitive-Behavioral Therapy (CBT) with Hypnotically-Induced Dissociation(HID)[h]
		An Integration of CBT and Psychodynamic Therapy[k]
		An Integration of Cognitive-Behavioral Therapy (CBT) and Transactional Analysis[r]
		Mindfulness Integrated Cognitive Therapy[s]
		An Integration of Hypnosis and Positive Psychology[t]
		Schema therapy (ST): An Integrated or Unified Approach[u,v,w,x]
		An Integrated Existential Approach[y]

[a]Comer (2015). [b]Marsh et al. (2014). [c]Nicolini, Arnold, Nestadt, Lanzagorta, and Kennedy (2009). [d]Bokor and Anderson (2014). [e]Spooren, Lesage, Lavreysen, Gasparini, and Steckler (2010). [f]Alexopoulos (2004). [g]Frederick (2002, 2007). [h]Meyerson and Konichezky (2011). [i]Mancini (2019). [j]Fenichel (1945). [k]Woon, Kanapathy, Zakaria, and Alfonso (2017). [l]Tenore and Basile (2019).[m] Wolfe (2005). [n]Doron and Kryios (2005). [o]Doron, Kyrios, and Moulding (2007). [p]Doron, Mikulincer, Sar-El, and Kyrios (2015). [q]Tolin and Maltby, (2008). [r]Fields (1998). [s]Mathur, Sharma, and Reddy (2016). [t]Zahi and Meyerson (2010). [u] Bamelis, Evers, Spinhoven, and Arntz (2014). [v]Legra, Verhey, and van Alphen (2017). [w] Young, Klosko, and Weishaar (2005). [x]Basile, Luppino, Mancini, and Tenore (2018). [y]Wolfe (2008).

2014). Individuals with OCD, however, have obsessions or unwanted thoughts and/or compulsions, repetitive behaviors, e.g., checking more than once that the door is locked, that take up a lot of time every day and/or cause them a lot of internal distress (APA, 2013). When individuals with OCD have intrusive thoughts, they employ rituals in an attempt to neutralize the perceived threat (Ingersoll & Marquis, 2014). Compulsions frequently are a reaction to obsessive ideation (Comer, 2015). It is common for the symptoms of OCD to wax and wane (Rasmussen & Eisen, 1991; Sherman, Ellison, & Iwamoto, 1996), and symptoms can increase as a result of the stressors of life (Abramowitz & Jacoby, 2013). What themes comprise obsessive thoughts? Obsessions can include preoccupations with contamination, uncertainty, and themes of a religious or sexual nature (Comer, 2015; Tolin & Meunier, 2008; Torres et al., 2013). Primary groupings of obsessions involve the avoidance of contamination, the presence of aggressive urges, sexual thoughts, themes of morality, order, and somatic concepts (Ray, 2018). Whereas obsessions that are autogenous can occur without an external provocation, reactive obsessions can be triggered because of an external occurrence (Abramowitz & Jacoby, 2015; Ray, 2018). Individuals with OCD are convinced that they must perform a ritual in an exact way or something negative will occur (Dougherty, Rauch, & Jenike, 2015). Checking rituals are common. For example, a college student who has conflicts with his roommate may check his roommate's computer a few times a day.

Diagnosis of Obsessive-Compulsive Disorder (OCD)

Whereas many individuals, throughout the course of their lives, experience periods of obsessive incidents or tendencies that are subclinical in nature that do not decrease their quality of life, others endure obsessive and compulsive symptoms that compromise their ability to achieve school and occupational goals, and in the latter case, comprise a pervasive part of their personality and warrant a diagnosis of obsessive-compulsive disorder (OCD) (Mancini, 2019). Individuals receive a diagnosis of the common psychological disorder, obsessive-compulsive disorder (OCD), when they perceive their obsessions and compulsions to be extreme, take up a lot of time (longer than one hour a day), cause them a lot of distress, and interfere with their functioning on a day to day basis (APA, 2013).

Prevalence of Obsessive-Compulsive Disorder (OCD)

Prevalence

Approximately 2.5% to 3% of individuals suffer with obsessive-compulsive disorder, a neurobiological disorder that holds their sufferers hostage if they do not fulfill their rituals (Mahoney & Wilke, 2012). Whereas the adult prevalence ranges from approximately 2% to 3%, the child and adolescent prevalence ranges from 1% to 2% (Ray, 2018). In the U.S., APA (2013) reports the estimate for the 12-month to be 1.2%. Worldwide, it is reported that 3 of 200 individuals have OCD (Mancini, 2019).

The prevalence of obsessive-compulsive disorder is the same for women and men and among individuals of various races (Comer, 2015; Matsunaga & Seedat, 2011). Whereas some researchers report that the prevalence of obsessive-compulsive ideation varies depending upon the culture (Comer, 2015; Matsunaga & Seedat, 2011), others report that there is no difference between cultures (Mancini, 2019).

Whereas anxiety disorders are prevalent in the elderly, OCD is not common (Beekman et al., 1998; Mancini, 2019). In fact, after age 54, OCD will develop in fewer than 1% of people (Kessler et al., 2005; Wolitzky-Taylor, Castriotta, Lenze, Stanley, & Craske, 2010). OCD in the elderly is strongly related to the death of a significant other and chronic sickness (Beekman, et al., 1998).

Onset

When do the symptoms of obsessive-compulsive disorder begin to emerge? Although OCD can begin in childhood, for the most part, it begins gradually in adolescence with a symptomatic deterioration as time goes on (Mancini, 2019). The symptoms of OCD usually begin in males when they are approximately 21 years of age and in females when they are approximately 21 to 24 (Abramowitz & Jacoby, 2013).

Heritability and Comorbidity

Evidence from twin studies demonstrates that anxiety and perfectionism can be inherited (Moser, Slane, Burt, & Klump, 2012). Different obsessive-compulsive thought types have shown to be associated with specific comorbid disorders (Leckman et al., 2010). For example, obsessive-compulsive religious thought types have been shown to be related to comorbid depression and anxiety (Leckman et al., 2010; Ray, 2018).

An Integrative Etiology of Obsessive-Compulsive Disorder (OCD): Focus, Underpinnings, and Causes of OCD

Different approaches have characterized the etiology of obsessive-compulsive disorder (OCD). Several theories of etiology and their variables have been implicated in the development of OCD (e.g. psychological, genetic, neuropsychological, environmental, biological) (Doron, Mikulincer, Sar-El, & Kyrios, 2015; Ingersoll & Marquis, 2014). Similarly, Meyerson & Konichezky (2011) categorized the subtypes of OCD into cognitive, biological, and emotional dimensions. They explain that whereas proponents of the cognitive subtype suggest that information-processing impairments may be implicated (e.g., Chamberlain, Blackwell, Fineberg, Robbins, & Sahakian, 2005), the biological subtype includes genetic components that emphasize heredity (e.g., Hettema, Neale, & Kendler, 2001; Jonnal, Gardner, Prescott, & Kendler, 2000), and the emotional subtype can include the existential etiology (e.g., Yalom, 1980). Ingersoll and Marquis (2014) point out that an integral psychotherapy model is consistent with Barlow's (2000, 2002) triple vulnerability perspective (discussed in Chapter 6) in recognizing that both biological predispositions and psychological vulnerabilities, general as well as specific, can be implicated in the unfolding of OCD.

Impairment to the attachment system can further exacerbate sensitivities and can impair individuals' abilities to cope, thereby further promoting the development of OCD, replete with its obsessions and compulsions (Doron et al., 2015). The lack of security in attachments revolves around the elements of anxiety (the extent to which an individual is concerned that a significant other will be unresponsive) and avoidance (the degree to which an individual does not have trust in the kindness of a significant other and seeks detachment) (Brennan, Clark, & Shaver, 1998; Doron et al., 2015). Anxiety and avoidant attachment insecurities are associated with beliefs such as perfectionism and an inflated sense of danger (Doron et al., 2015; Doron, Moulding, Kyrios, Nedeljkovic, & Mikulincer, 2009). Doron et al.'s (2015) diathesis-stress model suggests that challenges to sensitive domains of the self along with a lack of security in attachments interact, thereby increasing an individual's tendency to develop OCD. Doron et al. (2015) suggest that treatment for OCD needs to include sensitive domains of the self and the attachment system to increase effectiveness.

Obsessive-Compulsive Disorder (OCD) from a Neurological, Biological, and Genetic Perspective

What are the neurological, biological, and genetic influences related to obsessive-compulsive disorder (OCD)? Viewing OCD from a neurological perspective posits that the cause may be biochemical or that there is an anatomical change in the central nervous system, and in this case, hereditary and autoimmune variables may play a part (Mancini, 2019). Although a genetic association for OCD has not been established, it has been found that members of the same family have OCD (Ray, 2018). It has been suggested that genetic inheritance may contribute to the serotonin and brain circuit irregularities, e.g., abnormalities of the caudate nuclei and orbitofrontal cortex, that are found in individuals with OCD (Comer, 2015; Marsh et al., 2014; Nicolini, Arnold, Nestadt, Lanzagorta, & Kennedy, 2009). Neuroimaging results for OCD have demonstrated malfunctioning in the orbitofrontal cortex and the anterior cingulate cortex (Chamberlain et al., 2005). Mahoney and Wilke (2012) explain that individuals with OCD have a larger cortex, as demonstrated by magnetic resonance imaging (MRI). Individuals with OCD suffer from neurobiological dysregulation (Hyman & Pedrick, 2005).

Is there a connection between pharmacotherapy and the etiology of OCD? The finding that the antidepressants, clomipramine and fluoxetine (Anafranil and Prozac), drugs that elevate serotonin activity, decrease the symptoms of OCD, have led researchers to assert that low serotonin is implicated in the onset of OCD (Bokor & Anderson, 2014; Comer, 2015; Stein & Fineberg, 2007). Proponents of a biological explanation of the development of OCD assert that whereas serotonin is implicated most frequently, the neurotransmitters, dopamine, GABA, and glutamate, have contributed to the onset of OCD (Bokor & Anderson, 2014; Comer, 2015; Spooren, Lesage, Lavreysen, Gasparini, & Steckler, 2010).

The Interaction of Biological and Environmental Variables in the Development of Obsessive-Compulsive Disorder (OCD)

What is the connection between biological and environmental influences? An integrative stress diathesis model that includes both biological and socio-psychological factors can explain the complex etiology of OCD in its recognition that both intrapsychic and external issues can contribute to symptoms in clients with vulnerabilities (Alexopoulos, 2004; Frederick, 2002, 2007; Meyerson & Konichezky, 2011). Stressful experiences have been shown to precede the beginning of OCD, and it is genetic and biological variables that predispose some individuals to respond strongly to experiences of stress (De Loof, Zandbergen, Lousberg, Pols, & Griez, 1989; Ingersoll & Marquis, 2014; Jones & Menzies, 1998). Ingersoll and Marquis (2014) point out that environmental factors such as caregivers who emphasize that a child's intrusive thoughts are wrong and those who place demands on young children to be perfect can contribute to an individual's development of OCD.

Psychological Approaches to Obsessive-Compulsive Disorder (OCD)

Although Mancini (2019) recognizes that obsessive-compulsive disorder (OCD) has been viewed from a neurological, neuropsychological, dispositional, purely psychological, and/or a biopsychosocial perspective, he takes the position that OCD is purely psychological, that individuals with OCD manifest obsessions and compulsions because they fear guilt and believe that guilt must be avoided. The concepts of responsibility, the fear of guilt, and avoiding contact with disgusting material are implicated in the etiology of OCD (Mancini & Gangemi, 2011; Tenore & Basile, 2019;).

How do the family members of individuals with OCD contribute to an individual's development and maintenance of OCD? Individuals with obsessions describe their parents as displaying responses that were neither proportionate to the seriousness of their faults nor expected (Tenore & Basile, 2019). Parents of individuals with OCD find it difficult to convey an adequate perspective towards responsibility and may induce shame in relation to their children's small errors (Tenore & Basile, 2019; Wolfe, 2005). Individuals' experiences of parents' reactions that are neither consistent nor proportionate are correlated with elevated levels of responsibility (Careau, O'Connor, Turgeon, & Freeston, 2012; Tenore & Basile, 2019). Tenore and Basile (2019) explain that family members of individuals with OCD tend to criticize and to emphasize guilt, and when faced with a threatening event, this family points a finger at someone that they can label responsible. They suggest that individuals with OCD learn to seek perfection in order to avoid guilt, particularly in a situation where a warm relationship with a close figure is threatened (Tenore & Basile, 2019). Individuals with OCD are deeply affected by the displays of disapproval of family members that further trigger the obsessions and compulsions, and those affected with OCD frequently feel that they cannot be forgiven (Tenore & Basile, 2019).

Psychoanalytic or Psychodynamic Approaches to Obsessive-Compulsive Disorder (OCD)

A psychoanalytic orientation views obsessive-compulsive disorder in relation to the ambivalence that emerges from the imbalance between a severe superego linked to hypercritical parents and aggressive drives that derive from anger that is repressed (Fenichel, 1945; Woon, Kanapathy, Zakaria, & Alfonso, 2017). When individuals have a problem with the integration of the aforementioned contradictory self-characteristics, they may employ defense mechanisms, e.g., magical ideation, undoing, isolation of emotion, that result in the development of OCD (Woon et al., 2017). Proponents of psychodynamic theories point out that the defenses of isolation or disowning one's intrusive ideation, undoing or performing behaviors with the intention of erasing one's impulses, and reaction formation or adopting a way of living that is the opposite of one's unwanted impulses, are frequently found in individuals who have obsessive-compulsive disorder (Comer, 2015).

Self-Psychology Approaches to Obsessive-Compulsive Disorder (OCD)

Mahoney and Wilke (2012) demonstrate how a self-psychology treatment approach recognizes the internal torment of patients with obsessive-compulsive disorder (OCD). They explain that theorists who are intersubjective (e.g., Stolorow, Brandchaft, & Atwood, 1987) extend Kohut's (1971, 1977) notion of self-objects (objects that service the self) while recognizing that when an individual's central affect states frequently lack attunement from parents, the affect states are not integrated, and the individual experiences fragmentation. According to a self-psychology approach, the obsessive thoughts represent an attempt to cope with the distress of fragmentation, and the rituals serve to keep the thoughts (e.g., murder) away while reducing the anxiety (Mahoney & Wilke, 2012). Whereas Mahoney and Wilke (2012) are aware of the need for neuroscience and cognitive-behavioral approaches in understanding the etiology and treating the symptoms of OCD, they recommend the integrated application of self-psychology, developmental, and relational treatment models to enhance the understanding of the etiology of OCD to include a view beyond symptoms, thereby promoting the opportunity for a more durable treatment outcome.

Self-Wounds

Chapter 5 discussed Wolfe's (2003) integrative approach to the anxiety disorders with its emphasis on self-wounds. Individuals with OCD have internalized the shame and the idea that they, in reality, are bad people (Tenore &

Basile, 2019; Wolfe, 2005). The self-wounds related to the shame of individuals with OCD can generate obsessions, the merging of thoughts and actions in the minds of individuals with OCD can result in anxiety, and the compulsions that ensue are attempts to ward off the anxiety (Salkovskis, 1985; Wolfe, 2005). Avoidance of thoughts about anxiety, compulsions, and persistent self-wounds maintain the obsessive-compulsive disorder (Wolfe, 2005).

Cognitive-Behavioral Perspectives and Obsessive-Compulsive Disorder (OCD)

How do cognitive-behavioral frameworks explain the etiology of obsessive-compulsive disorder (OCD)? The cognitive-emotional schemas that include the need for control, perfectionism, thought–action fusion, and difficulty with uncertainty, hypothesized by cognitive-behavioral theory, are similar to psychodynamic conceptualizations of OCD, e.g., magical thinking of the psychoanalytic orientation and the notion of ambivalent self-representations suggested by the object relations perspective that pertain to criticism of the self, rigidity, and the need for control (Blatt, Auerbach, & Levy, 1997; Obsessive Compulsive Cognitions Working Group, OCCWG, 1997; Woon et al., 2017). OCD schemas aim to decrease ambivalence, and individuals with OCD have contrasting self and other representations, which derive from attachment deficits (Woon et al., 2017). Whereas a cognitive framework delineates a picture of the causes and maintenance of OCD, the schemas offer a dynamic understanding of the daily mental state of an individual with OCD (Basile et al., 2018).

With respect to a cognitive approach to OCD, the focus is on the ideas that perpetuate the obsessive-compulsive symptoms (Mahoney & Wilke, 2012). Individuals with OCD attribute threatening meanings to their intrusive thoughts (Mahoney & Wilke, 2012). Comer (2015) explains that proponents of cognitive theories propose that individuals with obsessive-compulsive disorder tend to self-blame (e.g., Grayson, 2014), have elevated standards of morality (e.g., Whitton, Henry, & Grisham, 2014), possess an inflated sense of responsibility (e.g., Lawrence & Williams, 2011), and seek to neutralize their intrusive thoughts by checking for danger (e.g., Jacob, Larson, & Storch, 2014). According to cognitive researchers, the attempts of individuals to recognize and avoid objectionable cognitions can lead to obsessive-compulsive features (Comer, 2015).

Proponents of behavioral theories propose that individuals with obsessive-compulsive disorder have encountered several accidental connections whereby their compulsions have emerged as a way to avoid or decrease anxiety (Comer, 2015; Frost, Steketee, & Williams, 2001; Grayson, 2014). Neutral items such as knives may start to trigger an uncomfortable feeling because they were originally associated with an anxiety-inducing incident, and the compulsions are employed to decrease the anxiety that was generated during the original association, and, then, are maintained by the satisfaction of decreasing such anxiety (Mahoney & Wilke, 2012; McGinn & Sanderson, 1999).

Clinical Practice Applications of Single-School, Integrated, and Unified Psychotherapy Treatment Models for Obsessive-Compulsive Disorder (OCD)

This section focuses on several integrated and unified psychotherapy treatment models for obsessive-compulsive disorder (OCD). First, the response of individuals with OCD to single-school approaches, e.g., cognitive behavioral therapy, is discussed, and, then, integrated and unified models for the treatment of OCD is presented. With respect to a comparison between the aforementioned approaches to treatment, when a transdiagnostic unified protocol (UP) was compared with single-disorder protocols (SDPs) for obsessive-compulsive disorder (OCD), it was found that the UP was as effective a treatment as the SDPs; however, the dropout rate for UP was lower than for the SDPs (Barlow et al., 2017; Kennedy and Barlow, 2018).

Single-School Cognitive-Behavioral Approaches to Obsessive-Compulsive Disorder (OCD)

How do single-school therapy approaches affect patients with obsessive-compulsive disorder? Although cognitive-behavioral therapy (CBT) has been shown to be an effective evidence-based treatment approach for obsessive-compulsive disorder (OCD), only 40% to 70% percent of clients respond to treatment (Meyerson & Konichezky, 2011). Exposure and response prevention (EX/RP) (Foa & Kozak, 1986) is a psychosocial intervention for obsessive-compulsive disorder (OCD) that has much empirical support (Ray, 2018). Exposure and response prevention (ERP), first developed by Meyer (1966), is considered the gold standard intervention for the treatment of OCD (Chambless et al., 1998; van Balkom et al., 1994); however, it has been found that the high rate of noncompliance (30% to 60%) of cognitive-behavioral approaches, has prompted some clinicians to use other psychotherapeutic interventions (Pallanti et al., 2002; Schruers, Koning, Luermans, Haack, & Griez, 2005; Zahi & Meyerson, 2010). Approximately a quarter of individuals with OCD do not engage with suggested CBT methods, and CBT homework engagement is found to be approximately 50% (Detweiler & Whisman, 1999; Franklin & Foa, 2002).

Although CBT/ERP is highly efficacious in the treatment of OCD, CBT is not as effective when a patient with OCD has obsessions without compulsions (Christensen, Hadzi-Pavlovic, Andrews, & Mattick, 1987; Rosa-Alcázar, Sánchez-Meca, Gómez-Conesa, & Marín-Martínez, 2008). Whereas cognitive-behavioral approaches to OCD stress cognitive components and treat OCD symptoms with CBT methods, they fail to include the developmental, emotional (e.g., shame), transference, and countertransference aspects of OCD (Mahoney & Wilke, 2012).

In summary, obsessive-compulsive disorder has not historically responded well to single-school therapies (Norcross, 2005). For example, Franklin & Foa

(2014) show that 25% of patients with obsessive-compulsive disorder who have been treated with ERP fail to improve at all, and few patients who have been treated with ERP are free from all of their symptoms.

An Integration of a Cognitive Approach with Self Theories for Obsessive- Compulsive Disorder (OCD)

In light of the aforementioned findings and in an attempt to service a more comprehensive group of individuals, clinicians need to be open to seeking integrative or unified psychotherapy approaches. In response to the fact that a large number of clients do not benefit from cognitive-behavioral therapy (Fisher & Wells, 2005), researchers such as Doron, Kyrios, and Moulding (2007) integrated self-theories within a cognitive framework in order to treat obsessive-compulsive disorder. The aforementioned multidimensional model relies on both psychodynamic and cognitive-behavioral perspectives as it enhances a recognition of the etiology and promotion of obsessive-compulsive disorder (OCD). The integrated model suggests that the likelihood of developing obsessions increases when individuals experience sensitivity in self-domains such as morality and relations, two domains perceived to be critical for self-worth (Doron & Kryios, 2005; Doron et al., 2015). The conversion of intrusive thoughts into obsessions is regulated by the degree to which these thoughts challenge essential self-perceptions (Doron et al., 2015). Not every individual who experiences a negative incident that challenges sensitive self-domains (e.g., performance at work, relationships) is subject to negative self-worth and obsessions despite the fact that challenges to sensitive self-domains (e.g., relationships, morality) have been linked to vulnerability for OCD (Doron & Kryios, 2005; Doron et al., 2015; Doron, Moulding, Kyrios, & Nedeljkovic, 2008).

An Integration of Cognitive-Behavioral Therapy (CBT) with Motivational Interviewing (MI) for Obsessive-Compulsive Disorder (OCD)

How has motivational interviewing (MI) been integrated with cognitive-behavioral therapy (CBT)? Motivational interviewing underscores the following principles: Showing empathy, pointing out discrepancy, moving with resistance, and facilitating self-effectiveness (Miller & Rollnick, 2002). Why integrate motivational interviewing with other treatments? Although research has shown that patients who are recipients of motivational interviewing at the inception of an intervention achieve a more effective outcome than patients who do not receive motivational interviewing, motivational interviewing can be used throughout the therapy process (Miller & Rollnick, 2002). Tolin and Maltby (2008) used motivational interviewing (MI) with patients with obsessive-compulsive disorder (OCD) who refused exposure and response prevention (ERP) interventions. They employed MI in order to engage the aforementioned patients in treatment.

An Integration of Cognitive-Behavioral Therapy (CBT) with Hypnotically-Induced Dissociation (HID) for Obsessive-Compulsive Disorder (OCD)

Whereas cognitive-behavioral therapy (CBT) helps patients with obsessive-compulsive disorder (OCD) cope with external stressors, it does not often help with intrapsychic and developmental issues (Meyerson and Konichezky, 2011). It is important for clinicians to consider integrated or unified psychotherapy treatments for OCD in order to address in-depth issues that may remain untreated with CBT methods. For example, Meyerson and Konichezky (2011) suggest complementing CBT with a hypnotically induced dissociation (HID) treatment for patients with OCD, and they propose that the ability to access underlying psychological issues is a primary goal of HID. Meyerson and Konichezky (2011) demonstrated how HID can enhance the treatment of patients with OCD by addressing intrapsychic issues, e.g., developmental issues, existential fears, and the uncovering of repressed trauma.

An Integration of CBT and Psychodynamic Therapy for Obsessive-Compulsive Disorder (OCD)

For obsessive-compulsive disorder (OCD) that is resistant to treatment or comorbid OCD, Woon et al. (2017) proposed the integration of cognitive-behavioral therapy (CBT) and psychodynamic therapy with an emphasis on a good therapeutic relationship, specifically for patients who do not do well with medication. Psychodynamic therapy can benefit patients with OCD who have interpersonal problems and low self-esteem (Chlebowski & Gregory, 2009; Woon et al., 2017).

An Integration of Cognitive-Behavioral Therapy (CBT) and Transactional Analysis for Obsessive-Compulsive Disorder (OCD)

Fields (1998) used an integrative framework that includes transactional analysis and cognitive behavioral therapy (CBT) methods to treat obsessive-compulsive disorder (OCD). For example, transactional analysis ideas were employed to relate how the adult ego state of a patient with OCD can challenge the irrational thoughts of the ego state of the child (cognitive psychotherapy), and how the adult ego state can teach the child ego state to alter behaviors (behavioral instruction) (Fields, 1998). By integrating transactional analysis with cognitive therapy and response prevention, Fields (1998) showed how the integration empowered a patient to hold responsibility for ritual prevention and to offer the patient a way to hypothesize issues from an intrapsychic perspective.

An Integrated Framework for Obsessive-Compulsive Disorder (OCD): Mindfulness Integrated Cognitive Therapy (MICT)

Recent integrated psychotherapy approaches that address the suffering of patients with obsessive-compulsive disorder (OCD) who do not benefit from single-school approaches include Mindfulness Integrated Cognitive Therapy (MICT) which has been shown to decrease the severity of obsessive-compulsive symptoms in individuals with moderate to severe symptoms of obsessive-compulsive disorder (Mathur, Sharma, & Reddy, 2016). The mindfulness portion of the aforementioned integrated approach encourages clients with OCD to be less ruminative, more psychologically flexible, and facilitates entry into a mode of being, thereby offering an opportunity to validate one's own perceptions (Didonna, 2009; Mathur et al., 2016).

An Integration of Hypnosis and Positive Psychology for Obsessive-Compulsive Disorder (OCD)

Whereas the behavioral approach (e.g., ERP) to obsessive-compulsive disorder (OCD) emphasizes the resistance of compulsive behaviors, integrated psychotherapy approaches may focus on joining the symptoms and reframing the thoughts as positive rather than on symptom removal (Seligman, Rashid, & Parks, 2006; Zahi & Meyerson, 2010). For example, Zahi and Meyerson (2010) used an integrated approach, a hypnotic intervention along with a positive psychology approach, in the treatment of OCD. The suggestion here is that psychotherapists combine the aforementioned two approaches in an effort to join patients in their obsessive thoughts and reframe the thoughts as positive rather than to attempt to remove the thoughts (Zahi & Meyerson, 2010). Zahi and Meyerson's (2010) strategically oriented treatment that utilizes hypnosis is consistent with Seligman et al.'s (2006) positive therapy approach that the goal of emotional health is not symptom removal but the attainment of positive emotional existence that engages a life of purpose and meaning.

Schema therapy (ST): An Integrated and Unified Approach for Obsessive-Compulsive Disorder (OCD) and Obsessive-Compulsive Personality (OCPD) Disorder

What is schema therapy, and when has it been used? Schema therapy, an integrative or unified flexible approach that integrates gestalt, object relations, cognitive-behavioral, and psychodynamic therapy into one systematic framework, has been shown to be more effective than standard interventions in the treatment of obsessive-compulsive personality disorder and has been used to treat other anxiety disorders as well (Bamelis, Evers, Spinhoven, & Arntz, 2014; Legra, Verhey, & van Alphen, 2017; Young, Klosko, & Weishaar, 2005). Schema therapy offers more than eclecticism as it comprises a system that integrates from different orientations that practitioners can apply by using a coherent model (Edwards & Arntz, 2012).

Basile et al. (2018) proposed an integrated model that combines cognitive therapy (CT) and schema therapy (ST) in the treatment of OCD. Whereas cognitive methods can be applied to treat obsessive-compulsive disorder (OCD), experiential methods that are emotion-focused can help patients to examine variables that they experienced when they were younger that might have contributed towards a constellation of obsessive schema that lead to obsessive symptoms (Basile et al., 2018). Whereas the imagery and chair work of the integrated, experiential emotion-focused therapy can help individuals with OCD to heal negative affect linked to early experiences replete with stress, cognitive techniques can help those with OCD to accept guilt and disgust while learning to nurture a compassionate view towards themselves (Basile et al., 2018).

According to Legra and colleagues (2017), a schema can comprise a persistent dysfunctional theme or a frustrated emotional need that exists throughout an individual's life, and early trauma, e.g., constant abuse or neglect, can result in the development and maintenance of dysfunctional schemas, e.g., standards that are inflexible. They explain that schemas can wax and wane, can emerge as different domains during an individual's life, and when forgotten, can return when an individual is older. Legra and colleagues (2017) suggest that the more intense or the longer the trauma that an individual experiences, the lower the tendency for the dysfunctional schema to change, and biological, psychological, social, and cultural variables can influence the stability of a schema. They assert that if therapists recognize patients' trauma and how the trauma recapitulates when the patient is older (e.g., choosing a spouse that matches the dysfunctional schema), therapists can be aware of the essence of the schema and plan their interventions accordingly. The aforementioned conceptualization is consistent, for example, with the suggestion that spouses have opposite defense mechanisms (Goldenberg & Goldenberg, 1980; Scaturo, 1994) discussed in the section on an integration of individual and couples therapy for panic disorder (PD) in Chapter 6.

The therapeutic relationship is important in schema therapy given that it can facilitate the possibility for reparenting for a client (van Vreeswijk et al., 2012). Therapists and patients who engage in a working alliance during schema therapy explore the schemas that contribute to the makeup of patients (van Vreeswijk et al., 2012). To confront difficult schemas, therapists use chair dialogues that offer patients corrective and healthy alternatives to schemas that are filled with pain (Kellogg, 2012).

Integrated Existential Approaches for Obsessive-Compulsive Disorder (OCD)

How can integrated existential therapy approaches benefit individuals with OCD? Reliance on cognitive processes in reaction to the existential recognition of one's eventual death is related to higher phobic and obsessive-compulsive symptoms (Strachan et al., 2007). Wolfe (2008) developed an existential integrated approach to the anxiety disorders that demonstrates how obsessive-compulsive disorder can be explained from the vantage point of the theme of death anxiety. The primary diagnostic tool for uncovering the implicit underpinnings of anxiety symptoms is Wolfe's Focusing Technique, a type of exposure that is imaginal (Wolfe, 2003; Wolfe & Sigl, 1998). This technique is a method for discovering the meaning of obsessive and compulsive symptoms, and for patients with obsessive-compulsive disorder, it involves a meticulous attention on the obsessive thought (Wolfe, 2003).

Medication and CBT for Obsessive-Compulsive Disorder (OCD)

Cognitive therapy, behavioral therapy (exposure and response prevention, ERP), and medications such as serotonin reuptake inhibitors have been shown to be empirically supported in the treatment of OCD (Ingersoll & Marquis, 2014; Mathur et al., 2016). The evidence-based research that substantiates pharmacotherapy's effectiveness for OCD is greater than pharmacotherapy's evidence for other anxiety disorders (Pelligrino, Pierce, & Walkup, 2011). The SSRI, sertraline (Zoloft), has been shown to be effective in the treatment of OCD (Allgulander et al., 2004; March et al., 1998). The serotonin-norepinephrine reuptake inhibitor (SNRI), venlafaxine (Effexor), can serve as an alternate medication to the SSRIs for OCD (Julien, 2013; Sansone & Sansone, 2011). Whereas CBT can increase the efficacy of psychotropics, adding medication may not necessarily enhance a patient's outcome with CBT (Abramowitz & Jacoby, 2013).

The tricyclics were first introduced in the 1950s for adults with anxiety, and clomipramine (Anafranil) was approved by the FDA for children with OCD (Pelligrino et al., 2011). Although today the use of the tricyclic antidepressants (TCAs) is restricted, in general, the TCA, clomipramine (Anafranil), continues to be used for the treatment of OCD (Julien, 2013).

Whereas individuals with social anxiety disorder were almost two times more likely to refuse medication over therapy and individuals with panic disorder were almost three times more likely to refuse medication over therapy as an intervention, no differences were found in rates of refusal between pharmacotherapy and psychotherapy for individuals with OCD (Swift, Greenberg, Tompkins, & Parkin, 2017). The existence of comorbid emotional disorders with OCD suggest combined pharmacotherapy and therapy (e.g., Hohagen et al., 1998); however, it has been demonstrated that half of clients do not adequately improve with a combined intervention of CBT and medication (Sookman & Steketee, 2007).

How to Implement Integrative Psychotherapy in Practice for Obsessive-Compulsive Disorder (OCD)

The following case study demonstrates the implementation of an integrated emotional schema therapy model with cognitive therapy in the treatment of an adult with obsessive-compulsive disorder (OCD). Basile and colleagues (2018) proposed an integrated model that combines cognitive therapy (CT) and schema therapy (ST) for the treatment of OCD. The integrated psychotherapy treatment approach of an individual with OCD presented in the following case study relies on Basile et al.'s (2018) integrative framework of schema therapy to help a patient understand the emotional schemas comprising her OCD, and the treatment draws on the integrative model of schema treatment of Sookman and Steketee (2007), an approach that can combine with exposure and response prevention (ERP) to reinforce learning that is meaningful.

Emma is a 42-year-old math professor who terminated therapy after receiving one year of exposure response prevention (ERP) for obsessive-compulsive disorder (OCD). She said that ERP therapy with her prior therapist did not help much, and, after a year of therapy, she had as many obsessions and compulsions as before entering treatment. At present, she reported feeling exhausted from her rituals, somewhat depressed, angry at her friends who have been hostile towards her, and the quality of her life has decreased significantly. Emma tends to check and recheck her math work excessively, and she checks tires, doors, ovens, windows, locks, and her car repeatedly. Emma admits that her approach is not rational, but has difficulty discontinuing her checking rituals. At this time, Emma refuses ERP or medication.

Sookman, Pinard, and Beck (2001) suggest that the existence of schemas linked to felt vulnerability comprises the features of some individuals who refuse ERP. Various subtypes of OCD are represented within the framework of an emotional schema therapy model (Sookman & Pinard, 2007; Sookman, Pinard, & Beauchemin, 1994; Sookman & Steketee, 2007). The emotional schema framework includes notions of schemas (e.g., Beck & Freeman, 1990), developmental concepts (e.g., Piaget, 1960), and a conceptualization of attachment theory (Bowlby, 1985), ideas that pertain to OCD (Sookman and Steketee, 2007).

The therapist used an integrative framework of schema therapy to help Emma understand the emotional schemas comprising her OCD. Whereas experiential methods can help individuals become aware of negative affect and to change its related dysfunctional schemas (Basile et al., 2018), cognitive methods can reduce the obsessive symptoms of guilt and disgust (Basille et al., 2018; Berle & Phillips, 2006; Mancini, 2019).

As part of the integrative model of schema-based psychotherapy (Basile et al., 2018), the therapist included a psychoeducational process. During this process, the therapist informed Emma about the emotional schemas that comprise her dysfunctional beliefs that include her inflated sense of responsibility on the job and at home (e.g., her thoughts that she is responsible for her obsessions and that she needs to eradicate them as soon as possible), her tendency towards perfectionism (e.g., if what she plans is not materializing, she is not performing as effectively as possible), and other schemas.

It has been shown that cognitive therapy alone, which addresses patients' faulty interpretations related to beliefs, without an exposure portion, can help to decrease the symptoms of obsessive-compulsive disorder when a patient feels that exposure therapy is intrusive or experiences side effects of the SSRIs (Muse, Moore, & Stahl, 2013; Wilhelm et al., 2009). In fact, research has shown that cognitive therapy (CT) has been demonstrated to assist patients with dysfunctional thoughts (Wilhelm & Steketee, 2006). Van Oppen and colleagues (1995) found that there might be a slight advantage to cognitive therapy over ERP when the subtype is checking.

The therapist used cognitive therapy to introduce Emma to alternatives to her dysfunctional beliefs. For example, with respect to the dysfunctional belief of perfectionism, the therapist suggested that rather than constructing a scenario that events must go right at every moment, Emma consider an alternative scenario where unexpected events will occur because folks are imperfect, and, that at the same time, in this new reality, Emma is sufficiently resourceful to devise resolutions for the unexpected events that may go awry. Emma was able to accept this alternative thought, particularly when the therapist helped her get in touch with the healthy part of herself that she knew to be competent and resourceful. Emma reported that she found the cognitive portion of the therapy less stressful than the exposure therapy that she had experienced in the past.

The therapist helped Emma to understand her past attachment to her grandmother who raised her and to develop present schemas that work better for her. Emma related that her grandmother who had raised her used to criticize her when she engaged in endeavors such as learning to play soccer, learning to ski, and when doing her homework. Emma developed a sense that she could not do things right. When she was an adolescent, Emma began to use checking as a way to be more perfect so that she could please her grandmother. Her checking reinforced her hope that her grandmother would praise her. The therapist helped Emma to alter the schema where she feels that she is not successful to a feeling that she is as able and resourceful as her fellow mathematicians.

Emma's emotional schemas include the subtype, shame or humiliation, feeling humiliated about her need to be so conscientious in taking care of her property that she sometimes returned to her house close to eight times to see if she locked the door. The therapist fostered a strong interpersonal working alliance with Emma, offered empathy and understanding, and began to more deeply explore the theme of humiliation. The therapist encouraged Emma to more meaningfully explore her feelings of anxiety and helped her to identify a past experience that had previously been beyond her awareness. One day, upon feeling confident within the therapeutic relationship, Emma revealed that when she was nine years old, an intruder had entered her house when her sister had inadvertently left the door ajar. Terror ensued as it was Emma who attempted to protect herself, her grandmother, and her sister. Fortunately, her neighbor rang the doorbell at that time, realized that something was awry, called the police, and the intruder fled. Once this memory became conscious, Emma was able to see herself as a resourceful and brave individual for having endured a threatening experience that would terrify most adults. At this point, Emma gave up one of her core features that she was a loser for checking the doors several times before leaving her house. The therapist reinforced the idea that Emma's anxiety and accompanying door checks functioned, in her mind, as a way to shield herself and others from harm. The therapist helped Emma to identify the effect of this past experience upon her present functioning. Experiential approaches to psychotherapy underscore an integrative perspective that include themes of agency and survival, and when a client attends internally and is supported by a therapist, meaning can be created within the context of a new adaptive awareness (Angus et al., 2015; Elliott et al., 2013).

The integrative model of schema treatment can combine with ERP to reinforce learning that is meaningful (Sookman & Steketee, 2007). Although Emma was averse to ERP with her prior therapist, soon after disclosing the intruder experience and attaching meaning to it, Emma felt able to engage in ERP, started to postpone her checks, and the number of checks decreased. With respect to the urge to check, whenever Emma had an urge, the therapist invited her to envision herself as a young girl who won a medal of honor for enduring a life altering experience, for succeeding at a developmental task way beyond her years. After a year and a half of therapy, Emma's checking compulsions decreased. Emma began to accept that she, like others, would not be completely without intrusions and that although the checking of her math work decreased, it did not completely remit. At the same time, the quality of Emma's life, despite a few regressions, particularly when she became burdened at work, improved. Although Emma's compulsions decreased and she felt somewhat better after approximately a year and a half, she decided to continue further work in experiential therapy for her depression.

References

Abramowitz, J. S., & Jacoby, R. J. (2013). Obsessive-compulsive disorder. In S. M. Stahl & B. A. Moore (Eds.), *Anxiety disorders: A guide for integrating psychopharmacology and psychotherapy* (pp. 133–154). New York, NY: Routledge.

Abramowitz, J. S., & Jacoby, R. J. (2015). Obsessive-compulsive and related disorders: A critical review of the new diagnostic class. *Annual Review of Clinical Psychology, 11*(1), 165–186. doi: 10.1146/annurev-clinpsy-032813-153713

Alexopoulos, G. S. (2004). On the "infallibility" of psychopathology and its implications for action. *American Journal of Psychiatry, 161*(12), 2151–2154. doi: 10.1176/appi.ajp.161.12.2151

Allgulander, C., Dahl, A. A., Austin, C., Morris, P. L., Sogaard, J. A., Fayyad, R., … Clary, C. M. (2004). Efficacy of sertraline in a 12-week trial for generalized anxiety disorder. *The American Journal of Psychiatry, 161*(9), 1642–1649. doi: 10.1176/appi.ajp.161.9.1642

American Psychiatric Association. (2013). *Diagnostic and statistical manual of mental disorders* (5th ed.). Washington, DC: Author.

Angus, L., Watson, J. C., Elliott, R., Schneider, K., & Timulak, L. (2015). Humanistic psychotherapy research 1990–2015: From methodological innovation to evidence-supported treatment outcomes and beyond. *Psychotherapy Research, 25*(3), 330–347. doi: 10.1080/10503307.2014.989290

Bamelis, L. L. M., Evers, S. M. A. A., Spinhoven, P., & Arntz, A. (2014). Results of a multicenter randomized controlled trial of the clinical effectiveness of schema therapy for personality disorders. *American Journal of Psychiatry, 171*(3), 305–322. doi: 10.1176/appi.ajp.2013.12040518

Barlow, D. H. (2000). Unraveling the mysteries of anxiety and its disorders from the perspective of emotion theory. *American Psychologist, 55*(11), 1247–1263. doi: 10.1037/0003-066X.55.11.1247

Barlow, D. H. (2002). *Anxiety and its disorders: The nature and treatment of anxiety and panic* (2nd ed.). New York, NY: Guilford Press.

Barlow, D. H. (2004). *Anxiety and its disorders: The nature and treatment of anxiety and panic* (2nd ed.). New York, NY: Guilford Press.

Barlow, D. H., Farchione, T. J., Bullis, J. R., Gallagher, M. W., Murray-Latin, H., Sauer-Zavala, S., … Cassiello-Robbins, C. (2017). The unified protocol for transdiagnostic treatment of emotional disorders compared with diagnosis-specific protocols for anxiety disorders: A randomized clinical trial. *JAMA Psychiatry, 74*(9), 875–884. doi: 10.1001/jamapsychiatry.2017.2164

Basile, B., Luppino, O. I., Mancini, F., & Tenore, K. (2018). A theoretical integration of schema therapy and cognitive therapy in OCD treatment: Experiential techniques and cognitive-based interventions in action (Part III). *Psychology, 9*(9), 2296–2311. doi: 10.4236/psych.2018.99131

Beck, A. T., & Freeman, A. (1990). *Cognitive therapy of personality disorders*. New York, NY: Guilford Press.

Beekman, A. T., Bremmer, M. A., Deeg, D. J., van Balkom, A. J., Smit, J. H., de Beurs, E., … van Tilburg, W. (1998). Anxiety disorders in later life: A report from the Longitudinal Aging Study Amsterdam. *International Journal of Geriatric Psychiatry, 13*(10), 717–726. doi: 10.1002/(SICI)1099-1166(1998100)13:10<717::AID-GPS857>3.0.CO;2-M

Berle, D., & Phillips, E. S. (2006). Disgust and obsessive-compulsive disorder: An update. *Psychiatry, 69*(3), 228–238. doi: 10.1521/psyc.2006.69.3.228

Blatt, S. J., Auerbach, J. S., & Levy, K. N. (1997). Mental representations in personality development, psychopathology, and the therapeutic process. *Review of General Psychology*, 351–374. doi: 10.1037/1089-2680.1.4.351

Bokor, G., & Anderson, P. D. (2014). Obsessive-compulsive disorder. *Journal of Pharmacy Practice, 27*(2), 116–130. doi: 10.1177/0897190014521996

Bowlby, J. (1985). The role of childhood experience in cognitive disturbance. In M. J. Mahoney & A. Freeman (Eds.), *Cognition and psychotherapy* (pp. 181–200). New York, NY: Plenum Press.

Brennan, K. A., Clark, C. L., & Shaver, P. R. (1998). Self-report measurement of adult attachment. In J. A. Simpson & W. S. Rholes (Eds.), *Attachment theory and close relationships* (pp. 46–76). New York, NY: Guilford Press.

Careau, Y., O'Connor, K. P., Turgeon, L., & Freeston, M. H. (2012). Childhood experiences and adult beliefs in obsessive-compulsive disorder: Evaluating a specific etiological model. *Journal of Cognitive Psychotherapy, 26*(3), 236–256. doi: 10.1891/0889-8391.26.3.236

Chamberlain, S. R., Blackwell, A. D., Fineberg, N. A., Robbins, T. W., & Sahakian, B. J. (2005). The neuropsychology of obsessive compulsive disorder: The importance of failures in cognitive and behavioural inhibition as candidate endophenotypic markers. *Neuroscience and Biobehavioral Reviews, 29*(3), 399–419. doi: 10.1016/j.neubiorev.2004.11.006

Chambless, D. L., Baker, M. J., Baucom, D. H., Beutler, L. E., Calhoun, K. S., Crits-Christoph, P., … Woody, S. R. (1998). Update on empirically validated therapies, II. *The Clinical Psychologist, 51*(1), 3–16.

Chlebowski, S., & Gregory, R. J. (2009). Is a psychodynamic perspective relevant to the clinical management of obsessive–compulsive disorder? *American Journal of Psychotherapy, 63*(3), 245–256. doi: 10.1176/appi.psychotherapy.2009.63.3.245

Christensen, H., Hadzi-Pavlovic, D., Andrews, G., & Mattick, R. (1987). Behavior therapy and tricyclic medication in the treatment of obsessive-compulsive disorder: A quantitative review. *Journal of Consulting and Clinical Psychology, 55*(5), 701–711. doi: 10.1037/0022-006X.55.5.701

Comer, R. J. (2015). *Abnormal psychology*. New York, NY: Worth Publisher.

De Loof, C., Zandbergen, J., Lousberg, H., Pols, H., & Griez, E. (1989). The role of life events in the onset of panic disorder. *Behaviour Research and Therapy, 27*(4), 461–463. doi: 10.1016/0005-7967(89)90017-X

Detweiler, J. B., & Whisman, M. A. (1999). The role of homework assignments in cognitive therapy for depression: Potential methods for enhancing adherence. *Clinical Psychology: Science and Practice, 6*(3), 267–282. doi: 10.1093/clipsy.6.3.267

Didonna, F. (2009). Mindfulness and obsessive-compulsive disorder: Developing a way to trust and validate one's internal experience. In F. Didonna (Ed.), *Clinical handbook of mindfulness-integrated* (pp. 189–219). New York, NY: Springer.

Doron, G., & Kyrios, M. (2005). Obsessive compulsive disorder: A review of possible specific internal representations within a broader cognitive theory. *Clinical Psychology Review, 25*(4), 415–432. doi: 10.1016/j.cpr.2005.02.002

Doron, G., Kyrios, M., & Moulding, R. (2007). Sensitive domains of self-concept in obsessive- compulsive disorder (OCD): Further evidence for a multidimensional model of OCD. *Journal of Anxiety Disorders, 21*(3), 433–444. doi: 10.1016/j.janxdis.2006.05.008

Doron, G., Mikulincer, M., Sar-El, D., & Kyrios, M. (2015). Integrating psychodynamic and cognitive approaches to obsessive compulsive disorder–attachment insecurities and self-related sensitivities in morality and relational domains. In P. Luyten, L. C. Mayes, P. Fonagy, M. Target & S. J. Blatt (Eds.), *Handbook of contemporary psychodynamic approaches to psychopathology* (pp. 199–215). New York, NY: Guilford Press.

Doron, G., Moulding, R., Kyrios, M., & Nedeljkovic, M. (2008). Sensitivity of self-beliefs in obsessive compulsive disorder (OCD). *Anxiety and Depression, 25*(10), 874–884. doi: 10.1002/da.20369

Doron, G., Moulding, R., Kyrios, M., Nedeljkovic, M., & Mikulincer, M. (2009). Adult attachment insecurities are related to obsessive compulsive phenomena. *Journal of Social and Clinical Psychology, 28*(8), 1022–1049. doi: 10.1521/jscp.2009.28.8.1022

Dougherty, D. D., Rauch, S. L., & Jenike, M. A. (2015). Treatment of obsessive compulsive disorder. In P. E. Nathan & J. M. Gorman (Eds.), *A guide to treatments that work* (pp. 545–570). New York, NY: Oxford University Press.

Edwards, D., & Arntz, A. (2012). Schema therapy in historical perspective. In M. van Vreeswijk, J. Broersen & M. Nadort (Eds.), *The Wiley-Blackwell handbook of schema therapy: Theory, research, and practice* (pp. 3–26). Oxford: Wiley-Blackwell.

Elliott, R., Watson, J., Greenberg, L. S., Timulak, L., & Freire, E. (2013). Research on humanistic-experiential psychotherapies. In M. J. Lambert (Ed.), *Bergin & Garfield's handbook of psychotherapy and behavior change* (6th ed.) (pp. 495–538). New York, NY: Wiley.

Fenichel, O. (1945). *The psychoanalytic theory of neurosis*. New York, NY: Norton.

Fields, L. (1998). An integrative brief treatment approach for obsessive-compulsive disorder. *Journal of Psychotherapy Integration, 8*(3), 161–172. doi: 10.1023/A:1023237529718

Fisher, P. L., & Wells, A. (2005). How effective are cognitive and behavioral treatments for obsessive-compulsive disorder? A clinical significance analysis. *Behavior Research and Therapy*, *43*(12), 1543–1558. doi: 10.1016/j.brat.2004.11.007

Foa, E., & Kozak, M. (1986). Emotional processing of fear: Exposure to corrective information. *Psychological Bulletin*, *99*(1), 20–35. doi: 10.1037/0033-2909.99.1.20

Franklin, M. E., & Foa, E. B. (2002). Cognitive behavioral treatments for obsessive–compulsive disorder. In P. E. Nathan & J. M. Gorman (Eds.), *A guide to treatments that work* (2nd ed., pp. 367–386). London: Oxford University Press.

Franklin, M. E., & Foa, E. B. (2014). Obsessive-compulsive disorder. In D. H. Barlow (Ed.), *Clinical handbook of psychological disorders: A step-by-step treatment manual* (5th ed., pp. 155–205). New York, NY: Guilford Press.

Frederick, C. (2002). Liberating Sisyphus: Hypnotically facilitated therapy for obsessive-compulsive disorder. *Hypnos*, XXIX, 99–105.

Frederick, C. (2007). Hypnotically facilitated treatment of obsessive-compulsive disorder: Can it be evidence-based? *International Journal of Clinical and Experimental Hypnosis*, *55*(2), 189–206. doi: 10.1080/00207140601177913

Frost, R. O., Steketee, G., & Williams, L. (2001). Obsessive-compulsive disorder. In H. S. Friedman (Ed.), *Specialty articles from the encyclopedia of mental health* (pp. 277–290). San Diego, CA: Academic Press.

Goldenberg, I., & Goldenberg, H. (1980). *Family therapy. An overview.* Monterey, CA: Brooks/Cole.

Grayson, J. (2014). *Freedom from obsessive-compulsive disorder: A personalized recovery program for living with uncertainty* (Updated ed.). Berkley, MI: Berkley Book Company Trade.

Hettema, J. M., Neale, M. C., & Kendler, K. S. (2001). A review and meta-analysis of the genetic epidemiology of anxiety disorders. *American Journal of Psychiatry*, *158*(10), 568–578. doi: 10.1176/appi.ajp.158.10.1568

Hohagen, F., Winkelmann, G., Rasche-Räuchle, H., Hand, I., König, A., Münchau, N., … Berger, M. (1998). Combination of behaviour therapy with fluvoxamine in comparison with behaviour therapy and placebo: Results of a multicentre study. *The British Journal of Psychiatry*, *173*(Suppl. 35), 71–78. doi: 10.1037/t57982-000

Hyman, B. M., & Pedrick, C. (2005). *The OCD workbook* (2nd ed.). Oakland, CA: New Harbinger Press.

Ingersoll, R. E., & Marquis, A. (2014). *Understanding psychopathology: An integral exploration.* Upper Saddle River, NJ: Pearson Education.

Jacob, M. L., Larson, M. J., & Storch, E. A. (2014). Insight in adults with obsessive–compulsive disorder. *Comprehensive Psychiatry*, *55*(4), 896–903. doi: 10.1016/j.comppsych.2013.12.016

Jones, M. K., & Menzies, R. G. (1998). The relevance of associative learning pathways in the development of obsessive–compulsive washing. *Behaviour Research and Therapy*, *36*(3), 273–283. doi: 10.1016/S0005-7967(98)00021-7

Jonnal, A. H., Gardner, C. O., Prescott, C. A., & Kendler, K. S. (2000). Obsessive and compulsive symptoms in a general population sample of female twins. *American Journal of Medical Genetics*, *96*(6), 791–796. doi: 10.1002/1096-8628(20001204)96:6<791::aid-ajmg19>3.0.co;2-c

Julien, R. M. (2013). Pharmacological treatment of anxiety disorders across the lifespan. In S. M. Stahl & B. A. Moore (Eds.), *Anxiety disorders: A guide for integrating psychopharmacology and psychotherapy* (pp. 51–70). New York, NY: Routledge.

Kellogg, S. (2012). On speaking one's mind: Using chairwork dialogues in schema therapy. In M. van Vreeswijk, J. Broersen & M. Nadort (Eds.), *The Wiley-Blackwell handbook of schema therapy: Theory, research, and practice* (pp. 197–208). Oxford: Wiley-Blackwell.

Kennedy, K. A., & Barlow, D. (2018). The unified treatment for transdiagnostic treatment of emotional disorders: An introduction. In D. H. Barlow & T. J. Farchione (Eds.), *Applications of the unified protocol for transdiagnostic treatment of emotional disorders* (pp. 1–16). New York, NY: Oxford University Press.

Kessler, R. C., Berglund, P., Demler, O., Jin, R., Merikangas, K. R., & Walters, E. E. (2005). Lifetime prevalence and age-of-onset distributions of DSM-IV disorders in the National Comorbidity Survey Replication. *Archives of General Psychiatry, 62*(6), 593–602. doi: 10.1001/archpsyc.62.6.593

Kohut, H. (1971). *The analysis of the self.* New York, NY: International Universities Press.

Kohut, H. (1977). *The restoration of the self.* New York, NY: International Universities Press.

Lawrence, P. J., & Williams, T. I. (2011). Pathways to inflated responsibility beliefs in adolescent obsessive-compulsive disorder: A preliminary investigation. *Behavioral and Cognitive Psychotherapy, 39*(2), 229–234. doi: 10.1017/S1352465810000810

Leckman, J. F., Denys, D., Simpson, H., Mataix-Cols, D., Hollander, E., Saxena, S., ... Stein, D. J. (2010). Obsessive–compulsive disorder: A review of the diagnostic criteria and possible subtypes and dimensional specifiers for DSM-V. *Depression and Anxiety, 27*(6), 507–527. doi: 10.1002/da.20669

Legra, M. J. H., Verhey, F. R. J., & van Alphen, S. P. J. (2017). A first step toward integrating schema theory in geriatric psychiatry: A Delphi study. *International Psychogeriatrics, 29*(7), 1069–1076. doi: 10.1017/S1041610217000412

Mahoney, D. M., & Wilke, D. L. (2012). The self psychological view of the obsessive-compulsive disorder: Treating the tormented self. *Annals of Psychotherapy and Integrative Health, 15*(1), 26–34.

Mancini, F. (2019). Introduction. In F. Mancini (Ed.), *The obsessive mind* (pp. 1–4). Abingdon-on-Thames: Routledge.

Mancini, F., & Gangemi, A. (2011). Fear of deontological guilt and fear of contamination in obsessive-compulsive disorder. *Psicoterapia Cognitiva e Comportamentale, 17*(3), 395–404.

March, J. S., Biederman, J., Wolkow, R., Safferman, A., Mardekian, J., Cook, E. H., ... Steiner, H. (1998). Sertraline in children and adolescents with obsessive-compulsive disorder: A multicenter randomized controlled trial. *JAMA, 280*(20), 1752–1756.

Marsh, R., Horga, G., Parashar, N., Wang, Z., Peterson, B. S., & Simpson, H. B. (2014). Altered activation in fronto-striatal circuits during sequential processing of conflict in unmedicated adults with obsessive-compulsive disorder. *Biological Psychiatry, 75*(8), 615–622. doi: 10.1016/j.biopsych.2013.02.004

Mathur, S., Sharma, M. P., & Reddy, J. Y. (2016). Preliminary findings of efficacy of Mindfulness Integrated Cognitive Therapy (MICT) for Obsessive-Compulsive Disorder (OCD). *Archives of Mental Health, 17*(1), 65–69.

Matsunaga, H., & Seedat, S. (2011). Obsessive-compulsive spectrum disorders: Cross-national and ethnic issues. In E. Hollander, J. Zohar, P. J. Sirovatka & D. A. Regier (Eds.), *Obsessive-compulsive spectrum disorders: Refining the research agenda for DSM-V* (pp. 205–221). Washington, DC: American Psychiatric Publishing.

McGinn, L., & Sanderson, W. (1999). *Treatment of obsessive-compulsive disorder.* Northvale, NJ: Jason Aronson.

Meyer, V. (1966). Modification of expectations in cases with obsessional rituals. *Behaviour Research and Therapy, 4*(4), 273–280. doi: 10.1016/0005-7967(66)90083-0

Meyerson, J., & Konichezky, A. (2011). Hypnotically induced dissociation (HID) as a strategic intervention for enhancing OCD treatment. *American Journal of Clinical Hypnosis, 53*(3), 169–181. doi: 10.1080/00029157.2011.10401755

Miller, W. R., & Rollnick, S. (2002). *Motivational interviewing: Preparing people for change* (2nd ed.). New York, NY: Guilford Press.

Moser, J. S., Slane, J. D., Burt, S. A., & Klump, K. L. (2012). Etiologic relationships between anxiety and dimensions of maladaptive perfectionism in young adult female twins. *Depression and Anxiety, 29*(1), 47–53. doi: 10.1002/da.20890

Muse, M. D., Moore, B. A., & Stahl, S. M. (2013). Benefits and challenges of integrative treatment. In S. M. Stahl & B. A. Moore (Eds.), *Anxiety disorders: A guide for integrating psychopharmacology and psychotherapy* (pp. 3–24). New York, NY: Routledge.

Nicolini, H., Arnold, P., Nestadt, G., Lanzagorta, N., & Kennedy, J. L. (2009). Overview of genetics and obsessive–compulsive disorder. *Psychiatry Research, 170*(1), 7–14. doi: 10.1016/j.psychres.2008.10.011

Norcross, J. C. (2005). A primer on psychotherapy integration. In J. C. Norcross & M. R. Goldfried (Eds.), *Handbook of psychotherapy integration* (2nd ed., pp. 3–23). New York, NY: Oxford University Press.

Obsessive Compulsive Cognitions Working Group (OCCWG). (1997). Cognitive assessment of obsessive-compulsive disorder. *Behavior Research and Therapy, 35*(7), 667–681. doi: 10.1016/S0005-7967(97)00017-X

Pallanti, S., Hollander, E., Bienstock, C., Koran, L., Leckman, J., Marazziti, D., ... Zohar, J. (2002). Treatment non-response in OCD: Methodological issues and operational definitions. *International Journal of Neuropsychopharmacology, 5*(2), 181–191. doi: 10.1017/S1461145702002900

Pelligrino, L., Pierce, C., & Walkup, J. T. (2011). Pharmacological management of childhood and adolescent anxiety disorders. In W. K. Silverman & A. P. Field (Eds.), *Anxiety disorders in children and adolescents* (2nd ed., pp. 367–391). New York, NY: Cambridge University Press.

Piaget, J. (1960). *The child's conception of the world* (J. & A. Tomilson, Trans.). Totowa, NJ: Littlefield, Adams. (Original work published 1926).

Rasmussen, S. A., & Eisen, J. L. (1991). Phenomenology of OCD: Clinical subtypes, heterogeneity and coexistence. In J. Zohar, T. Insel & S. Rasmussen (Eds.), *The psychobiology of obsessive-compulsive disorder* (pp. 13–43). New York, NY: Springer.

Ray, W. J. (2018). *Abnormal psychology*. Thousand Oaks, CA: Sage.

Rosa-Alcázar, A. I., Sánchez-Meca, J., Gómez-Conesa, A., & Marín-Martínez, F. (2008). Psychological treatment of obsessive–compulsive disorder: A meta-analysis. *Clinical Psychology Review, 28*(8), 1310–1325. doi: 10.1016/j.cpr.2008.07.001

Salkovskis, P. M. (1985). Obsessional-compulsive problems: A cognitive-behavioural analysis. *Behaviour Research and Therapy, 23*(5), 571–583. doi: 10.1016/0005-7967(85)

Sansone, R. A., & Sansone, L. A. (2011). SNRIs pharmacological alternatives for the treatment of obsessive compulsive disorder? *Innovations in Clinical Neuroscience, 8*(6), 10–14.

Scaturo, D. J. (1994). Integrative psychotherapy for panic disorder and agoraphobia in clinical practice. *Journal of Psychotherapy Integration, 4*(3), 253–272. doi: 10.1037/h0101261

Schruers, K., Koning, K., Luermans, J., Haack, M. J., & Griez, E. (2005). Obsessive-compulsive disorder: A critical review of therapeutic perspectives. *Acta Psychiatrica Scandinavica, 111*(4), 261–271. doi: 10.1111/j.1600-0447.2004.00502.x

Seligman, M. E. P., Rashid, T., & Parks, A. C. (2006). Positive psychotherapy. *American Psychologist, 61*(8), 774–788. doi: 10.1037/0003-066X.61.8.774

Sherman, A., Ellison, J. M., & Iwamoto, S. (1996). Obsessive-compulsive disorder: The integration of cognitive behavioral treatment with pharmacotherapy. In J. M. Ellison

(Ed.), *Integrative treatment of anxiety disorders* (pp. 153–197). Washington, DC: American Psychiatric Press.

Sookman, D., & Pinard, G. (2007). Specialized cognitive behavior therapy for resistant obsessive-compulsive disorder: Elaboration of a schema-based model. In L. P. Riso, P. L. du Toit, D. J. Stein & J. E. Young (Eds.), *Cognitive schemas and core beliefs in psychological problems: A scientist-practitioner guide* (pp. 93–103). Washington, DC: American Psychological Association.

Sookman, D., Pinard, G., & Beauchemin, N. (1994). Multidimensional schematic restructuring treatment for obsessions. Theory and practice. *Journal of Cognitive Psychotherapy*, *8*(3), 175–194. doi: 10.1891/0889-8391.8.3.175

Sookman, D., Pinard, G., & Beck, A. T. (2001). Vulnerability schemas in obsessive-compulsive disorder. *Journal of Cognitive Psychotherapy: An International Quarterly*, *15*(2), 109–130. doi: 10.1891/0889-8391.15.2.109

Sookman, D., & Steketee, G. (2007). Directions in specialized cognitive behavior therapy for resistant obsessive-compulsive disorder: Theory and practice of two approaches. *Cognitive and Behavioral Practice*, *14*(1), 1–17. doi: 10.1016/j.cbpra.2006.09.002

Spooren, W., Lesage, A., Lavreysen, H., Gasparini, F., & Steckler, T. (2010). Metabotropic glutamate receptors: Their therapeutic potential in anxiety. In M. B. Stein & T. Steckler (Eds.), *Behavioral neurobiology of anxiety and its treatment. Current topics in behavioral neurosciences* (pp. 391–413). New York, NY: Springer Science + Business Media.

Stein, D. J., & Fineberg, N. A. (2007). *Obsessive-compulsive disorder.* Oxford, England: Oxford University Press.

Stolorow, R. D., Brandchaft, B., & Atwood, G. E. (1987). *Psychoanalytic treatment: An intersubjective approach.* Hillsdale, NJ: The Analytic Press.

Strachan, E., Schimel, J., Arndt, J., Williams, T., Solomon, S., Pyszczynski, T., & Greenberg, J. (2007). Terror mismanagement: Evidence that mortality salience exacerbates phobic and compulsive behaviors. *Personality and Social Psychology Bulletin*, *33*(8), 1137–1151. doi: 10.1177/0146167207303018

Swift, J. K., Greenberg, R. P., Tompkins, K. A., & Parkin, S. R. (2017). Treatment refusal and premature termination in psychotherapy, pharmacotherapy, and their combination: A meta-analysis of head-to-head comparisons. *Psychotherapy*, *54*(1), 47–57. doi: 10.1037/pst0000104

Tenore, K., & Basile, B. (2019). Vulnerability in obsessive-compulsive disorder. In F. Mancini (Ed.), *The obsessive mind* (pp. 133–148). Abingdon-on-Thames: Routledge.

Tolin, D. F., & Maltby, N. (2008). Motivating treatment-refusing patients with obsessive-compulsive disorder. In H. Arkowitz, H. A. Westra, W. R. Miller & S. Rollnick (Eds.), *Motivational interviewing in the treatment of psychological problems* (pp. 85–108). New York, NY: Guilford Press.

Tolin, D. F., & Meunier, S. A. (2008). Contamination and decontamination. In J. S. Abramowitz, D. McKay & S. Taylor (Eds.), *Obsessive-compulsive disorder: Subtypes and spectrum conditions* (pp. 3–18). Oxford, England: Elsevier. doi: 10.1016/B978-008044701-8/50002-4

Torres, A. R., Shavitt, R. G., Torresan, R. C., Ferrão, Y. A., Miguel, E. C., & Fontenelle, L. F. (2013). Clinical features of pure obsessive-compulsive disorder. *Comprehensive Psychiatry*, *54*(7), 1042–1052. doi: 10.1016/j.comppsych.2013.04.013

van Balkom, A. J., van Oppen, P., Vermeulen, A. W., van Dyck, R., Nauta, N. C., & Vorst, H. (1994). A meta-analysis on the treatment of obsessive compulsive disorder: A comparison of antidepressants, behaviour and cognitive therapy. *Clinical Psychology Review*, *14*(5), 359–381. doi: 10.1016/0272-7358(94)90033-7 van Oppen, P., de Haan, E., van Balkom, A. J., Spinhoven, P., Hoogduin, K., & van Dyck, R. (1995). Cognitive therapy and exposure in vivo in the treatment of obsessive compulsive disorder. *Behaviour Research and Therapy*, *33*(4), 379–390. doi: 10.1016/0005-7967(94)00052-l

van Vreeswijk, M., Broersen, J., Bloo, J., & Haeyen, S. (2012). Techniques within schema therapy. In M. van Vreeswijk, J. Broersen & M. Nadort (Eds.), *The Wiley-Blackwell handbook of schema therapy: Theory, research, and practice* (pp. 185–195). Oxford: Wiley-Blackwell.

Whitton, A. E., Henry, J. D., & Grisham, J. R. (2014). Moral rigidity in obsessive-compulsive disorder: Do abnormalities in inhibitory control, cognitive flexibility and disgust play a role? *Journal of Behavior Therapy and Experimental Psychiatry*, *45*(1), 152–159. doi: 10.1016/j.jbtep.2013.10.001

Wilhelm, S., & Steketee, G. (2006). *Cognitive therapy of obsessive-compulsive disorder: A guide for professionals*. Oakland, CA: New Harbinger.

Wilhelm, S., Steketee, G., Fama, J. M., Buhlmann, U., Teachman, B. A., & Golan, E. (2009). Modular cognitive therapy for obsessive-compulsive disorder: A wait-list controlled trial. *Journal of Cognitive Psychotherapy*, *23*(4), 294–305. doi: 10.1891/0889-8391.23.4.294

Wolfe, B. E. (2003). Integrative psychotherapy of the anxiety disorders. In J. C. Norcross & M. R. Goldfried (Eds.), *Handbook of psychotherapy integration* (2nd ed., pp. 263–280). New York, NY: Oxford University Press.

Wolfe, B. E. (2005). *Understanding and treating anxiety disorders: An integrative approach to healing the wounded self*. Washington, DC: American Psychological Association.

Wolfe, B. E. (2008). Existential issues in anxiety disorders and their treatment. In K. I. Schneider (Ed.), *Existential-integrative psychotherapy* (pp. 204–216). New York, NY: Routledge.

Wolfe, B. E., & Sigl, P. (1998). Experiential psychotherapy of the anxiety disorders. In L. S. Greenberg J. C. Watson & G. Lietaer (Eds.), *Handbook of experiential psychotherapy* (pp. 272–294). New York, NY: Guilford Press.

Wolitzky-Taylor, K. B., Castriotta, N., Lenze, E. J., Stanley, M. A., & Craske, M. G. (2010). Anxiety disorders in older adults: A comprehensive review. *Depression and Anxiety*, *27*(2), 190–211. doi: 10.1002/da.20653

Woon, L. S. C., Kanapathy, A., Zakaria, H., & Alfonso, C. A. (2017). An integrative approach to treatment-resistant obsessive-compulsive disorder. *Psychodynamic Psychiatry*, *45*(2), 237–257. doi: 10.1521/pdps.2017.45.2.237

Yalom, I. D. (1980). *Existential psychotherapy* (1st ed.). New York, NY: Basic Books.

Young, J. E., Klosko, J. S., & Weishaar, M. E. (2005). *Schemagerichte therapie. Handbook voor therapeutin*. Houten: Bohn Stafleu van Loghum.

Zahi, A., & Meyerson, J. (2010). Application of hypnotic strategies sustained by a positive psychology orientation in treating OCD patients. *Contemporary Hypnosis*, *27*(3), 177–183.

10 Posttraumatic Stress Disorder (PTSD)

Introduction

Although posttraumatic stress disorder used to be classified as an anxiety disorder, the DSM-5 no longer classifies PTSD as an anxiety disorder (APA, 2013). Chapter 10 focuses on an integrated etiology of posttraumatic stress disorder (PTSD) and clinical practice applications of integrated, integrative, and unified psychotherapy treatment models for posttraumatic stress disorder (PTSD). At the end of the chapter, a case study is presented to demonstrate the implementation of an integrated psychotherapy approach for posttraumatic stress disorder (PTSD). The case study relies on Wolfe's (2005) integrative model of psychotherapy, and the psychotherapy integration includes cognitive-behavioral, hypnosis, interpersonal, and self-psychology themes in the treatment of a patient who returned from Vietnam with PTSD.

Symptoms of Posttraumatic Stress Disorder (PTSD)

Which symptoms characterize posttraumatic stress disorder (PTSD)? Posttraumatic stress disorder (PTSD) is characterized by an individual's experience of a threat of a serious event (e.g., rape or a threat of death from combat or a natural disaster), symptoms that are intrusive where an individual perceives that the trauma is repeating itself, avoidance, negative changes in thought or affect, and aggressive or hypervigilant behaviors (Comer, 2015; American Psychiatric Association, 2013). Rape was found to be the traumatic event with the most elevated risk (Kessler, Sonnega, Bromet, Hughes, & Nelson, 1995).

A psychobiology of trauma approach asserts that a human being is integrated, a mind–body unit with several levels of data interacting in an involved manner (Walker, 1989). Walker (1989), whose interacting psychobiology model of trauma focuses on the relationship between the body and the mind, explains that traumatic events and the experience of stress that these events produce can have an effect on individuals at the following interrelated levels: Biological, psychological, relational, and cultural.

Symptoms of posttraumatic stress disorder that correspond to the biological level include hyperarousability or hypervigilance (Walker, 1989). In addition to hyperarousal, PTSD symptoms include re-experience, negative mood, thought changes, and avoidance (APA, 2013; Pyszczynski & Kesebir, 2011). Many individuals with posttraumatic stress disorder report that they have difficulty sleeping (Colvonen, Ellison, Haller, & Norman, 2019). Symptoms of PTSD that correspond to the psychological include disturbing flashbacks or depression (Walker, 1989). Symptoms at the social level of being include difficulties in attaching to others or isolation, and at the cultural level, individuals with symptoms of PTSD can become estranged from their culture, depending upon the culture's stance on how it reacts to people who are mistreated (Walker, 1989).

Research on PTSD has demonstrated that stress in relationships is correlated with the severity of symptoms (Riggs, Byrne, Weathers, & Litz, 1998). Symptoms such as avoidance and hyperarousal tend to have the worst effect on interactions with significant others (Cook, Riggs, Thompson, Coyne, & Sheikh, 2004; Riggs et al., 1998; Solomon, Dekel, & Zerach, 2008). The symptom cluster, avoidance, is harmful for veterans because it promotes social isolation, overall, and distance in the interactions between the couple (Blow, Curtis, Wittenborn, & Gorman, 2015; Sherman, Zanotti, & Jones, 2005).

Diagnosis of Posttraumatic Stress Disorder (PTSD)

What characterizes a diagnosis of posttraumatic stress disorder (PTSD), and is the diagnosis for PTSD different than for acute stress disorder? Disorders that result from stress include adjustment disorder and acute stress disorder as well as posttraumatic stress disorder; however, the magnitude of the stressor is the greatest for PTSD and the least for adjustment disorder (Ray, 2018). Whereas acute stress disorder and PTSD are characterized by specific symptoms, adjustment disorder can be diagnosed without the presence of particular symptoms (Ray, 2018). According to DSM-5 (APA, 2013), whereas individuals are diagnosed with acute stress disorder (ASD) if the onset of their symptoms occur within a month from the trauma and endure for less than a month, individuals are diagnosed with posttraumatic stress disorder (PTSD) if the distress cannot be attributed to a different condition (e.g., medical) and ensue for longer than one month (APA, 2013; Comer, 2015). Westfall and Nemeroff (2016) assert that a diagnosis of posttraumatic stress disorder fits for individuals who develop pervasive intrusive and avoidance symptoms in addition to negative thoughts and affect. They assert that these symptoms tend to be accompanied by alterations in arousal after a traumatic incident triggers deleterious consequences within the contexts of systems that are involved in cognitive, affective, and biological processes, e.g., limbic system. Acute stress disorder can occur both when a patient experiences traumatic events as well as when a patient views traumatic events happening to another individual (Ray, 2018). Symptoms of ASD after the traumatic event can include flashbacks, negative emotions, dissociative symptoms, avoidance, and arousal. It has been found that approximately 80% of individuals with acute stress disorder (ASD) develop posttraumatic stress disorder (Bryant, Moulds, Guthrie, & Nixon, 2005; Comer, 2015); however, it is suggested that if patients receive therapy early in time, the occurrence of PTSD can be decreased (Bryant, Friedman, Spiegel, Ursano, & Strain, 2011; Ray, 2018). Nickerson and Bryant (2013) point out that although many individuals with ASD receive a diagnosis of PTSD, there are many individuals who experience trauma who receive a diagnosis of PTSD, but do not display the symptoms of ASD within four weeks post trauma. They attribute the aforementioned finding to the criteria of symptoms of dissociation needed for a diagnosis of ASD.

Prevalence of Posttraumatic Stress Disorder (PTSD)

Prevalence

How prevalent is posttraumatic stress disorder (PTSD)? Posttraumatic stress disorder is a public health issue given its elevated level of impairment and its high risk of suicide (Gallagher, 2018; Gradus et al., 2010; Holowka & Marx, 2012). The percent of adults who have been shown to experience posttraumatic stress disorder after a trauma is 8% (Kilpatrick et al., 2013). In the U.S., the prevalence for 12 months for PTSD is approximately 3.5% (APA, 2013; Ray, 2018). Hispanic Americans have been shown to be more predisposed to posttraumatic stress than other cultures (Comer, 2015; Galea, Ahern, Resnick, Vlahov, 2006; Koch & Haring, 2008). PTSD has been shown to be twice as likely in females than in males, and the symptoms of PTSD last longer in females (Kessler et al., 1995; Ray, 2018).

Onset

When does posttraumatic stress disorder begin? Whereas phobias and separation anxiety disorder emerge when an individual is a child, posttraumatic stress disorder, similar to generalized anxiety disorder and panic disorder, commences later, rarely prior to early adolescence (Paus, Keshavan, & Giedd, 2008). Some researchers, however, assert that acute or posttraumatic stress disorder may emerge in childhood, adolescence, or adulthood (Alisic et al., 2014; Comer, 2015; Monson, Resick, & Rizvi, 2014). When PTSD occurs in children and adolescents, it is frequently a result of early trauma (Julien, 2013).

Comorbidity

Is PTSD comorbid with other psychiatric and physical disorders? There is a high comorbidity with other disorders as evidenced by the finding that other disorders accompany PTSD in more than 80% of veterans with PTSD (Sharpless & Barber, 2011). There is a relationship between PTSD and a greater risk of other emotional disorders such as major depressive disorder (MDD), anxiety disorders (e.g., OCD, social anxiety disorder, panic disorder), and use of substances, and between PTSD and medical diseases such as heart disease and diabetes (Ray, 2018; Ross et al., 2017; Westfall & Nemeroff, 2016). Depression is a comorbid syndrome that can accompany PTSD (Gallagher, 2018), and individuals with PTSD are at a greater risk for suicide than are individuals with other types of anxiety disorders (Galovski & Lyons, 2004). The aforementioned comorbidity pattern suggests the need for more than one treatment type (Ray, 2018).

An Integrative Etiology of Posttraumatic Stress Disorder (PTSD): Focus, Underpinnings, and Causes of PTSD

What are the factors that characterize posttraumatic stress disorder (PTSD) and individuals with PTSD? Posttraumatic stress disorder can be thought of as the lack of affect regulation after a traumatic incident (Seligowski, Lee, Bardeen, & Orcutt, 2015). The disorder can develop when threatening traumatic events that occur to an individual are not processed (Gilbert & Orlans, 2011). Gallegos and Hillbrand (2016) explain that individuals with trauma histories share the features of dysfunctional attachments, stressed relatedness, a maladaptive capacity to self-soothe, and impaired functioning.

Rather than relying on purely physiological or intrapsychic explanations, Wilson (1989) developed an integrative model that implicates complex person (e.g., genetic inclinations to traumatic events, personality) and environmental (e.g., trauma dimensions, the context post trauma) interactions that can influence the way in which patients react to trauma. The characteristics of the person and environmental elements have an impact on the patient's adaptation after the trauma, and coping responses can range from dysfunctional to progressive growth (Wilson, 1989). The aforementioned model can serve as a template for the study of traumatic stress responses and includes complex person–environmental interactions which influence how different people will respond to traumatic events (Wilson, 1989).

What is the cause of PTSD? The cause of PTSD is the trauma itself; however, some individuals may be more predisposed than others to develop PTSD (Elhai, Ford, & Naifeh, 2010; Ingersoll & Marquis, 2014). An individual's predisposition to developing PTSD subsequent to a traumatic event needs to take into consideration an interaction of factors, e.g., physiological, genetic, and psychological variables (Ingersoll & Marquis, 2014). In addition to the relevance of neuroscience themes such as dysregulated circuits, genetic factors, and epigenetics to PTSD, other variables have been shown to be relevant. For example, it is possible that the disruption of sleep affects PTSD; however, findings have not been consistent (Ross, 2014; Ross et al., 2017).

Neuroscience and Posttraumatic Stress Disorder (PTSD)

What is the nature of the experience of trauma? What is the feeling of being stuck? When individuals experience excessive fear, powerlessness, and feel threatened by disintegration, they are experiencing trauma (Gilbert & Orlans, 2011). It has been shown that an individual's history of attachment affects one's ability to cope with trauma that may occur later (Gilbert & Orlans, 2011; Schore, 1994; Siegel, 1999). Past stressors and trauma related to attachment issues have an effect on the brain circuitry that is implicated in the processing of emotions, thereby making it more likely to develop an emotional disorder (Puetz et al., 2014). It is the right hemisphere that is involved in the dysregulated emotional arousal system of individuals with PTSD (Gilbert & Orlans, 2011). Attachment interactions structure the coping mechanisms of the right hemisphere in infants, and the lack of empathic responses by caregivers have been found to generate trauma, which is stored in memory (Gilbert & Orlans, 2011). For example, human beings who need to bond, but are afraid to trust, may end up feeling stuck (Cozolino, 2006; Gilbert & Orlans, 2011).

How does neuroscience play a role in the development and maintenance of PTSD? The sympathetic nervous system (a portion of the autonomic nervous system that controls basic functions of the body), the hypothalamic-pituitary-adrenocortical (HPA) axis (the connection between the hypothalamus, pituitary, and adrenal gland), fear conditioning, and the startle reflex have been shown to play a role in PTSD (Ingersoll & Marquis, 2014; Schnurr et al., 2002). Both the hippocampus and a hyperactive amygdala have been implicated in posttraumatic stress disorder (Comer, 2015; Greene, Bailey & Neumeister, 2013; Rauch, Shin, & Phelps, 2006). Research has shown that too much stress on the hippocampus can lead to memory deficits linked to trauma and that a malfunctioning amygdala can generate the intense memories experienced by individuals with posttraumatic stress disorder (Ingersoll & Marquis, 2014; McEwan et al., 1992; Protopopescu et al., 2005). Results of fMRI investigations demonstrated that the prefrontal cortex of patients with PTSD is underactivated and fails to block reactions of fear from the amygdala with increased rational thought processes (Greene et al., 2013; Kent & Rauch, 2003). In contrast, the amygdala is overactivated in individuals with stress disorders (Chattarji, Tomar, Suvrathan, Ghosh, & Rahman, 2015; Ray, 2018). In short, individuals with stress disorders have been found to have changes in brain systems such as the amygdala, prefrontal cortex, and hippocampus (Chattarji et al., 2015).

Ross and colleagues (2017) proposed an integrated neuroscience treatment plan for PTSD that includes neuroscience themes, e.g., dysregulated circuits, genetic factors, epigenetics, and others, to illustrate how a biopsychosocial approach intersects with neuroscience. For example, an approach based on brain circuits includes the reciprocal inhibitory relationship between the amygdala and the medial prefrontal cortex (mPFC), and it has been suggested that there may be a tendency for patients with PTSD to have an imbalance such that prefrontal cortex function is decreased while the activation of the amygdala is increased (Ross et al., 2017).

Genetic Variables and Posttraumatic Stress Disorder (PTSD)

What is the relationship between genetic variables and the development of posttraumatic stress disorder (PTSD)? Today's etiological approaches underscore internal and external factors in the acquisition of the anxiety disorders (Greene et al., 2013). Integrative diathesis-stress models are associated with PTSD (Bowman & Yehuda, 2004; McKeever & Huff, 2003). Elwood and colleagues (2009) explain that for these models, although the traumatic event is the key stressor that triggers PTSD symptoms, there is individual variation before the trauma that may trigger PTSD symptoms, and that individuals with considerable psychological vulnerability (either inborn or learned) before the trauma may carry a higher risk of the occurrence of PTSD than individuals with a lesser amount of vulnerability. Given that only some individuals who have experienced a traumatic event develop PTSD, it is possible that it is not only stress that is implicated in the acquisition of PTSD (Greene et al., 2013). It is suggested that genetics may influence the development of PTSD, with some individuals being more likely than others to succumb to PTSD after a traumatic event (Greene et al., 2013; Yehuda & Seckl, 2011).

With respect to genetic factors, it has been shown that there are genetic differences related to whether an individual who experiences a stressor will develop PTSD (Friedman & Karam, 2008; Ingersoll & Marquis, 2014; Koenen et al., 2002). The finding that the cortisol levels of both the women with PTSD who were pregnant during the attacks on the World Trade Center and their babies who were born after the terrorist attacks were found to be more elevated than average suggests that the offspring inherited a propensity towards posttraumatic stress disorder (Comer, 2015; Yehuda & Bierer, 2007).

With respect to an approach based on epigenetics or heritable modifications in gene expression, researchers found that an early traumatic event experienced in childhood can result in irregularity in the HPA axis and impaired reactions to stressors experienced in adulthood (Ross et al., 2017). Furthermore, the traumatic events that individuals experience may have an impact on the gene expression of their children and may affect predisposition to trauma (Dias, Maddox, Klengel, Ressler, 2015; Ross et al., 2017; Yehuda et al., 2014). In short, abuse suffered in childhood can have a lasting epigenetic impact (McGowan et al., 2009; Ray, 2018).

Psychological Factors and Posttraumatic Stress Disorder (PTSD)

There are psychological factors that can influence the development of PTSD. For example, researchers have demonstrated that psychological variables such as cognitive vulnerabilities may predispose individuals to posttraumatic stress disorder (Epstein, 1991; Ingersoll & Marquis, 2014; McCann & Pearlman, 1990). Cognitive vulnerabilities, e.g., rumination, anxiety sensitivity, or the apprehension of anxiety (Reiss, 1991), may be related to the development and continuation of PTSD (Elwood, Hahn, Olatunji, & Williams, 2009). With respect to cognitive frameworks of PTSD, the kind of trauma, a trauma's severity, the traumatic event's cultural setting, and one's understanding of the trauma can influence the occurrence of PTSD (Ross et al., 2017).

The Total Ecological System (Magnavita & Anchin, 2014) and Posttraumatic Stress Disorder (PTSD)

According to Magnavita and Anchin (2014), a diathesis can endure at many different levels (e.g., intrapsychic, sociocultural, and others) and can persist both for current and future episodes of emotional disorders. The first level of the total ecological system (TES), the intrapsychic-biological, emphasizes the mind or brain, and the processes at this level include neurotransmitter activity and the limbic system (Magnavita & Anchin, 2014). In traumatic situations, the limbic system of humans, unlike that of animals, persists, and, thus, it is harder for humans to return to a state of balance after a traumatic event (Magnavita & Anchin, 2014; Sapolsky, 2004). Given the higher level of humans' relationships, humans are more prone to trauma than many animals, and individuals who have experienced many traumatic situations can endure persistent limbic hyperarousal resulting in anxiety (Magnavita & Anchin, 2014). Read, Perry, Moskowitz, and Connolly's (2001) traumagenic neurodevelopmental model supports the findings that early traumatic events can elicit neurobiological sensitivity, change brain structures, and lead to psychological disorders such as posttraumatic disorder (PTSD) (Grawe, 2007; Magnavita & Anchin, 2014).

Magnavita and Anchin's (2014) second level of the total ecological system (TES), the interpersonal-dyadic level, includes self–other dyads. There are large traumas, those that place a patient's life in danger, and small traumas, which are characterized by enduring relational damages at the interpersonal-dyadic level (Magnavita & Anchin, 2014; Neborsky & Solomon, 2001). The different types of traumas invariably include an interpersonal component, e.g., an environmental type of trauma that involves the death of a family member or an exploitative type of trauma that is concerned with physical abuse (Magnavita and Anchin, 2014).

With respect to sociocultural factors, it has been demonstrated that variations in PTSD in individuals from different cultures are linked to whether a particular culture focuses on independence or on a group stance, e.g. a Western versus a Middle Eastern culture (Ingersoll & Marquis, 2014; Jobson & O'Kearney, 2008). The severity of the trauma, a low degree of social and family support, and other life stressors are strong predictors of acute stress disorder or PTSD (Brewin, Andrews, & Valentine, 2000; DiGangi et al., 2013; Uchino & Birmingham, 2011).

Death Anxiety and Posttraumatic Stress Disorder (PTSD)

What is the association between death anxiety and the development and maintenance of posttraumatic stress disorder (PTSD)? Anger buffer disruption theory

(ABDT) is an extension of terror management theory (TMT) (Greenberg, Pyszczynski, & Solomon, 1986), an integrative theory that describes the contribution of the knowledge of mortality to behavior (Solomon, Greenberg, & Pyszczynski, 1991). Anger buffer disruption theory (ABDT) can explain responses to trauma as well as the origin and maintenance of PTSD (Pyszczynski & Kesebir, 2011). When an individual's mechanisms that offer a buffer or protection against general anxiety and, more specifically, against death anxiety are disrupted, PTSD can ensue, and the individual is left without defenses and is flooded with anxiety (Pyszczynski & Kesebir, 2011).

Clinical Practice Applications of Single-School, Integrated, and Integrative Psychotherapy Treatment Models for Posttraumatic Stress Disorder (PTSD)

Can individuals adjust after experiencing trauma, and do they tend to seek psychotherapy? Several factors can determine an individual's adjustment after the experience of a traumatic event. The quality and accessibility of social support and the amount of psychological tension experienced during recovery can determine an individual's psychological outcome post trauma (Greenberg, Brooks, & Dunn, 2015). Individuals tend to seek psychotherapy more or less depending upon the emotional disorder. It is not usual for individuals with posttraumatic stress disorder to seek psychotherapy; however, individuals with PTSD are less likely to seek help than individuals with depression (Corrigan & Hull, 2015; Westfall & Nemeroff, 2016). Frequently, PTSD is not reported and not treated, and few individuals with PTSD experience a total remission of symptoms (Westfall & Nemeroff, 2016). The goal of most treatments for PTSD is to facilitate the experience of the original trauma in a controlled setting or to facilitate catharsis (Ray, 2018).

CBT, Psychodynamic, and Interpersonal Approaches for Posttraumatic Stress Disorder (PTSD)

Psychotherapy interventions derived from CBT with the most empirical support and found to be the most effective with veterans include prolonged exposure (PE) (Foa & Kozak, 1986), cognitive processing therapy (CPT) (Resick & Schnicke, 1992), and eye movement desensitization and reprocessing (EMDR) (Shapiro, 1995) (Sharpless & Barber, 2011). Whereas, generally, posttraumatic stress disorder has not historically responded well to single-school therapies (Norcross, 2005), imaginal exposure has been shown to be effective in the treatment of posttraumatic stress disorder (Abramowitz, Deacon, & Whiteside, 2011; Keane & Kaloupek, 1996). Psychotherapy interventions such as dialectical behavioral therapy (DBT) and other treatments that target trauma have been utilized to treat individuals with histories of trauma and have worked; however, there are several patients for whom the aforementioned treatments have not been effective (Gallegos & Hillbrand, 2016). Patients with posttraumatic stress disorder have been shown to drop out of effective trauma-focused therapies such as the prolonged exposure of Foa, Hembree, and Rothbaum (2007) and Resick, Monson, and Chard's (2017) cognitive processing therapy (Varkovitzky, Sherill, & Reger, 2018).

What treatments have been employed with patients who select not to engage in exposure therapy? For patients with PTSD who do not wish exposure methods, psychodynamic therapy is warranted, and interpersonal therapy (IPT) has been used to treat PTSD as well (Sharpless & Barber, 2011). Hypnosis has been utilized alone and along with other treatments, and has been found to decrease the symptoms of PTSD (Abramowitz, Barak, Ben-Avi, Knobler, 2008; Sharpless & Barber, 2011).

An Integrated Behavioral, Psychodynamic and Attribution Model for Survivors of Trauma

Researchers have developed a psychotherapy approach that integrates behavioral, psychodynamic, and attribution perspectives to treat survivors of trauma who enact self-injurious and violent behaviors (Gallegos & Hillbrand, 2016). To address the needs of survivors of trauma for whom treatment aimed at symptom reduction and a quick return to community did not work, it is suggested that clinicians use an integrated behavioral, psychodynamic, and attribution model that focuses on the establishment of a therapeutic milieu, the reward of positive behaviors, the development of trust in the intervention team, and the use of individual therapy (Gallegos & Hillbrand, 2016). The aforementioned integrated model is not a new approach, but a combination of already extant and empirically supported treatments (Gallegos & Hillbrand, 2016). Such an integrated approach considers training staff to develop long-term strategies to teach survivors of trauma who enact violent behaviors to work on controlling their impulses, soothing themselves, and developing empathy (Gallegos & Hillbrand, 2016). Gallegos and Hillbrand (2016) assert that their integrative model is innovative in its employment of in vivo strategies for rewarding adaptive responses in total care contexts with the goal of facilitating new skills, and, in turn, offering individuals with trauma the opportunity to define themselves anew.

Are there other models that integrate CBT methods and psychodynamic treatment for patients with PTSD? Alternative approaches that include CBT and psychodynamic interventions in the treatment of PTSD include the use of brief eclectic psychotherapy (BEPP), an evidence-based intervention that combines cognitive-behavioral methods, psychodynamic interventions, and directive therapy, for patients with PTSD (Gersons & Schnyder, 2013).

An Integration of CBT and Motivational Interviewing (MI) for Posttraumatic Stress Disorder (PTSD)

Are there other alternate treatments to monotherapy? Chapter 5 discussed an integration of CBT with motivational interviewing for generalized anxiety disorder (GAD). This integrated treatment can be utilized for patients with posttraumatic stress disorder (PTSD) (Murphy, Thompson, Murray, Rainey, & Uddo, 2009). Whereas treatment programs for PTSD that are confrontational may lead to resistance and result in ineffectiveness, supportive interventions such as motivational interviewing (MI) may apply to the treatment of PTSD (Miller, Benefield, & Tonigan, 1993; Miller & Rollnick, 2002; Murphy, 2008). Murphy (2008) instituted a program that included motivational interviewing (MI) for individuals suffering from PTSD. MI targeted the identification of problems, facilitated change, and engaged veterans diagnosed with PTSD in treatment (Murphy, 2008).

Emotionally Focused Therapy (EFT): An Integrated Treatment for Posttraumatic Stress Disorder (PTSD)

Emotionally Focused Therapy (EFT), an evidence-based treatment with low rates of dropout, which integrates experiential therapy and family systems, can be used to work with couples who struggle with PTSD (Blow et al., 2015; Johnson, Hunsley, Greenberg, & Schindler, 1999). EFT is well suited for veterans with PTSD and relies on attachment theory while targeting the expression of emotions in an adaptive manner (Blow et al., 2015). Individuals with PTSD have difficulty regulating their emotions because of what they suffered in combat, and frequently experience hyperarousal and affect numbing, resulting in distressed relationships (Greenman & Johnson, 2012; Johnson, 2002). The purpose of this integrated psychotherapy is to create a safe environment where couples can discuss their vulnerabilities in order to build a deeper relationship (Blow et al., 2015). Methods that EFT therapists utilize to address trauma that is complex include chair tasks (Paivio & Pascual-Leone, 2010). Chapter 5 discussed the use of chair conversations within the context of EFT for individuals with generalized anxiety disorder.

An Existential Integrative Model That Incorporates a Behavioral Approach for Posttraumatic Stress Disorder (PTSD)

How can an existential integrative model be used to treat individuals with posttraumatic stress disorder (PTSD)? Recently, Sotskova and Dossett (2017) proposed an integrative model for the treatment of PTSD, an example of assimilative integration that describes an existential integrative framework. This approach is similar to Schneider's (2008) existential integrative psychotherapy (IEP) discussed in Chapter 3. Sotskova and Dossett's (2017) existential integrative approach to treatment is an example of assimilative integration in that it encourages the therapist whose primary theoretical orientation is existential to borrow from a behavioral perspective by using exposure in order to treat PTSD. In this case, a therapist with an existential orientation can conceptualize the behavioral portion, the exposure, from the vantage point of an existential approach by helping the patient to tolerate painful feelings and facilitating the broadening of a patient's range of experiential feelings (Sotskova and Dossett, 2017). Whereas the exposure is interpreted from the position of the therapist's primary theoretical orientation, an existential perspective, the therapist understands that the exposure can be interpreted from a cognitive-behavioral approach as well, an orientation that links exposure to learning and memory (Sotskova and Dossett, 2017). A therapist who uses an existential integrative model can maintain the different approaches simultaneously without the need to remove or resolve the differences (Sotskova and Dossett, 2017). Sotskova and Dossett (2017) explained that whereas the existential approach is the main theoretical orientation, both psychodynamic and cognitive-behavioral perspectives were integrated with a reliance upon the values of assimilative integration.

Integrated Existential Treatment, Death Anxiety, and Trauma

What is the relationship between an integrated existential treatment, death anxiety, and trauma? Lewis (2014) proposed a brief existential treatment, a terror management theory (TMT) existential integrated treatment (TIE) collaboration, with a focus on mortality salience (MS), the state of recognition of an individual's eventual death, to assist patients to find meaning in their fear or anxiety related to death. Lewis (2014) cautions about the suitability of TMT TIE with certain patients. For example, therapists need to consider whether talking about death will help a patient or elevate a patient's risk, or whether a patient will become more positive or defensive when talking about a particular traumatic event (Lewis, 2014; Greenberg, Koole, & Pyszczynski, 2004).

An Integrated Neuroscience Treatment Plan for Posttraumatic Stress Disorder (PTSD)

The section on the integrated etiology of posttraumatic stress disorder (PTSD) in this chapter discussed the association between neuroscience and PTSD. According to Ross et al.'s (2017) integrated neuroscience treatment plan for PTSD, which illustrates how a biopsychosocial approach intersects with neuroscience, it is proposed that a broad scope of interventions for PTSD may have a common therapeutic plan to restore equilibrium between the amygdala and the prefrontal cortex. For example, selective serotonin reuptake inhibitors (SSRIs) may be effective in reducing overactivity in the amygdala, and therapy may help control anxiety and arousal (Ross et al., 2017; Shin, Rauch, & Pitman, 2006).

With respect to epigenetics and posttraumatic stress disorder (discussed in the etiology section of this chapter), it has been demonstrated that therapy has helped to undo a number of DNA methylation patterns related to PTSD, indicating that epigenetic alterations, although robust, are not absolute (Ross et al., 2017; Yehuda et al., 2013). Given an epigenetic model, treatments that preclude early trauma along with those that lessen the enduring effect of early trauma are recommended (Kaufman, Gelernter, Hudziak, Tyrka, & Coplan, 2015; Ross et al., 2017).

An Integrative Diathesis Approach for Posttraumatic Stress Disorder (PTSD)

How does an integrative approach that incorporates the notion of vulnerability apply to posttraumatic stress disorder? An integrative diathesis perspective compares several vulnerability aspects at the same time while investigating the interactions among the vulnerabilities with the goal of providing a comprehensive understanding of the emergence of PTSD (Elwood et al., 2009). During the course of an individual's lifetime, a variety of stressors may occur, and the focus of therapeutic interventions needs to be on working on the vulnerability so as to reduce future episodes of an emotional disorder (Magnavita & Anchin, 2014). According to Elwood et al. (2009), treatment that underscores vulnerabilities that are cognitive, e.g., anxiety sensitivity, are associated with a decrease in cognitive vulnerability and anxiety (e.g., Schmidt et al., 2007). Given that cognitive style can increase an individual's risk towards developing anxiety because of thoughts that magnify danger, it is suggested that clinicians use an integrative approach of cognitive vulnerability in their treatment of PTSD (Elwood et al., 2009; Ingersoll & Marquis, 2014).

Psychopharmacological Treatment, Monotherapy, and Medication Combined with Therapy for Posttraumatic Stress Disorder (PTSD)

Is medication or medication combined with therapy effective for the treatment of posttraumatic stress disorder (PTSD)? Although the trauma-focused therapies have resulted in more enduring benefits than nontrauma-focused therapy or medication (Lee et al., 2016), medication for the treatment of PTSD has been found to be beneficial (Williams, Richardson, & Galovski, 2013), and psychopharmacological treatments for PTSD have included antianxiety and antidepressant medications (Comer, 2015; Morgan, Lockwood, Steinke, Schleenbaker, & Botts, 2012; Writer, Meyer, & Schillerstrom, 2014). Although trauma-focused treatments are considered interventions that are first-line, the effects of stress inoculation therapy were reduced over time (Lee et al., 2016). Whereas exposure and cognitive trauma-focused therapy aim to extinguish fear reactions that are conditioned, medications blunt the expression of PTSD symptoms, but do not act on the underlying mechanisms (Lee et al., 2016).

There have been many studies that investigated medication for PTSD. Williams and colleagues (2013) point out that whereas the SSRIs and the SNRIs have been implicated in the treatment of PTSD (e.g., Benedek, Friedman, Zatzick, & Ursano, 2009), the Institute of Medicine (IOM, 2007) asserts that there is insufficient evidence to recommend that the SSRIs are effective for PTSD. Recently, venlafaxine (Effexor XR) and sertraline (Zoloft) were shown to be more effective than other medications (Lee et al., 2016).

The antidepressant, mirtazapine (Remeron), has been shown to be useful in the treatment of PTSD (VA/DoD, 2010). Whereas some research shows that antiepileptic medication is not an effective treatment for PTSD (Lee et al., 2016), other research shows that antiepileptic medication helps with PTSD-related nightmares (Ahern, Juergens, Cordes, Becker, & Krahn, 2011; Julien, 2013;). Prazosin (Minipres) has been suggested for PTSD related-nightmares as well (Aurora et al., 2010; Julien, 2013). Whereas the benzodiazepines may be useful for reducing anxiety and stress in the short run, caution needs to be taken against their use for a long period of time because of the risk for addiction (Nickerson & Bryant, 2013).

A combination of psychotherapy and medication was not shown to be more effective than monotherapy alone in the treatment of PTSD (Hetrick, Purcell, Garner, & Parslow, 2010). No treatment or combination of treatments for PTSD have been found to either prevent PTSD or to guarantee remission (Westfall & Nemeroff, 2016). The norm in the majority of therapeutic settings is to combine psychotherapy with pharmacotherapy in the treatment of PTSD; however, the aforementioned approach needs to target patients with PTSD who do not show improvement with psychotherapy by itself (Muse, Moore, & Stahl, 2013).

What is the difference between treatment for PTSD and interventions for acute stress disorder (ASD)? Medication that has been used for PTSD may not help that much for acute stress disorder (ASD) (Nikerson & Bryant, 2013). Whereas psychological debriefing post trauma has not been shown to prevent the emergence of PTSD, both CBT and time have been shown to be helpful in the reduction of symptoms of acute stress disorder (ASD) and in preventing PTSD from developing (Nickerson & Bryant, 2013).

How does PTSD compare to other emotional disorders with respect to therapy and medication refusal? Chapters 5 and 9 discuss rates of refusal for GAD and OCD respectively. Similar to the findings for GAD and OCD, no differences were found in rates of refusal between pharmacotherapy and psychotherapy for individuals with PTSD (Swift, Greenberg, Tompkins, & Parkin, 2017).

Clinical Practice Applications of Integral Treatment and a Unified Approach for Posttraumatic Stress Disorder (PTSD)

The section on the integrated etiology of posttraumatic stress disorder discussed the relationship between the total ecological system (Magnavita and Anchin, 2014) and posttraumatic stress disorder (PTSD). How does this integral or unified treatment approach apply to posttraumatic stress disorder, and how does an integral therapist navigate when treating an individual with PTSD? An integral approach to PTSD takes into account four quadrants, levels and lines of development, and a patient's minute-to-minute states (Ingersoll & Marquis, 2014). Psychotherapists who use an integral approach facilitate interventions for PTSD sufferers in these quadrants (Ingersoll & Marquis, 2014).

For example, integral therapists who treat patients with PTSD encourage good physical health, e.g., regular sleep patterns, in the Upper Right (UR) quadrant (Ingersoll & Marquis, 2014). Psychotherapists who treat clients with PTSD focus on a patient's sense of self and ideology, e.g., a plan for the universe, in the Upper Left (UL), on the patient's social system in the Lower Right, (LR), e.g., living in a setting where there are buses and trains, and on the patient's community of friends in the Lower Left quadrant (LL) (Ingersoll & Marquis, 2014).

How can a unified psychotherapy approach facilitate change for a client with PTSD? A therapist working within the first level of the client's total ecological system (TES), the intrapsychic-biological with its emphasis on the mind or brain, may choose to point out to patients with PTSD that their overly sensitive limbic systems may be contributing to their difficulties in overcoming the effects of trauma (Magnavita & Anchin, 2014). The aforementioned approach, which does not pathologize the experiences of patients who self-blame, can serve as a way for patients to develop empathy for themselves and can serve to dispel patients' dysfunctional beliefs that they caused the trauma that they endured (Magnavita & Anchin, 2014).

Magnavita and Anchin (2014) emphasize that a unified approach to psychotherapy treatment requires that therapists empower their patients by educating them about neurobiological concepts. An explanation of epigenetic mechanisms serves as a unifying concept that can facilitate the value of psychotherapy in that the learning that takes place during therapy may generate changes in gene expression and strengthen synapses (Gabbard, 2000; Magnavita & Anchin, 2014). Magnavita and Anchin (2014) suggest that a unified psychotherapist incorporate neurobiological instruments such as biofeedback and electroencephalogram (EEG) technology into their repertoires to restore a sense of balance. They propose that measures of biofeedback can offer patients feedback about their state of arousal, and EEG technology can record and change brain activity.

What is the relationship between trauma and the cognitive domain of a client's total ecological system (TES)? The cognitive domain, another critical portion of the intrapsychic-biological level of the TES, is critical for a unified psychotherapist (Magnavita & Anchin, 2014). For example, the tendency for individuals to recall more emotionally charged material is reflected in the interaction between cognition and emotion (Magnavita & Anchin, 2014; Siegel, 1999). Magnavita and Anchin (2014) explain that the damaging effects of early trauma are engraved in the cognitive-emotional schema of a patient's neural network, are projected into a patient's daily relational interactions (at the interpersonal-dyadic level), and are difficult for a therapist to treat. In addition to offering exposure or EMDR to treat trauma, they suggest the use of anxiety-reducing techniques such as biofeedback, relaxation training, mindfulness, and self-soothing.

This section offered examples of integral therapy for the treatment of PTSD from the perspective of the quadrants (e.g., Ingersoll & Marquis, 2014). How do therapists who practice integral therapy employ lines of development in the treatment of individuals suffering from PTSD? A focus of an integral therapist needs to be on safety and stabilization (Ingersoll & Marquis, 2014). The integrally informed therapist who treats trauma recognizes that the interpersonal line of development is crucial for developing an atmosphere of safety and stability, particularly when working with patients with relational trauma (Briere, 2006; Ingersoll & Marquis, 2014). The theme of attachment injuries can contribute to a therapist's understanding of a patient's interpersonal line of development, and it is important for therapists to recognize that patients who have sustained early childhood relational trauma may have a lot of difficulty attaching to others, thereby affecting the patient's ability to form a therapeutic bond with a therapist (Ingersoll & Marquis, 2014).

A Transdiagnostic Unified Protocol (UP) for Posttraumatic Stress Disorder (PTSD)

Are there other unified treatments for posttraumatic stress disorder (PTSD)? Another unified treatment approach for PTSD is the transdiagnostic unified protocol (UP) of Varkovitzky and colleagues (2018) who presented a UP for veterans who were diagnosed with posttraumatic stress disorder and different comorbidities. The UP, in harmony with prolonged exposure and cognitive processing therapy, can address emotion regulation in patients with several disorders such as anxiety and posttraumatic stress disorder (Barlow, Farchione et al., 2011; Varkovitzky et al., 2018). The aforementioned transdiagnostic treatment may suit clients and mental health professionals who wish to select a psychotherapy approach that is not trauma-focused in order to target a broad spectrum of symptoms and general dissatisfaction with life (Varkovitzky et al., 2018). The UP consists of an integration of approaches employed in cognitive-behavioral treatments that are empirically supported (Norton & Paulus, 2016; Varkovitzky et al., 2018). It was found that at the end of UP treatment, patients reported that they had fewer problems with emotion regulation, a decreased number of symptoms of posttraumatic stress disorder than they had prior to being treated with the UP, an increase in quality of life, and that the improvements in anxiety endured for at least a year and a half following UP treatment (Bullis, Fortune, Farchione, & Barlow, 2014; Carl, Gallagher, Sauer-Zavala, Bentley, & Barlow, 2014; Varkovitzky et al., 2018).

Since the transdiagnostic UP focuses on transdiagnostic aspects of vulnerability (such as neuroticism) that are common to several disorders, the UP may be considered to be a potentially advantageous intervention for PTSD (Barlow, Sauer-Zavala, Carl, Bullis, & Ellard, 2014; Gallagher, 2018). The UP highlights motivation and engagement, which can help with patient retention, and it focuses on adaptive affect regulation strategies that can help patients with PTSD as they experience exposure for a comorbid depressive disorder (Gallagher, 2018).

How to Implement Integrated Psychotherapy in Practice for Posttraumatic Stress Disorder (PTSD)

The following case study of an individual with posttraumatic stress disorder after the Vietnam War relies on Wolfe's (2005) integrative model of psychotherapy. The psychotherapy integration includes the use of self psychology themes, cognitive-behavioral therapy (CBT), hypnosis, and interpersonal therapy to treat a patient who returned from Vietnam with a diagnosis with PTSD.

The use of integrated psychotherapy that combines self psychology themes, CBT, hypnosis, and interpersonal therapy is illustrated in the case of Roberta, age 23, adult child, of her survivor parents, Hannah, and Alex. Roberta reported that her mother suffered from symptoms of PTSD, and when Roberta was a child, her mother did not often speak of her traumatic experiences at Bergen-Belsen concentration camp. According to Roberta, her mother was depressed, defended against her past traumatic experiences during WWII, and she displayed overprotective behaviors towards Roberta. Roberta reported that when she was a child her mother was often withdrawn and spoke to her infrequently; however, her father related stories about his service with the army during WWI and with the resistance movement during WWII.

Roberta reported that she remembers that her mother's nightmares were severe and that her father took care of many of her daily needs. Roberta identified with the stories that her father told about the wars, and she sought to emulate her father's career path. She related to the therapist that she deployed as a nurse to Vietnam after her boyfriend broke up with her. While in Vietnam, Roberta developed severe symptoms of stress trauma and was sent back to the U.S. for treatment. When Roberta met the therapist, she reported that she had trouble concentrating because of intrusive thoughts, flashbacks, low self-esteem, irritability, increased symptoms of severe stress, anxiety, and self-blame.

At the outset, Roberta's therapist utilized empathic attunement and an open listening approach to establish and maintain a therapeutic relationship with Roberta. Initially, Roberta refused CBT methods, e.g., exposure. When the traumatic event prevents an individual with PTSD from trusting interpersonal relationships, interpersonal psychotherapy (IPT) can decrease feelings of demoralization and help with social skills (Markowitz et al., 2009). The therapist used interpersonal therapy to help Roberta cope with her stress and difficulty relating to her former friends in the U.S.

After several months, Roberta was willing to try CBT methods for her intrusive thoughts and flashbacks. It has been shown that an integrated treatment of hypnosis and cognitive-behavioral therapy is helpful in alleviating symptoms of PTSD (Bryant et al., 2006). The therapist utilized CBT methods, e.g., imaginal exposure, along with relaxation techniques and hypnosis to decrease Roberta's severe symptoms of stress and intrusive thoughts related to her deployment.

After 10 sessions of CBT along with relaxation methods and hypnosis for Roberta's PTSD symptoms, Roberta reported some relief from her symptoms;

however, she related that she continued to feel troubled. The therapist shifted to a self-psychology approach. For the self-psychology portion of the integrative therapy approach, the therapist relied on Kohut's (1984) selfobject themes as illustrated by Freyberg's (1989) explanation of the difficulties with self cohesion that children of holocaust survivors confront during their lives.

Solomon, Kotler, and Mikulincer (1988) utilize the term, PTSD latency, to characterize a greater propensity towards PTSD among the offspring of holocaust survivors, particularly when faced with serious stressors. The therapist, although cognizant of Roberta's early history, related to Roberta by focusing on difficulties that were idiosyncratic to her own particular lifestyle in the present, e.g., a recent breakup with her boyfriend and her difficult deployment to Vietnam.

Roberta displayed resilience and seemed to rely on the values that her parents instilled in her prior to her deployment to Vietnam. It appears that Roberta did not sustain deeper damage to the self because the trauma that she endured after her boyfriend left her and during deployment in Vietnam was mitigated by the values imparted to her during her childhood and adolescent years as well as the supportive relationship that Roberta had with her father.

Empathy allows a therapist to understand what is going on in a client's mind, to prepare a client for psychological interpretations, repairs the disruptions that take place in the therapeutic relationship, and is the essence of therapeutic engagement (Gilbert & Orlans, 2011; Kohut, 1984; Peri et al., 2015). When a therapist uses emotional attunement to understand the emotional being of patients, patients can more easily become aware of their own thoughts and feelings (Peri, Gofman, Tal, & Tuval-Mashiach, 2015; Stern, 1985). The therapist was able to empathically feel herself into Roberta's difficult circumstances. According to Kohut (1971, 1977), if the parent, in this case, Roberta's mother, is unable to offer sufficient empathy to meet the needs of the child, the child may not develop sufficient coping abilities to self-soothe and maintain self-esteem. Although Roberta reported that she felt somewhat better after CBT, Roberta continued to report difficulties, which could be attributed to the empathic failures that she experienced during childhood when her mother was not receptive to her selfobject needs. When Roberta was growing up, she felt that something was wrong with her when, in reality, her mother was too depressed to respond to her. Roberta learned to internalize her mother's distraught state, and it took her a long time to trust her buddies in Vietnam, while she was away from home.

Several months into the self-psychology portion of the therapy, Roberta was able to share with the therapist some dreadful memories about her mother's experiences during WWII. Roberta seemed to live and protect her silent mother's history during WWII as if it were her own. During the course of therapy, after listening to Roberta's recollections when she was a child and Roberta's narratives of her more recent Vietnam experiences, the therapist developed a countertransference reaction and sought consultation to address the jarring experiences of war.

In contrast to research that projects pathology onto the offspring of holocaust survivors, Albeck (1994) proposes that parents who survived the holocaust transmit trauma to their children; however, their children have the potential to be fully functioning adults. The offspring of holocaust survivors tend to keep their connection with their families by integrating their parents' experiences (Albeck, 1994). Throughout the therapy, the therapist worked on developing trust by empathically attuning to Roberta's subjective world. Roberta informed the therapist several times that the therapist was not one of her family's close friends who had survived the war and that the therapist was an outsider who could not relate to the experiences of her family of origin, nor did she know what Roberta endured in Vietnam. The therapist understood that Roberta's current feelings about her interrupted deployment in Vietnam and the loss of her relationship with her boyfriend may be retraumatizing her. Roberta's present situation regarding her difficult deployment may have reactivated her early anxiety, stress reactions, and sorrow.

During the self-psychology portion of the therapy, Roberta periodically reported a few mild symptoms, and, during these times, the therapist did not hesitate to intersperse CBT methods to help Roberta cope better. Roberta reported that she was doing somewhat better after about a year and a half of therapy. She attended a party given by one of her Vietnam buddies, and she expressed pride that she had been with them. The therapist validated by smiling and encouraging Roberta to talk about her friends.

Developing a client's arrested self-structures and facilitating a client's ability to make use of interpretive material requires that a therapist empathically understand a client's worldview (Gilbert & Orlans, 2011; Kohut, 1977). After two years of the self-psychology part of the therapy, Roberta expressed a wish to continue further self-exploration in therapy. During the self-psychology phase, the therapist helped Roberta to work on individuation and self-compassion, and to rid herself of the guilty feelings that somehow she was responsible for the bad events that befell her. Roberta began to understand her need for a selfobject to validate her unique experiences and challenging past, and how her own experiences are distinct from her mother's history of trauma. As she continued to recover, Roberta felt less vulnerable, less stressed, more able to connect with friends, and her flashbacks receded. At the end of the third year of therapy, Roberta, although somewhat vulnerable to anxiety, blamed herself less for the events of her life, and seemed to develop a more cohesive and strengthened sense of self, with her self-esteem spiraling downward less frequently.

Summary

Trauma, from an integrative point of view, involves a multi-faceted perspective that includes a focus on the physiological, the psychological, and the contribution of attachment processes as well as patterns of patient regulation and a view of the present dyadic relationship between patient and therapist (Gilbert & Orlans, 2011). This chapter discussed the integrated and unified etiology and psychotherapy treatment frameworks for posttraumatic stress disorder (PTSD) (see Table 10.1). Rather than rely on a manualized, unitary treatment approach for PTSD, the therapist in the case study presentation

Table 10.1 Posttraumatic Stress Disorder (PTSD)

Etiology: Neuroscience	*Etiology*	*Integrated and Unified Psychotherapy*
Biological Individuals with stress disorders have been found to have changes in brain systems such as the amygdala, prefrontal cortex, and hippocampus.[a]	Psychological Cognitive vulnerabilities, e.g., rumination, anxiety sensitivity, the apprehension of anxiety linked to PTSD[e,f]	An Integrated Behavioral, Psychodynamic and Attribution Model[k]
Genetic[b,c]	The Total Ecological System (TES)[g]	An Integration of CBT and Motivational Interviewing[l,m,n,o]
Epigenetics or Heritable Modifications in Gene Expression Irregularity in the HPA axis[d]	Death Anxiety Anger buffer disruption theory (ABDT), an extension of TMT, can explain responses to trauma as well as the origin and maintenance of PTSD.[h,i,j]	Emotionally Focused Therapy (EFT)[p,q]
		An Existential Integrative Model That Incorporates a Behavioral Approach[r] Integrated Existential Treatment, Death Anxiety, and Trauma[s] An Integrated Neuroscience Treatment Plan[t,u] An Integrative Diathesis Approach[e] An Integral Approach to PTSD[v] A Transdiagnostic Unified Protocol (UP) for Posttraumatic Stress Disorder (PTSD)[w]

[a] Chattarji, Tomar, Suvrathan, Ghosh, and Rahman (2015). [b]Greene, Bailey, and Neumeister (2013). [c]Yehuda & Seckl (2011). [d]Ross et al. (2017). [e]Elwood, Hahn, Olatunji, and Williams (2009). [f]Reiss (1991). [g]Magnavita and Anchin (2014). [h]Greenberg, Pyszczynski, and Solomon (1986). [i]Pyszczynski and Kesebir (2011). [j]Solomon, Greenberg, and Pyszczynski (1991). [k]Gallegos and Hillbrand (2016). [l]Miller, Benefield, and Tonigan (1993). [m]Miller and Rollnick (2002). [n]Murphy (2008). [o]Murphy, Thompson, Murray, Rainey, and Uddo (2009). [p]Blow, Curtis, Wittenborn, and Gorman (2015). [q]Johnson, Hunsley, Greenberg, and Schindler (1999). [r]Sotskova and Dossett (2017). [s]Lewis (2014). [t]Ross et al. (2017). [u]Shin, Rauch, and Pitman (2006). [v]Ingersoll and Marquis (2014). [w]Varkovitzky, Sherill, and Reger (2018).

demonstrated how a therapeutic response needs to involve the consideration of the unique issues of an individual client. In considering integrated treatment, the therapist needs to consider the scope of the trauma and whether its nature involves a response to a situational incident and/or a dysregulated self-structure with early insecure attachment (Gilbert & Orlans, 2011).

References

Abramowitz, E. G., Barak, Y., Ben-Avi, I., & Knobler, H. Y. (2008). Hypnotherapy in the treatment of chronic combat-related PTSD patients suffering from insomnia: A randomized, zolpidem-controlled clinical trial. *International Journal of Clinical and Experimental Hypnosis, 56*(3), 270–280. doi: 10.1080/00207140802039672

Abramowitz, J. S., Deacon, B. J., & Whiteside, S. P. H. (2011). *Exposure therapy for anxiety: Principles and practices*. New York, NY: Guilford Press.

Ahern, E. P., Juergens, T., Cordes, T., Becker, T., & Krahn, D. (2011). A review of atypical antipsychotic medications for posttraumatic stress disorder. *International Clinical Psychopharmacology, 26*(4), 193–200. doi: 10.1097/YIC.0b013e3283473738

Albeck, J. H. (1994). Intergenerational consequences of trauma: Reframing traps in treatment theory — A second-generation perspective. In E. B. Williams & J. F. Sommer, Jr. (Eds.), *Handbook of post-traumatic therapy* (pp. 106–125). Westport, CT: Greenwood Publishing Group.

Alisic, E., Zalta, A. K., van Wesel, F., Larsen, S. E., Hafstad, G. S., Hassanpour, K., & Smid, G. E. (2014). Rates of post-traumatic stress disorder in trauma-exposed children and adolescents: Meta-analysis. *The British Journal of Psychiatry, 204*(5), 335–340. doi: 10.1192/bjp.bp.113.131227

American Psychiatric Association. (2013). *Diagnostic and statistical manual of mental disorders* (5th ed.). Washington, DC: Author.

Aurora, R. N., Zak, R. S., Auerbach, S. H., Casey, K. R., Chowdhuri, S., Karippot, A., … Morgenthaler, T. I. (2010). Best practice guide for the treatment of nightmare disorder in adults. *Journal of Clinical Sleep Medicine, 6*(04), 389–401.

Barlow, D. H., Farchione, T. J., Fairholme, C. P., Ellard, K. K., Boisseau, C. L., Allen, L. B., & Ehrenrecih-May, J. (2011). *Unified protocol for transdiagnostic treatment of emotional disorders: Therapist guide*. New York, NY: Oxford University Press.

Barlow, D. H., Sauer-Zavala, S., Carl, J. R., Bullis, J. R., & Ellard, K. K. (2014). The nature, diagnosis, and treatment of neuroticism: Back to the future. *Clinical Psychological Science, 2*(3), 344–365. doi: 10.1177/2167702613505532

Benedek, D. M., Friedman, M. J., Zatzick, D., & Ursano, R. J. (2009). Guideline watch (March 2009): Practice guideline for the treatment of patients with acute stress disorder and posttraumatic stress disorder. *Focus*, 7(2), 204–213. doi: 10.1176/foc.7.2.foc204

Blow, A. J., Curtis, A. F., Wittenborn, A. K., & Gorman, L. (2015). Relationship problems and military related PTSD: The case for using emotionally focused therapy for couples. *Contemporary Family Therapy, 37*(3), 261–270. doi: 10.1007/s10591-015-9345-7

Brewin, C. R., Andrews, B., & Valentine, J. D. (2000). Meta-analysis of risk factors for posttraumatic stress disorder in trauma-exposed adults. *Journal of Consulting and Clinical Psychology, 68*(5), 748–766. doi: 10.1037/0022-006X.68.5.748

Bowman, M. L., & Yehuda, R. (2004). Risk factors in the adversity-stress model. In G. M. Rosen (Ed.), *Posttraumatic stress disorder: Issues and controversies* (pp. 15–38). New York, NY: John Wiley and Sons, Ltd.

Briere, J. (2006). Dissociative symptoms and trauma exposure: Specificity, affect dysregulation, and posttraumatic stress. *The Journal of Nervous and Mental Disease, 194*(2), 78–82. doi: 10.1097/01.nmd.0000198139.47371.54

Bryant, R. A., Friedman, M. J., Spiegel, D., Ursano, R., & Strain, J. (2011). A review of acute stress disorder in DSM-5. *Depression and Anxiety, 29*(9), 802–817. doi: 10.1002/da.20737

Bryant, R. A., Moulds, M. L., Guthrie, R. M., & Nixon, R. D. V. (2005). The additive benefit of hypnosis and cognitive-behavioral therapy in treating acute stress disorder. *Journal of Consulting and Clinical Psychology, 73*(2), 334–340. doi: 10.1037/0022-006X.73.2.334

Bryant, R. A., Moulds, M. L., Nixon, R. D., Mastrodomenico, J., Felmingham, K., & Hopwood, S. (2006). Hypnotherapy and cognitive behaviour therapy of acute stress disorder: A 3- year follow-up. *Behaviour Research and Therapy, 44*(9), 1331–1335. doi: 10.1016/j.brat.2005.04.007

Bullis, J. R., Fortune, M. R., Farchione, T. J., & Barlow, D. H. (2014). A preliminary investigation of the long-term outcome of the unified protocol for transdiagnostic treatment of emotional disorders. *Comprehensive Psychiatry, 55*(8), 1920–1927. doi: 10.1016/j.comppsych.2014.07.016

Carl, J. R., Gallagher, M. W., Sauer-Zavala, S. E., Bentley, K. H., & Barlow, D. H. (2014). A preliminary investigation of the effects of the unified protocol on temperament. *Comprehensive Psychiatry, 55*(6), 1426–1434. doi: 10.1016/j.comp-psych.2014.04.015

Chattarji, A. S., Tomar, A., Suvrathan, A., Ghosh, S., & Rahman, M. M. (2015). Neighborhood matters: Divergent patterns of stress-induced plasticity across the brain. *Nature Neuroscience, 18*(10), 1364–1375. doi: 10.1038/nn.4115

Colvonen, P. J., Ellison, J., Haller, M., & Norman, S. B. (2019). Examining insomnia and PTSD over time in veterans in residential treatment for substance use disorders and PTSD. *Behavioral Sleep Medicine, 17*(4), 524–535. doi: 10.1080/15402002.2018.1425869

Comer, R. J. (2015). *Abnormal psychology*. New York, NY: Worth Publisher.

Cook, J. M., Riggs, D. S., Thompson, R., Coyne, J. C., & Sheikh, J. (2004). Posttraumatic stress disorder and current relationship functioning among World War II ex-prisoners of war. *Journal of Family Psychology, 18*(1), 36–45. doi: 10.1037/0893-3200.18.1.36

Corrigan, F. M., & Hull, A. M. (2015). Recognition of the neurobiological insults imposed by complex trauma and the implications for psychotherapeutic interventions. *The British Journal of Psychology Bulletin, 39*(2), 79–86. doi: 10.1192/pb.bp.114.047134

Cozolino, L. (2006). *The neuroscience of human relationships: Attachment and the developing social brain*. New York, NY: Norton.

Dias, B. G., Maddox, S. A., Klengel, T., & Ressler, K. J. (2015). Epigenetic mechanisms underlying learning and the inheritance of learned behaviors. *Trends in Neurosciences, 38*(2), 96–107. doi: 10.1016/j.tins.2014.12.003

DiGangi, J. A., Gomez, D., Mendoza, L., Jason, L. A., Keys, C. B., & Koenen, K. C. (2013). Pretrauma risk factors for posttraumatic stress disorder: A systematic review of the literature. *Clinical Psychology Review, 33*(6), 728–744. doi: 10.1016/j.cpr.2013.05.002

Elhai, J. D., Ford, J. D., & Naifeh, J. A. (2010). Assessing trauma exposure and posttraumatic morbidity. In G. M. Rosen & B. C. Frueh (Eds.), *Clinician's guide to posttraumatic stress disorder* (pp. 119–151). Hoboken, NJ: John Wiley and Sons.

Elwood, L. S., Hahn, K. S., Olatunji, B. O., & Williams, N. L. (2009). Cognitive vulnerabilities to the development of PTSD: A review of four vulnerabilities and the proposal of an integrative vulnerability model. *Clinical Psychology Review, 29*(1), 87–100. doi: 10.1016/j.cpr.2008.10.002

Epstein, S. (1991). Impulse control and self-destructive behavior. In L. P. Lipsitt & L. L. Mitnick (Eds.), *Self-regulatory behavior and risk-taking: Causes and consequences* (pp. 273–284). Norwood, NJ: Ablex.

Foa, E. B., Hembree, E. A., & Rothbaum, B. O. (2007). *Prolonged exposure therapy for PTSD: Emotional processing of traumatic experiences*. New York, NY: Oxford University Press.

Foa, E. B., & Kozak, M. J. (1986). Emotional processing of fear: Exposure to corrective information. *Psychological Bulletin, 99*(1), 20–35. doi: 10.1037/0033-2909.99.1.20

Freyberg, J. T. (1989). The emerging self in the survivor family. In P. Marcus & A. Rosenberg (Eds.), *Healing their wounds: Psychotherapy with Holocaust survivors and their families* (pp. 85–104). New York, NY: Praeger Publishers.

Friedman, M. J., & Karam, E. G. (2008). Posttraumatic stress disorder. In G. Andrews, D. S. Charney, P. J. Sirovatka & D. A. Regier (Eds.), *Stress-induced and fear circuitry disorders: Refining the research agenda for DSM-5* (pp. 3–29). Washington, DC: American Psychiatric Association.

Gabbard, G. O. (2000). A neurobiologcially informed perspective on psychotherapy. *British Journal of Psychiatry*, 177, 117–122. doi: 10.1192/bjp.177.2.117

Galea, S., Ahern, J., Resnick, H., & Vlahov, D. (2006). Post-traumatic stress symptoms in the general population after a disaster: Implications for public health. In Y. Nerea, R. Gross, R. D. Marshall & E. S. Susser (Eds.), *9/11: Mental health in the wake of terrorist attacks* (pp. 19–44). New York, NY: Cambridge University Press.

Gallegher, M. W. (2018). The unified protocol for posttraumatic stress disorder . In D. H. Barlow & T. J. Farchione (Eds.), *Applications of the unified protocol for transdiagnostic treatment of emotional disorders* (pp. 111–126). New York, NY: Oxford University Press.

Gallegos, R. A., & Hillbrand, M. (2016). Integrative treatment of complex trauma: Integrating behavioral, dynamic, and attribution models. *Journal of Psychotherapy Integration, 26*(3), 259–272. doi: 10.1037/a0040043

Galovski, T., & Lyons, J. A. (2004). Psychological sequelae of combat violence: A review of the impact of PTSD on the veteran's family and possible interventions. *Aggression and Violent Behavior, 9*(5), 477–501. doi: 10.1016/S1359-1789(03)00045-4

Gersons, B. P. R., & Schnyder, U. (2013). Learning from traumatic experiences with brief eclectic psychotherapy for PTSD. *European Journal of Psychotraumatology, 4*(1), 21369. doi: 10.3402/ejpt.v4i0.21369

Gilbert, M., & Orlans, V. (2011). *Integrative therapy: 100 key points and techniques*. New York, NY: Routledge.

Gradus, J. L., Qin, P., Lincoln, A. K., Miller, M., Lawler, E., Sørensen, H. T., & Lash, T. L. (2010). Posttraumatic stress disorder and completed suicide. *American Journal of Epidemiology, 171*(6), 721–727. doi: 10.1093/aje/kwp456

Grawe, K. (2007). *Neuropsychotherapy: How the neurosciences inform effective psychotherapy*. New York: Psychology Press.

Greenberg, J., Koole, S. L., & Pyszczynski, T. (2004). *Handbook of experimental existential psychology*. New York, NY: The Guilford Press.

Greenberg, J., Pyszczynski, T., & Solomon, S. (1986). The causes and consequences of a need for self-esteem: A terror management theory. In R. F. Baumeister (Ed.), *Public self and private self* (pp. 189–212). New York, NY: Springer-Verlag.

Greenberg, N., Brooks, S., & Dunn, R. (2015). Latest developments in post-traumatic stress disorder: Diagnosis and treatment. *British Medical Bulletin, 114*(1), 147–155. doi: 10.1093/bmb/ldv014

Greene, A. M., Bailey, C. R., & Neumeister, A. (2013). A biopsychosocial approach to anxiety. In S. M. Stahl & B. A. Moore (Eds.), *Anxiety disorders: A guide for integrating psychopharmacology and psychotherapy* (pp. 25–50). New York, NY: Routledge.

Greenman, P., & Johnson, S. (2012). United we stand: Emotionally focused therapy (EFT) for couples in the treatment of post-traumatic stress disorder. *Journal of Clinical Psychology, 68*(5), 561–569. doi: 10.1002/jclp.21853

Hetrick, S. E., Purcell, R., Garner, B., & Parslow, R. (2010). Combined pharmacotherapy and psychological therapies for post traumatic stress disorder (PTSD). *Cochrane Database of Systematic Reviews*, 7(7), CD007316. doi: 10.1002/14651858.CD007316.pub2

Holowka, D. W., & Marx, B. P. (2012). Assessing PTSD-related functional impairment and quality of life. In G. J. Beck & D. M. Sloan (Eds.), *Oxford handbook of traumatic stress disorders* (pp. 315–332). New York, NY: Oxford University Press.

Ingersoll, R. E., & Marquis, A. (2014). *Understanding psychopathology: An integral exploration*. Upper Saddle River, NJ: Pearson Education.

Institute of Medicine. (2007). *Treatment of PTSD: Assessment of the evidence*. Washington, DC: National Academic Press.

Jobson, L., & O'Kearney, R. (2008). Cultural differences in personal identity in post-traumatic stress disorder. *British Journal of Clinical Psychology, 47*(1), 95–109. doi: 10.1348/014466507X235953

Johnson, S. (2002). *Emotionally focused couple therapy with trauma survivors: Strengthening attachment bonds*. New York, NY: Guilford Press.

Johnson, S., Hunsley, J., Greenberg, L., & Schindler, D. (1999). Emotionally focused couples therapy: Status and challenges. *Clinical Psychology: Science and Practice, 6*(1), 67–79.

Julien, R. M. (2013). Pharmacological treatment of anxiety disorders across the lifespan. In S. M. Stahl & B. A. Moore (Eds.), *Anxiety disorders: A guide for integrating psychopharmacology and psychotherapy* (pp. 51–70). New York, NY: Routledge.

Kaufman, J., Gelernter, J., Hudziak, J. J., Tyrka, A. R., & Coplan, J. D. (2015). The Research Domain Criteria (RDoC) project and studies of risk and resilience in maltreated children. *Journal of the American Academy of Child and Adolescent Psychiatry, 54*(8), 617–625. doi: 10.1016/j.jaac.2015.06.001

Keane, T. M., & Kaloupek, D. G. (1996). Cognitive behavior therapy in the treatment of posttraumatic stress disorder. *The Clinical Psychologist, 49*(1), 7–8.

Kent, J. M., & Rauch, S. L. (2003). Neurocircuitry of anxiety disorders. *Current Psychiatry Reports, 5*(4), 266–273. doi: 10.1176/foc.2.3.402

Kessler, R. C., Sonnega, A., Bromet, E., Hughes, M., & Nelson, C. B. (1995). Posttraumatic stress disorder in the National Comorbidity Survey. *Archives of General Psychiatry, 52*(12), 1048–1060. doi: 10.1001/archpsyc.1995.03950240066012

Kilpatrick, D. G., Resnick, H. S., Milanak, M. E., Miller, M. W., Keyes, K. M., & Friedman, M. J. (2013). National estimates of exposure to traumatic events and PTSD prevalence using DSM-IV and DSM-5 criteria. *Journal of Traumatic Stress, 26*(5), 537–547. doi: 10.1002/jts.21848

Koch, W. J., & Haring, M. (2008). Posttraumatic stress disorder. In M. Hersen & J. Rosqvist (Eds.), *Handbook of psychological assessment, case conceptualization, and treatment, Vol. I: Adults* (pp. 263–290). Hoboken, NJ: John Wiley & Sons.

Koenen, K. C., Harley, R., Lyons, M. J., Wolfe, J., Simpson, J. C., Goldberg, J., ... Tsuang, M. (2002). A twin registry study of familial and individual risk factors for trauma exposure and posttraumatic stress disorder. *Journal of Nervous and Mental Disease, 190*(4), 209–218. doi: 10.1097/00005053-200204000-00001

Kohut, H. (1971). *The analysis of the self*. New York, NY: International Universities Press.

Kohut, H. (1977). *The restoration of the self*. New York, NY: International Universities Press.

Kohut, H. (1984). *How psychoanalysis cures*. Chicago, IL: University of Chicago Press.

Lee, D. J., Schnitzlein, C. W., Wolf, J. P., Vythilingam, M., Rasmusson, A. M., & Hoge, C. W. (2016). Psychotherapy versus pharmacotherapy for posttraumatic stress disorder:

Systemic review and meta-analyses to determine first-line treatments. *Depression and Anxiety*, *33*(9), 792–806. doi: 10.1002/da.22511

Lewis, A. M. (2014). Terror management theory applied clinically: Implications for existential-integrative psychotherapy. *Death Studies*, *38*(6), 412–417. doi: 10.1080/07481187.2012.753557

Magnavita, J. J., & Anchin, J. C. (2014). *Unifying psychotherapy: Principles, methods, and evidence from clinical science.* New York, NY: Springer.

Markowitz, J. C., Milrod, B., Bleiberg, K., & Marshall, R. D. (2009). Interpersonal factors in understanding and treating PTSD. *Journal of Psychiatric Practice*, *15*(2), 133–140. doi: 10.1097/01.pra.0000348366.34419.28

McCann, I. L., & Pearlman, L. A. (1990). *Psychological trauma and the adult survivor: Theory, therapy and transformation.* New York, NY: Brunner/Mazel.

McEwan, B. S., Angulo, J., Cameron, H., Chao, H. M., Daniels, D., Gannon, M. N., … Woolley, C. (1992). Paradoxical effects of adrenal steroids on the brain: Protection versus degeneration. *Biological Psychiatry*, *31*(2), 177–199. doi: 10.1016/0006-3223(92)90204-D

McGowan, P. O., Sasaki, A., D'Alessio, A. C., Dymov, S., Labonté, B., Szyf, M., … Meany, M. J. (2009). Epigenetic regulation of the glucocorticoid receptor in human brain associates with childhood abuse. *Nature Neuroscience*, *12*(3), 342–348. doi: 10.1038/nn.2270

McKeever, V. M., & Huff, M. E. (2003). A diathesis-stress model of posttraumatic stress disorder: Ecological, biological, and residual stress pathways. *Review of General Psychology*, 7, 237–250. doi: 10.1037/1089-2680.7.3.237

Miller, W. R., Benefield, R. G., & Tonigan, J. S. (1993). Enhancing motivation for change in problem drinking: A controlled comparison of two therapist styles. *Journal of Consulting and Clinical Psychology*, *61*(3), 455–461. doi: 10.1037/0022-006X.61.3.455

Miller, W. R., & Rollnick, S. (2002). *Motivational interviewing: Preparing people for change* (2nd ed.). New York, NY: Guilford Press.

Monson, C. M., Resick, P. A., & Rizvi, S. L. (2014). Post-traumatic stress disorder. In D. H. Barlow (Ed.), *Clinical handbook of psychological disorders: A step-by-step treatment manual* (5th ed., pp. 62–113). New York, NY: Guilford Press.

Morgan, M., Lockwood, A., Steinke, D., Schleenbaker, R., & Botts, S. (2012). Pharmacotherapy regimens among patients with posttraumatic stress disorder and mild traumatic brain injury. *Psychiatric Services*, *63*(2), 182–185. doi: 10.1176/appi.ps.201000531

Murphy, R. T. (2008). Enhancing combat veterans' motivation to change posttraumatic stress disorder symptoms and other problem behaviors. In H. Arkowitz, H. A. Westra, W. R. Miller & S. Rollnick (Eds.), *Motivational interviewing in the treatment of psychological problems* (pp. 57–84). New York, NY: Guilford Press.

Murphy, R. T., Thompson, K. E., Murray, M., Rainey, Q., & Uddo, M. M. (2009). Effect of a motivation enhancement intervention on veterans' engagement in PTSD treatment. *Psychological Services*, *6*(4), 264–278. doi: 10.1037/a0017577

Muse, M. D., Moore, B. A., & Stahl, S. M. (2013). Benefits and challenges of integrative treatment. In S. M. Stahl & B. A. Moore (Eds.), *Anxiety disorders: A guide for integrating psychopharmacology and psychotherapy* (pp. 3–24). New York, NY: Routledge.

Neborsky, R. J., & Solomon, M. F. (2001). Attachment bonds and intimacy: Can the primary imprint of love change? In M. F. Solomon, R. J. Neborsky, L. McCullough, M. Alpert, F. Shapiro, & D. Malan (Eds.), *Short-term therapy for long-term change* (pp. 155–185). New York: Norton.

Nickerson, A., & Bryant, R. A. (2013). Acute stress disorder. In S. M. Stahl & B. A. Moore (Eds.), *Anxiety disorders: A guide for integrating psychopharmacology and psychotherapy* (pp. 155–175). New York, NY: Routledge.

Norcross, J. C. (2005). A primer on psychotherapy integration. In J. C. Norcross & M. R. Goldfried (Eds.), *Handbook of psychotherapy integration* (2nd ed., pp. 3–23). New York, NY: Oxford University Press.

Norton, P. J., & Paulus, D. J. (2016). Toward a unified treatment for emotional disorders: Update on the science and practice. *Behavior Therapy*, *47*(6), 854–868. doi: 10.1016/j.beth.2015.07.002

Paivio, S. C., & Pascual-Leone, A. (2010). *Emotion-focused therapy for complex trauma: An integrative approach.* Washington, DC: American Psychological Association.

Paus, T., Keshavan, K., & Giedd, J. N. (2008). Why do many psychiatric disorders emerge during adolescence? *Nature Reviews: Neuroscience*, *9*(12), 947–957. doi: 10.1038/nrn2513

Peri, T., Gofman, M., Tal, S., & Tuval-Mashiach, R. (2015). Embodied simulation in exposure-based therapies for posttraumatic stress disorder—A possible integration of cognitive behavioral theories, neuroscience, and psychoanalysis. *European Journal of Psychotraumatology*, *6*(1), 29301. doi: 10.3402/ejpt.v6.29301

Protopopescu, X., Pan, H., Tuescher, O., Cloitre, M., Goldstein, M., Engelien, W., … Stern, E. (2005). Differential time courses and specificity of amygdala activity in posttraumatic stress disorder subjects and normal control subjects. *Biological Psychiatry*, *57*(5), 464–473. doi: 10.1016/j.biopsych.2004.12.026

Puetz, V. B., Kohn, N., Dahmen, B., Zvyagintsev, M., Schüppen, A., Schultz, R. T. … Konrad, K. (2014). Neural response to social rejection in children with early separation experiences. *Journal of the American Academy of Child and Adolescent Psychiatry*, *53*(12), 1328–1337.e8. doi: 10.1016/j.jaac.2014.09.004

Pyszczynski, T., & Kesebir, P. (2011). Anxiety buffer disruption theory: A terror management account of posttraumatic stress disorder. *Anxiety, Stress, and Coping*, *24*(1), 3–26. doi: 10.1080/10615806.2010.517524

Rauch, S. L., Shin, L. M., & Phelps, E. A. (2006). Neurocircuitry models of posttraumatic stress disorder and extinction: Human neuroimaging research—Past, present, and future. *Biological Psychiatry*, *60*(4), 376–382. doi: 10.1016/j.biopsych.2006.06.004

Ray, W. J. (2018). *Abnormal psychology*. Thousand Oaks, CA: Sage.

Read, J., Perry, B., Moskowitz, A., & Connolly, J. (2001). The contribution of early traumatic events to schizophrenia in some patients: A traumagenic neurodevelopmental model. *Psychiatry*, *64*, 319–345. doi: 10.1521/psyc.64.4.319.18602

Reiss, S. (1991). Expectancy model of fear, anxiety, and panic. *Clinical Psychology Review*, *11*(2), 141−153. doi: 10.1016/0272-7358(91)90092-9

Resick, P. A., Monson, C. M., & Chard, K. M. (2017). *Cognitive processing therapy for PTSD: A comprehensive manual.* New York, NY: Guilford Press.

Resick, P. A., & Schnicke, M. K. (1992). CPT for sexual assault victims. *Journal of Consulting and Clinical Psychology*, *60*(5), 748–756. doi: 10.1037/0022-006X.60.5.748

Riggs, D. S., Byrne, C. A. , Weathers, F. W., & Litz, B. T. (1998). The quality of the intimate relationships of male Vietnam veterans: Problems associated with posttraumatic stress disorder. *Journal of Traumatic Stress*, *11*(1), 87–101.

Ross, D. A., Arbuckle, M. R., Travis, M. J., Dwyer, J. B., van Schalkwyk, G. I., & Ressler, K. J. (2017). An integrated neuroscience perspective on formulation and treatment planning for posttraumatic stress disorder: An educational review. *JAMA Psychiatry*, *74*(4), 407–415. doi: 10.1001/jamapsychiatry.2016.3325

Ross, R. J. (2014). The changing REM sleep signature of posttraumatic stress disorder. *Sleep, 37*(8), 1281–1282. doi: 10.5665/sleep.3912

Sapolsky, R. (2004). *Why zebras don't get ulcers* (3rd ed.). New York: Holt.

Schmidt, N. B., Eggleston, A. M., Woolaway-Bickel, K., Fitzpatrick, K. K., Vasey, M. W., & Richey, J. A. (2007). Anxiety sensitivity amelioration training (ASAT): A longitudinal primary prevention program targeting cognitive vulnerability. *Journal of Anxiety Disorders, 21*(3), 302–319. doi: 10.1016/j.janxdis.2006.06.002

Schneider, K. J. (2008). *Theory of the existential-integrative (EI) approach. Existential-integrative psychotherapy: Guideposts to the core of practice.* New York, NY: Routledge.

Schnurr, P. P., Friedman, M. J., & Bernardy, N. C. (2002). Research on posttraumatic stress disorder: Epidemiology, pathophysiology, and assessment. *Journal of Clinical Psychology, 58*(8), 877–889. doi: 10.1002/jclp.10064

Schore, A. N. (1994). *Affect regulation and the origin of the self: The neurobiology of emotional development.* Hillsdale, NJ: Lawrence Erlbaum Associates, Inc.

Seligowski, A. V., Lee, D. J., Bardeen, J. R., & Orcutt, H. K. (2015). Emotion regulation and posttraumatic stress symptoms: A meta-analysis. *Cognitive Behaviour Therapy, 44*(2), 87–102. doi: 10.1080/16506073.2014.980753

Shapiro, F. (1995). *Eye movement desensitization and reprocessing: Basic principles, protocols and procedures.* New York, NY: Guilford Press.

Sharpless, B. A., & Barber, J. P. (2011). A clinician's guide to PTSD treatments for returning veterans. *Professional Psychology: Research and Practice, 42*(1), 8. doi: 10.1037/a0022351

Sherman, M., Zanotti, D., & Jones, D. (2005). Key elements in couples therapy with veterans with combat-related posttraumatic stress disorder. *Professional Psychology: Research and Practice, 36*(6), 626–633. doi: 10.1037/0735-7028.36.6.626

Shin, L. M., Rauch, S. L., & Pitman, R. K. (2006). Amygdala, medial prefrontal cortex, and hippocampal function in PTSD. *Annals of the New York Academy of Sciences, 1071*, 67–79. doi: 10.1196/annals.1364.007

Siegel, D. J. (1999). *The developing mind.* New York, NY: Guilford Press.

Solomon, S., Greenberg, J., & Pyszczynski, T. (1991). A terror management theory of social behavior: The psychological functions of self-esteem and cultural worldviews. In M. Zanna (Ed.), *Advances in Experimental Social Psychology, Vol. 24* (pp. 93–159). Orlando, FL: Academic Press.

Solomon, Z., Dekel, R., & Zerach, G. (2008). The relationships between posttraumatic stress symptom clusters and marital intimacy among war veterans. *Journal of Family Psychology, 22*(5), 659–666. doi: 10.1037/a0013596

Solomon, Z., Kotler, M., & Mikulincer, M. (1988). Combat-related posttraumatic stress disorder among second-generation Holocaust survivors: Preliminary findings. *The American Journal of Psychiatry, 145*(7), 865–868. doi: 10.1176/ajp.145.7.865

Sotskova, A., & Dossett, K. (2017). Teaching integrative existential psychotherapy: Student and supervisor reflections on using an integrative approach early in clinical training. *The Humanistic Psychologist, 45*(2), 122–133. doi: 10.1037/hum0000049

Stern, D. N. (1985). *The interpersonal world of the infant.* New York: Basic Books.

Swift, J. K., Greenberg, R. P., Tompkins, K. A., & Parkin, S. R. (2017). Treatment refusal and premature termination in psychotherapy, pharmacotherapy, and their combination: A meta-analysis of head-to-head comparisons. *Psychotherapy, 54*(1), 47–57. doi: 10.1037/pst0000104

Uchino, B. N., & Birmingham, W. (2011). Stress and support processes. In R. J. Contrada & A. Baum (Eds.), *The handbook of stress science: Biology, psychology, and health* (pp. 111–121). New York, NY: Springer Publishing.

VA/DoD (Department of Veterans Affairs/Department of Defense). (2010). VA/DoD clinical practice guideline for the management of posttraumatic stress, version 2.0. Washington, DC: Veterans Health Administration, Department of Defense.

Varkovitzky, R. L., Sherrill, A. M., & Reger, G. M. (2018). Effectiveness of the unified protocol for transdiagnostic treatment of emotional disorders among veterans with posttraumatic stress disorder: A pilot study. *Behavior Modification, 42*(2), 210–230. doi: 10.1177/0145445517724539

Walker, A. J. (1989). The psychobiology of trauma. In J. P. Wilson (Ed.), *Trauma, transformation, and healing: An integrated approach to theory research, and post- traumatic therapy* (No. 14, pp. 21–37). New York, NY: Brunner/Mazel.

Westfall, N. C., & Nemeroff, C. B. (2016). State-of-the-art prevention and treatment of PTSD: Pharmacotherapy, psychotherapy, and nonpharmacological somatic therapies. *Psychiatric Annals, 46*(9), 533–549. doi: 10.3928/00485713-20160808-01

Williams, A. M., Richardson, G., & Galovski, T. E. (2013). Posttraumatic stress disorder. In S. M. Stahl & B. A. Moore (Eds.), *Anxiety disorders: A guide for integrating psychopharmacology and psychotherapy* (pp. 176–200). New York, NY: Routledge.

Wilson, J. P. (1989). A person-environment approach to traumatic stress reactions. In J. P. Wilson (Ed.), *Trauma, transformation, and healing: An integrated approach to theory research, and post-traumatic therapy* (No. 14, pp. 3–20). New York, NY: Bruner/Mazel.

Wolfe, B. E. (2005). *Understanding and treating anxiety disorders: An integrative approach to healing the wounded self.* Washington, DC: American Psychological Association.

Writer, B. W., Meyer, E. G., & Schillerstrom, J. E. (2014). Prazosin for military combat-related PTSD nightmares: A critical review. *Journal of Neuropsychiatry and Clinical Neurosciences, 26*(1), 24–33. doi: 10.1176/appi.neuropsych.13010006

Yehuda, R., & Bierer, L. M. (2007). Transgenerational transmission of cortisol and PTSD risk. *Progress in Brain Research, 167*, 121–135. doi: 10.1016/S0079-6123(07)67009-5

Yehuda, R., Daskalakis, N. P., Desarnaud, F., Makotkine, I., Lehrner, A. L., Koch, E., … Bierer, L. M. (2013). Epigenetic biomarkers as predictors and correlates of symptom improvement following psychotherapy in combat veterans with PTSD. *Frontiers in Psychiatry, 4*, 118. doi: 10.3389/fpsyt.2013.00118

Yehuda, R., Daskalakis, N. P., Lehrner, A., Desarnaud, F., Bader, H. N., Makotkine, I., … Meaney, M. J. (2014). Influences of maternal and paternal PTSD on epigenetic regulation of the glucocorticoid receptor gene in Holocaust survivor offspring. *American Journal of Psychiatry, 171*(8), 872–880. doi: 10.1176/appi.ajp.2014.13121571

Yehuda, R., & Seckle, J. (2011). Minireview: Stress related psychiatric disorders with low cortisol levels: A metabolic hypothesis. *Endocrinology, 152*(12), 4496–4503. doi: 10.1210/en.2011-1218

11 Conclusion

Where can students and therapists learn about integrated and unified treatments for the anxiety disorders? The book, *Anxiety Disorders: Integrated Psychotherapy Approaches*, traces the history of integrated treatment frameworks from the early part of the twentieth century to the present. *Anxiety Disorders: Integrated Psychotherapy Approaches* portrays the complex etiology of the anxiety disorders and how they can be explained within the context of integrated and unified approaches. The book explains the need for integrated treatment, points out the unique and common aspects of the various psychotherapy models, delineates the concepts and themes that underlie integrated psychotherapy models for the anxiety disorders, and provides a wide range of case studies of integrated and unified psychotherapy approaches for the anxiety disorders.

Anxiety Disorders: Integrated Psychotherapy Approaches integrates material from biological, social, developmental, and psychological aspects of human nature. An integrated or a unified perspective that is applied to psychotherapy can help both beginning and seasoned therapists to realize the benefit of reflecting upon the complex interaction among intrapsychic/biological, environmental, interpersonal, family, systems, and cultural processes in the treatment of the anxiety disorders. Psychotherapy has been shown to intersect with neuroscience in that psychobiological treatment can alter the structure and function of the brain (Shapiro, 2018). A unifying psychobiological perspective includes relational and biological components that complement each other (Shapiro, 2018).

Today, many training programs have incorporated an integrative framework (Castonguay, Eubanks, Goldfried, Muran, & Lutz, 2015; Norcross & Halgin, 2005). The practice of integrated psychotherapy calls for therapists to design their unique approaches to fit the needs of individual clients. The design of integrative psychotherapy models needs to be approached with humility as the process of integrated and unified research and practice, although conceived decades ago, is far from complete. As therapists decide on their integrated plans, they can draw upon extant integrated and unified models of psychotherapy that are congruent with their unique backgrounds, and proceed to shape their approach according to the individual needs of their patients (Gilbert & Orlans, 2011). Whereas some therapists and researchers who are proponents of unified approaches may draw predominantly from one angle, e.g., psychodynamic, others may draw from other frameworks, e.g., cognitive-behavioral, existential, developmental, psychoanalytic, and others. What is woven through the fabric of integrated and unified psychotherapy models is the relational component and its prominence within the context of the integrated treatments. Whether the relational component is called the therapeutic alliance, the working relationship, the therapeutic relationship, the interpersonal behaviors of patient and therapist, or some other term, the idea that each therapeutic dyad constructs its own unique relationship and reality is not to be underestimated.

Commonalities characterize the different integrated and unified psychotherapy models. Psychodynamic theories, similar to behavioral views, share the notion that anxiety disorders emerge from traumatic or negative learning situations (Marquis, 2018). Whereas the anxiety disorders are comorbid, they are distinct in that they are characterized by specific kinds of objects or situations that cause concern for patients (American Psychiatric Association, 2013).

Although the book, *Anxiety Disorders: Integrated Psychotherapy Approaches*, does not include the entire gamut of therapeutic approaches for the anxiety disorders, it presents a broad scope of integrated and unified psychotherapy frameworks from which practitioners can draw to treat patients with anxiety. Integrative therapists can rely on a panoply of orientations related to the etiology of integrated and unified perspectives as they learn to design thoughtful and careful assessments. At the same time, therapists can feel comfortable innovating spontaneously, without rigid adherence to theories, as they attend to their patients experience of minute-to-minute turning points within the context of a therapeutic dyad, family therapy, and group therapy. Although case studies of different integrative and unified approaches are presented, therapists are encouraged to devise their own careful assessments and case formulations.

If the life of a human being is complex, it is understandable that therapy would be too (Mahoney, 1991). There have been several waves or currents of integration, e.g., technical eclecticism, theoretical, common factors, assimilated. Enter the fifth wave, an integral or a unified metatheory, the most recent wave. At the center of unification is the notion that human beings who are complex need to be considered from a holistic point of view (Anchin, 2012). Integrated and unified psychotherapies are not tied to a unitary school, but represent an ongoing process that seeks to view human beings from a multidimensional perspective whose distress has derived from a myriad of causes, e.g., genetic, physiological, impaired cognitions and behaviors, dysfunctional social systems and families, and others (Marquis, 2018). Unified psychotherapy is in its infancy. Metatheoretical approaches can offer researchers and therapists of the future opportunities to study and integrate already integrated therapies. In the future, transdiagnostic integrationists may wish to devise a unified therapy treatment protocol that integrates both the cognitive-behavioral unified protocols of Barlow, Allen, and Choate (2004) and Barlow et al. (2011, 2018) with the unified psychodynamic psychotherapy (UPP-ANXIETY) model of Leichsenring and Salzer (2014).

Henriques (2017) suggests that unified approaches address the need for maps that can organize broad systems of a discipline such as psychology in a clear way. Future research needs to focus on an analysis of case studies of integrated and unified treatments that are weaker and those that succeed and the reasons for the outcomes. One avenue of comparison may be to compare the case studies of therapists who are grounded in a particular theory and have integrated other approaches with the case studies of therapists who are similarly grounded, but who have not integrated other approaches. Sessions that fail and those that succeed comprise the integrated and unified treatment case studies presented in this book, and it may be useful to examine the broad and narrow views of the intricacies of these sessions. We may find that what unifies us is that we can learn equally from our failures and our successes.

References

American Psychiatric Association. (2013). *Diagnostic and statistical manual of mental disorders* (5th ed.). Washington, DC: Author.

Anchin, J. C. (2012). Prologue to unified psychotherapy and clinical science. *Journal of Unified Psychotherapy and Clinical Science, 1*(1), 1–20.

Barlow, D. H., Allen, L. B., & Choate, M. L. (2004). Toward a unified treatment for emotional disorders. *Behavior Therapy, 35*(2), 205–230. doi: 10.1016/S0005-7894(04)80036-4

Barlow, D. H., Farchione, T. J., Fairholme, C. P., Ellard, K. K., Boisseau, C. L., Allen, L. B., & Ehrenreich-May, J. T. (2011). *Unified protocol for transdiagnostic treatment of emotional disorders: Therapist guide.* New York, NY: Oxford University Press.

Barlow, D. H., Farchione, T. J., Sauer-Zavala, S., Murray-Latin, H., Ellard, K. K., Bullis, J. R., … Cassiello-Robbins, C. (2018). *Unified protocol for transdiagnostic treatment of emotional disorders: Therapist guide* (2nd ed.). New York, NY: Oxford University Press.

Castonguay, L. G., Eubanks, C. F., Goldfried, M. R., Muran, J. C., & Lutz, W. (2015). Research on psychotherapy integration: Building on the past, looking to the future. *Psychotherapy Research, 25*(3), 365–382. doi: 10.1080/10503307.2015.1014010

Gilbert, M., & Orlans, V. (2011). *Integrative therapy: 100 key points and techniques.* New York, NY: Routledge.

Henriques, G. R. (2017). Character adaptation systems theory: A new big five for personality and psychotherapy, *Review of General Psychology, 21*(1), 9–22. doi: 10.1037/gpr0000097

Leichsenring, F., & Salzer, S. (2014). A unified protocol for the transdiagnostic psychodynamic treatment of anxiety disorders: An evidence-based approach. *Psychotherapy, 51*(2), 224–245. doi: 10.1037/a0033815

Mahoney, J. (1991). *Human change processes: The scientific foundations of psychotherapy.* New York, NY: Basic Books.

Marquis, A. (2018). *Integral psychotherapy: A unifying approach.* New York, NY: Routledge.

Norcross, J. C., & Halgin, R. P. (2005). Training in psychotherapy integration. In J. C. Norcross & M. R. Goldfried (Eds.), *Handbook of psychotherapy integration* (2nd ed., pp. 439–458). New York, NY: Oxford University Press.

Shapiro, Y. (2018). Psychodynamic psychiatry in the 21st century: Constructing a comprehensive science of experience. *Psychodynamic Psychiatry, 46*(1), 49–79. doi: 10.1521/pdps.2018.46.1.49

Index

Page numbers in *italics* indicate figures; Page numbers in **bold** indicate tables.